Practical Issues in Anesthesia and Intensive Care 2013

Contents

Perioperative Fluid Therapy and Fluid Therapy in Patients with Sepsis in Search of Clarification

Biagio Allaria

1.1 Introduction

A vital part of addressing this question is that fluid therapy, whether perioperative or in critical conditions, should follow a single important factor: to maintain good perfusion and oxygenation of the tissue. However, the behavior of individual organs and regions varies greatly in response to different diseases and even from one patient to the next with the same disease.

It is therefore very difficult to obtain precise information about perfusion and peripheral oxygenation since it is not an overall phenomenon but the sum of many regional perfusions that behave differently. Thus SV^-O_2 (or, more simply, $ScVO_2$), which is a satisfactory mirror of perfusion and peripheral oxygenation, says nothing about the real situation in different regions: we do not know if a drop in SV^-O_2 is linked to an intestinal, muscular, or cutaneous perfusion defect, etc.

There are methods to assess the microcirculation but even these, if used statically, may not be helpful. Yet the Oxygen Challenge Test, based on the response to transcutaneous PO_2 (tPO_2) upon inhalation of O_2 at 100 % (FiO_2 100 %), may be of help.

The increase in FiO_2 to 100 % leads to an improvement in tPO_2 only when the transportation of hyperoxygenated blood to cells is possible. Therefore, a positive Oxygen Challenge Test leads to a favorable prognosis. In fact, while baseline tPO_2 measured in one region is not indicative of tPO_2 in all regions, it seems that a

B. Allaria (✉)
Former Director of the Critical Patient Department of the National Institute
for the Study and Treatment of Tumors, currently Consultant in Clinical Risk Management,
National Institute for the Study and Treatment of Tumors,
Via Venezian 1, 20133, Milan, Italy
e-mail: biagio.allaria@tiscali.it

B. Allaria (ed.), *Practical Issues in Anesthesia and Intensive Care 2013*,
DOI: 10.1007/978-88-470-5529-2_1, © Springer-Verlag Italia 2014

positive Oxygen Challenge Test for tPO$_2$ in one region is valid for all other regions in both hemorrhagic and septic patients [1].

Reduced baseline tPO$_2$ may be linked to a macrocirculation defect in the transportation of O$_2$ (such as hemorrhage or cardiac insufficiency) while in septic patients who have already undergone fluid resuscitation and with a high cardiac output, this is more likely to be due to microcirculation damage.

In all three cases hyperoxygenation increases tPO$_2$ when tissue perfusion is guaranteed and does not increase it when it is not [2], and while baseline tPO$_2$ varies from region to region, the positive response to hyperoxygenation assessed in one region seems to apply to all other regions (muscles, bladder, kidneys, skin, liver, etc.).

However, tPO$_2$ is still barely in use as a monitoring technique and therefore it cannot clearly be considered a standard technique for assessing the need for fluid support in the body.

We mention this in this introduction only as an example of one of the trends underway.

Furthermore, we cannot treat indifferently the monitoring of highly varied clinical situations since this must be personalized based on a range of requirements.

We have therefore decided to address the theme of fluid therapy in order to deepen knowledge of the strategies for control and optimization of the volemic status in two different clinical situations: perioperative conditions and sepsis.

1.2   Strategies for the Control and Optimization of the Perioperative Volemic Status

It should first be said that we are not only addressing the issues of absolute or relative perioperative hypovolemia but also cases of hypervolemia that are at least as dangerous as hypovolemia and are often overlooked.

It is very easy to administer excessive doses of fluid in perioperative situations, as a result of erroneous assumptions. The first is that fasting for 12 or more hours leads to dehydration of the patient. In reality it has been known for more than 30 years that fasting, even during open-abdomen surgery, leads to fluid loss of 1 ml/kg/h and is therefore of little importance [3]. Various assumptions have been compared with this precise assessment, namely that during open-abdomen surgery the loss of fluid is equal to 10 times as much (10 ml/kg/h). Based on these assumptions, the trend in recent decades has been for the perioperative hyperinfusion of fluids.

It is now, however, the case to drastically reduce infusions but more recent studies by Rehm, who has focused on perioperative volemic patterns, seems to show a negative perioperative balance of 3–6 liters using the restrictive criteria described [4, 5].

Yet Heckel asks in an interesting work from 2011 [6], considering that the patient has lost very little fluid and volemic findings show considerable perioperative losses that are not justified by the clinical reality, where does the missing fluid loss end, considering that this volemic loss lasts until 72 h after surgery?

The usual opinion is that it ends with the appearance of a "third space" and that it is generally divided into two parts: the anatomical third space that coincides with the interstice and the non-anatomical third space that comprises spaces that are normally free of fluid such as the peritoneal, pleural or pericardial cavities, the intestine, and injured or traumatized tissue.

In the perioperative phase the shift of fluids is predominantly toward the third anatomic space or interstice.

In an interesting study from 2008, Chappel [7] identified two types of fluid release toward the interstices. The first occurs in small quantities, even in normal patients, and can reach abnormal levels in specific situations in which it increases hydrostatic pressure and/or reduces oncotic pressure, as is often the case with perioperative fluid overloading.

The second is abnormal fluid release caused by changes to the endothelial barrier which, promoted by BNP, is released in the event of overloading but also by organ manipulation (primarily the intestines) due to surgery. The fluids that enter the interstice in this situation are rich in protein while those of the first type are devoid of it.

From these observations it is clear that perioperative fluid overloading is at least as important as under filling, to which we have always paid great attention. We can think of only two conditions influenced heavily by edema: intestinal peristalsis and alveolar-capillary distribution of O_2. When is postoperative paralytic ileus and when is O_2 desaturation secondary to underestimated interstitial edema? Interstitial edema is, in fact, caused by tissue perfusion disorders no more or less than hypovolemia. However, the phenomenon is anything but rare if Lowell's findings of 1990 [8] are true, namely that 40 % of patients undergoing major general surgery showed a 10 % increase in weight, which was correlated with mortality.

It is therefore clear that perioperative infusions are performed very cautiously, taking care to replace only the visible losses (urine, blood, possible loss due to diarrhea, etc.) and by controlling weight, daily if possible. Postoperative weight gain may be caused only by water retention, which is the result of fluid entering the interstice.

However, hypotension and oliguria may be confirmed in the perioperative phase, which are expressions of possible hypovolemia for which sufficient information is required.

Let us now move on to the second important aspect of the perioperative volemic status of patients, namely hypovolemia.

It is important not to confuse the concept of hypovolemia with that of extravascular dehydration. Diuresis and *perspiratio* counterbalanced by infusions first leads to a reduction in the amount of fluid that is free of proteins and electrolytes in the interstices and only later reduces the circulating volume. Therefore, extravascular dehydration is prevented by introducing crystalloids in proportion to the losses. It is clear that the crystalloids are infused in the intravascular space but the rapid equilibrium between the intravascular space and interstitial space means that the administered fluids are distributed where they are required, namely the interstices.

The situation of hypovolemia following sudden loss of mass due to hemorrhage or persistent extravascular dehydration which results in the removal of fluids from circulation is a completely different situation.

In such cases, in theory the crystalloids may have a short, volemic, expansive effect but rapidly enter the interstices therefore losing their expansive volemic aspect. Only one-fifth of infused crystalloids remain in circulation and to obtain the same volemic expansion produced by colloids, a quantity of crystalloids four times higher is required [9]. It is clear that these are only general concepts since they cannot predetermine the percentage of crystalloids that leave the circulation in each patient, considering that the endothelial barrier is not equal in every patient, and, even without serious damage to the barrier caused by sepsis, different patterns are possible in different patients and therefore different amounts of infused fluid loss from the circulation to the interstices. It remains true that theoretically the restoration of interstitial fluids occurs with crystalloids and that colloids are more effective for volemic restoration. However, some considerations must be made for colloids.

There is only one natural colloid that is available in clinical practice: albumin.

Much has been written on the real use of albumin as a volemic expansive agent. Omitting the numerous clinical trials that are often in disagreement with each other, we will refer to only two articles.

The first is a review by Cochrane of 30 randomized studies in a total of 1,419 critically hypovolemic patients in whom crystalloids and albumin were measured. Albumin did not enable a reduction in mortality, but tended to increase it [10].

The SAFE study in 6,997 patients compared fluid resuscitation with albumin and saline solutions [11] but did not show any advantage in patients treated with albumin in terms of either mortality or duration of stay in intensive care or duration of mechanical ventilation.

Today it therefore does not seem acceptable to use human albumin for plasma expansion.

We have only just ceased saying that crystalloids are not suitable for volemic expansion, if not for very short periods, and therefore there remains nothing that points toward artificial colloids. Leaving aside dextrans, which are always used to a lesser extent, we can see how and if gelatins and hydroxyethyl starch can be used. Gelatins, which are polypeptides produced from bovine collagen, have a molecular weight that varies from 30,000 to 35,000 Dα, and are usually well tolerated. They do not influence coagulation or cause organ damage other than to the kidneys, where gelatins may create problems, at least according to some authors [12].

In some patients, such as those aged over 80 who undergo heart surgery, Boldr et al. compared 6 % hydroxyethyl starch (HES) 130/0.4 and 4 % gelatin, revealing greater renal dysfunction in patients treated with gelatin [13].

Even with gelatin, therefore, there is confusion despite it being well tolerated.

HES are artificial polymers derived from maize or potato amylopectin and are available in low-molecular-weight versions (130 da) and lower degree of substitution (0.4) and high-molecular-weight versions (200 da) and higher degree of substitution (0.5). HES 200/0.5 have negative effects on coagulation and reduce platelet adhesion. 6 % HES 130/0.4 solutions do not have this type of effect, or do so only minimally. The use of HES 200/0.5 on renal function has also aroused concerns. The more modern 6 % HES 130/0.4 seem to provide better guarantees in terms of renal function, even if they are used in large quantities [14].

On the other hand, the SOAP study showed no differences between HES 130/0.4 and HES 200/0.5 in 3,000 critical patients in terms of renal damage. It is necessary, however, to note that in this study doses of 13 ml/kg HES were not exceeded while in the other studies doses as high as 70 ml/kg were administered and the use of these colloids did not last for more than 2 days [15].

In summary, therefore, the introduction of crystalloids is recommended to balance fluid loss (diuresis in particular, due to the poor consistence of perspiration) and maintain normal hydration of the interstices and introduce colloids (or blood) to expand volemia if necessary.

These concepts, though simple, are very important since the incorrect use of crystalloids either too conservatively or too liberally may be harmful in the perioperative phase, just as the use of colloids for different purposes from those of volemic expansion which is considered essential would be just as damaging.

At the beginning of this chapter we mentioned that both hypovolemia and hypervolemia damage the endothelium, leading to edema, and that edemas may be the cause of tissue oxygenation deficiency in various regions, not least the intestines. Especially in abdominal surgery, if endothelial damage due to surgery, resection, and sutures is accompanied by iatrogenic damage caused by incorrect treatment of hypovolemia and/or the creation of hypervolemia, postoperative paralytic ileus becomes a reality that is difficult to overcome.

Another argument is the daily bread of anesthetists, namely the identification of dysvolemic situations (dysvolemia referring to either hypovolemia or hypervolemia) that need to be corrected.

Much has been written about the diagnostic strategies used to reveal the presence of hypovolemia, especially in the search for a suitable parameter for measurement that makes it possible to indicate the need for refilling of the circulation.

Since in the operating room, especially in patients who are at risk, central venous catheters are fairly common, we shall begin to address the diagnostic possibilities offered by CVP.

There is no need to restate that the absolute mean values for CVP do not provide a clear diagnostic pretext. CVP is the filling pressure of the right ventricle and the body uses various mechanisms to maintain it as normal and to ensure filling of the heart. If one thinks only that at the beginning of acute hypovolemia, as can be verified during surgery with blood loss, the splanchnic is able to mobilize approximately 700 cc of blood with a high Htc level, thus maintaining CVP and heart filling, output values are consequently normal.

In the initial phase of acute hypovolemia, therefore, CVP does not give any alarm signals.

When the splanchnic has taken up the entire available mass, mean circulatory filling pressure (MCFP) decreases as does CVP, but since venous return (VR) is governed by the formula

$$VR = MCFP - CVP$$

reducing MCFP and CVP in equal measure, it remains normal, thus maintaining normal heart filling and cardiac output. In these conditions, blood pressure remains normal even without an increase in heart rate.

In this phase, however, the fall in CVP, although not caused by a reduction in heart filling, is of diagnostic significance.

Let us consider a patient under general anesthesia with mechanical ventilation and a stable CVP of around 8 mmHg. A sudden fall to 5 mmHg with normal blood pressure and heart rate probably means the following: hypovolemia is confirmed; the splanchnic has already used up its involvement potential; venous return is still normal.

If doctors are not attentive to this phase of hemodynamic equilibrium, which is maintained thanks to compensatory mechanisms, and if possible blood loss continues, heart rate will increase, maintaining normal cardiac output despite a reduction in venous return and stroke volume (SV).

At this point there have already been two signals for hypovolemia: the fall in CVP and the increase in heart rate. Blood pressure may still be normal. We should not expect that this phase will lead to changes in tissue perfusion, which we referred to at the beginning of the chapter.

Therefore the first compensatory mechanism, involvement of the splanchnic mass, occurs without observation. The second is a fall in CVP, which may be understood by the anesthetist even in the absence of hypotension and an increase in heart rate. The third is the increase in heart rate. If at this time the anesthetist has not yet begun to repair by introducing a colloid, the compensatory mechanisms are exhausted: cardiac output will fall and blood pressure too, with signs of reduced tissue perfusion emerging (beginning with lactacidemia). Even before anesthesia begins, CVP, if observed dynamically, may provide information on the patient's volemic status. By observing CVP trends on the monitor (or better, by recording it on a graph), a change can be seen in normovolemic patients, with respiration no greater than 1 mmHg. A greater change indicates the suspicion of hypovolemia, which is felt at the beginning of mechanical ventilation and under the vasodilatory effect of anesthesia.

It is this situation that justifies the use of a "filling test" to better assess the value of perioperative infusions.

We also refer to another important topic for anesthetists: the use and interpretation of the "filling test" (or Fluid Challenge).

The first problem to be resolved is linked to the quality of the fluid to be introduced: crystalloid or colloid? Both have advantages and disadvantages. Colloids have the benefit, like the infused volume, of enabling a greater hemodynamic effect; crystalloids do not interfere with coagulation mechanisms and do not lead to anaphylactic phenomena that, though rare, may be caused by colloids. Few years ago a study on the use of the "fluid challenge" in intensive care showed that colloids were used in 62 % of cases and crystalloids in 38 % [16].

The second problem is related to the quantity of fluid to be infused. The most commonly advised dosage is 250 ml of colloid in 10–15 min [17].

Having chosen the type of fluid, its quantity and infusion speed, it is necessary to know which parameters to observe to assess the response.

It should be remembered that the "fluid challenge" is a real "stress test" that makes it possible to observe the response of the heart to a rapid increase in filling. Theoretically, a heart that responds with a significant increase in SV and a moderate increase in filling pressure is a heart that may benefit functionally from mass administration. On the other hand, a heart that responds with no increase in SV or with an insignificant increase, compared with a clear increase in filling pressure (either CVP or Wedge Pressure) is a heart that probably will not benefit functionally from mass administration.

It is therefore clear that the better method to conduct the Fluid Challenge and observe its result is to measure CVP (or Wedge Pressure) and SV.

But even with CVP alone it is possible to obtain useful information, though not precise, by using the Venn protocol [18].

This protocol considers that, if the bolus fluid infusion (250 ml of colloid in 8–10 min) leads to an increase in CVP of less than 3 mmHg, a second bolus may be administered safely. If CVP rises by between 3 and 5 mmHg, a delay is justified as well as the possible repetition of the test after a short period. If the increase in CVP exceeds 5 mmHg, it is advised to stop infusions even if a repetition of the test is considered necessary later.

In any case, the more advisable Fluid Challenge is based on observing the response of CVP and cardiac output, as recommended by Vincent and Weil in their review of the subject [19].

It will not escape the reader's notice that by initially speaking of the Fluid Challenge we mentioned the response of the CVP-SV pairing. Another protocol, by Viencent and Weil, uses the CVP-CO pairing.

Theoretically the more correct response to filling would be SV, since CO is not affected merely by filling by also by heart rate. In reality, SV variations are often moderate and create interpretational difficulties while CO variations are greater and easier to observe.

In any case, if SV is used to assess the Fluid Challenge response, it must be borne in mind that only an increase of at least 10 % is interpreted positively. Smaller increases are not considered significant.

Without SV it is possible to use a parameter that is available in all operating rooms: $EtCO_2$. Capnography is used most to monitor respiratory function but it cannot be forgotten that $EtCO_2$ is also an expression of metabolic activity

(CO$_2$ production) and CO$_2$ transport from the periphery to the lungs (cardiac output). Since ventilation and metabolic activity in general anesthesia is constant, a sudden variation in EtCO$_2$ is closely linked to a change in cardiac output. In the event of a sudden fall in EtCO$_2$ that is not justified by respiratory or metabolic alterations, it is appropriate to consider a fall in cardiac output. In this case, a Fluid Challenge may be performed using CVP + EtCO$_2$. If the response to the fluid bolus is a clear increase in EtCO$_2$ with a moderate rise in CVP, the Fluid Challenge may be considered positive.

Finally, we should not forget a simple maneuver that may help to understand outside the operating room whether a perioperative hypotensive event is due to hypovolemia or other causes.

Raising the legs at right angles helps the force of gravity to promote venous return from the periphery to the heart. If blood pressure improves with this maneuver and heart rate falls it is probable that the "filling test" is positive. Venous return may later be promoted by increasing the trunk to 45°.

In this way the splanchnic is compressed and, since it is the most important venous reservoir in the body, there is considerable "squeezing out" of blood toward the heart.

This "text-book semi-closure" of the patient's body enables, where possible, a useful diagnostic test to assess the presence of hypovolemia as the cause of a hypotensive event.

Naturally this maneuver has a diagnostic value when it does not incite pain, as in the case of postoperative hip surgery. The unpredictable response to the algogenic stimulus (vagal?, adrenergic?) makes the test minimally reliable.

Once faced with the problem of identifying a hypovolemic status, it must also be clarified how the presence of volemic overload can be discovered which, as we have seen, is not any less dangerous than hypovolemia. We cannot expect to discover overloading by monitoring CVP or WP: an increase in these parameters is not so much a sign of overload but of cardiac dysfunction, whether systolic or diastolic.

Nor, on the other hand, can we expect to see the consequences of overload, namely peripheral or pulmonary edema. Discovering overload at the beginning is therefore not very simple and we can thus be satisfied with relatively uncertain signs, such as the appearance of signs of dilution (such as a fall in Htc that does not result from other causes) or to understand as quickly as possible the signs of edema that is nevertheless a result of overload. Two techniques may be used for this purpose: measuring pulmonary extravascular water (pulmonary edema) and intra-abdominal pressure (intestinal edema).

EVLW may be monitored using the transpulmonary thermodilution technique with a suitable level of accuracy, considering that data obtained in this way are positively correlated with those obtained with the gold standard technique of dilution with a double indicator [20]. This technique is able to demonstrate variations in EVLW of 10–20 %. The normal EVLW value is 5–7 ml/kg and it may reach 30 ml/kg in the event of severe pulmonary edema.

According to an interesting study by Sakka, EVLW values of >15 ml/kg increase the mortality rate for critical patients to 65 % compared to 33 % for those whose EVLW value is <10 ml/kg [21].

EVLW maintains its predictive value for risk even in patients with ARDS in whom EVLW is indicated based not on body weight but rather on BMI [22].

Since the instrument enabling EVLW monitoring is very widespread, it may be useful to use it as a monitoring method in patients in whom the potentially long-term administration of fluids is planned in order to regulate the body.

The other technique, as mentioned, enables monitoring of intra-abdominal pressure (IAP), which is often conducted with an intra-bladder balloon catheter connected to a transducer (zero at mid armpit) and by measuring pressure until exhalation, with the patient in a supine position. The diagnostic criteria for identifying intra-abdominal hypertension (IAH) were determined by the World Society of Abdominal Compartment Syndrome (WSACS) [23].

According to the WSACS conference agreement, IAH refers to values of >12 mmHg and abdominal compartment syndrome (ACS) is defined as characterized by IAP values of >20 mmHg with organ dysfunction.

There are many causes of IAH, but several may be present perioperatively, such as: abdominal surgery, abdominal trauma, long-term fluid infusion, massive transfusions, paralytic ileus, acute pancreatitis, and liver transplant.

Fluid overloading in particular is considered an independent predictive factor for the risk of IAH.

We cannot end our discussion of perioperative infusions without referring to the type of crystalloids used.

We have spoken at length of the use of colloids and which ones are preferable for volemic expansion. We have also said, however, that we cannot rule out perioperative crystalloids to balance losses (urine, sweat, diarrhea, perspiration). Too often, however, we talk in general about crystalloids without properly defining them. This is wrong because not all crystalloids are the same, as is too often said: we refer to so-called isotonic saline solutions (0.9 % NaCl) and Ringer's solution. Isotonic saline solutions are often defined as physiological solutions, although there is no organic fluid in this composition and they are most commonly used in medical environments, while Ringer's solution is mostly used in surgery. This is a peculiarity that has no scientific explanation, but is nevertheless a reality throughout the world [24].

A generalization that results in equating isotonic saline and Ringer's solution is an error. Today it is right to affirm that in most clinical situations Ringer's lactate is preferable to a physiological solution. Many studies have shown that isotonic saline solutions can cause hyperchloremic acidosis, in both healthy volunteers and patients receiving fluid resuscitation, and if iatrogenic acidosis from a saline solution occurs in addition to acidosis that often accompanies states of hypoperfusion, it can be understood how this is largely contraindicated in states of tissue hyperperfusion. In the same patients Ringer's lactate does not have the same effect since, by transforming itself into glucose in either the liver or kidneys, it consumes H^+ and, especially in the liver, generates HCO^{3-}. With both of these mechanisms

Ringer's lactate has an antacid action and therefore an opposite effect to saline solutions. The superficial conviction that Ringer's lactate can increase lactacidemia is therefore incorrect. Administering it certainly increases blood lactate levels at first, but the transformation into HCO^3 occurs immediately afterwards and persists with an antacid action.

There are studies that show that in fluid resuscitation in patients with hemorrhage, the blood + Ringer's acetate combination enables evidently higher levels of survival compared to blood + physiological solution [25].

At this point it is not understood how even today a solution containing 154 mEq/l of Na and 154 mEq/l of Cl with a pH < 6 is still called physiological, taking into account the fact that it is often used in the long term in states of tissue hypoperfusion, helping to create dangerous metabolic acidosis.

It is also necessary to consider signs of coagulopathy due to physiological solutions, especially when they are used in patients with hemorrhage, and the effects of solutions with a high Cl^- content on renal function (thus reducing glomerular filtration) [26].

We must conclude, however, that a contraindication to Ringer's lactate has been recorded: renal insufficiency with hyperpotassemia, in view of the fact that the solution also contains 4–5 mEq/l of potassium.

It is worth mentioning, at the end of this chapter, the perioperative infusion strategy in the case of oliguria.

If we rule out primitive renal diseases and obstructive nephropathies that are in an absolute minority perioperatively, the most common cause of oliguria is renal hypoperfusion. The resulting treatment is fluid resuscitation and perhaps furosemide, which is still seen far too often.

The use of a loop diuretic in such cases causes depletion of the intravascular volume with a reduction in glomerular filtration and an increase in azotemia, which raises creatinine higher, creating an increase in the azotemia/creatinemia ratio.

This is a ratio that it would be wise to control in patients with oliguria who are treated with furosemide, since an increase implies discontinuation of the drug. Marik defines furosemide in states of oliguria as "the medicine of the devil" and this certainly seems to be justified.

1.3   Strategies for the Control and Optimization of Patients with Sepsis

The infusion strategy in the management of patients with serious sepsis or septic shock, especially if accompanied by acute respiratory insufficiency (ALI = acute lung injury), is of fundamental importance.

The guidelines of the Surviving Sepsis Campaign of 2008 [27] fix the principles of infusion treatment, which consist of early fluid infusion that is adequate for achieving precise objectives, followed by a phase in which fluids are infused more cautiously.

An initially aggressive infusion strategy is recommended, followed by a conservative infusion strategy when the state of septic shock is over.

This strategy is confirmed by many parties but the recent work of Murphy et al. [28]. in 200 patients with septic shock and ALI is particularly convincing, as it analyzed the efficacy of four infusion strategies: (1) adequate infusion in the initial phase followed by a restrictive strategy in the later phase; (2) adequate infusion in the initial phase followed by a liberal infusion strategy in the later phase; (3) inadequate infusion in the initial phase with a restrictive strategy in the later phase; (4) inadequate strategy in the initial phase followed by a later liberal strategy. The term "adequate" is relative to the infusion strategy suggested by the Sepsis Campaign, and the subdivision into patients who are treated adequately and those who are not treated adequately is possible because the report was retrospective and was based on analyses of information from two important North American hospitals.

The results clearly favor the first infusion strategy.

The difference in mortality between Group 1 (<20 %) and Group 4 (80 %) is particularly striking.

This work does not confirm what is already maintained throughout the world, namely in patients with serious sepsis and septic shock aggressive fluid treatment is justified that must be abandoned, even with the help of amines (mainly norepinephrine and/or dopamine, and possibly dobutamine in the event of persistently low cardiac output) that is barely possible.

Endothelial damage is probably the largest cause of changes that require a liberal infusion strategy.

It is appropriate that in addressing the issue of endothelial damage we pause to consider the new acquisitions on the structure of the superficial layer of the endothelium that is in contact with the blood.

On the surface of the endothelium, lipids of the plasma membrane may link sugar chains by forming **GLYCOPEPTIDES**; proteins of the membrane may link short sugar chains forming **GLYCOPROTEINS** or long sugar chains forming **PROTEOGLYCANS**. Glycoproteins, glycopeptides, and proteoglycans form a superficial structure that is in contact with the blood: **GLYCOCALYX**. The glycocalyx protects the surface of endothelial cells from chemical or mechanical damage. Sugar chains absorb water, making the endothelial cell membrane "slippery": this characteristic helps mobile cells such as leukocytes in transendothelial migration and prevents erythrocytes from adhering to each other and to the vessel walls.

The transmembranal passage of fluids is regulated by the glycocalyx system which acts as a molecular filter that holds back proteins and increases oncotic pressure on the superficial layer of the endothelial walls. The small space between the anatomical part of the vessel and the superficial layer is free from proteins.

The loss of fluids from the vessel is therefore regulated by oncotic pressure on the superficial layer. The classic Starling endothelial barrier is modified according to new acquisitions: there is a "double barrier" with not only endothelial cells but also with an endothelial surface layer composed of a glycocalyx. Therefore, an intact superficial layer is a vital condition for regular circulation.

It should also be said that the absorption of water and proteins by the glycocalyx means that 800 cc of plasma remains adhered to the walls and thus does not contribute to the circulation.

There are many factors that may lead to glycocalyx dysfunction by promoting leukocyte adhesion and increasing transendothelial permeability with the formation of edema. Ischemia itself causes damage to the glycocalyx but perhaps the greatest cause of glycocalyx deterioration is sepsis, which, by harming this structure, promotes considerable transendothelial passage of water and proteins with the formation of edema.

A little known factor in damaging the glycocalyx is fluid overloading. Bruegger [29] has shown that the increased presence of BNP following fluid overload is a cause of glycocalyx damage and therefore at least in part a cause of edema.

The damage caused to the glycocalyx by acute hypovolemia is also little known. Therefore, not only the acute inflammatory event of sepsis is the cause of damage to the endothelial barrier and therefore edema, but also fluid overloading and, furthermore, acute hypovolemia. This new understanding makes it easier to comprehend the phenomenon of edema, which is so common in all critical patients.

The continuous passage of water and proteins from the circulation to the interstices justifies hypovolemia which accompanies sepsis and also justifies the great care required for the infusion strategy.

Damage to the barrier from the inflammatory noxa is in fact later enhanced, as has been said, by changes caused by BNP in the event of fluid overloading and by hypovolemia itself if it is not treated effectively.

The formation of edema is, however, not only due to changes to the endothelial membrane of the capillaries but also to changes that occur in the interstice. Normally if the passage of fluid in the interstice increases, lymphatic drainage also increases, and the aqueous content of the interstice remains normal. In sepsis even lymphatic drainage, if it is also increased, is altered and unsuited to the increased fluid load.

Lymphatic disease also contributes to the formation and gradual worsening of edema. Moreover, while the passage of fluid into the interstice normally increases hydrostatic pressure in the interstice, resulting in the pressure later blocking the passage of water from the capillaries, in inflammation (and therefore sepsis) interstitial hydrostatic pressure does not increase sufficiently, and therefore does not provide the useful contrast to the formation of edema that it usually guarantees. This mechanism, which is particularly used in burns units, though proven for years [30], is not yet common knowledge among doctors, just as the importance of CVP in forming edema is undervalued in clinical practice.

The increase in CVP in fact slows down lymphatic flow, thus contributing to the formation and worsening of edema [31].

At this point it is essential to know what the international literature advises to obtain maximum possible certainty when it is necessary to infuse liquids in a real "colander" such as capillary circulation in septic patients who more than anyone else have an interstice that is too compliant as well as insufficient lymphatic drainage.

The first point to address is whether there are targets to be reached in the first phase and what is meant by "adequate infusion".

In the first phase in the treatment of serious sepsis or septic shock, when the imperative is volemic expansion, it is beyond doubt that plasma expanders such as HES are preferable to crystalloids.

These enable global savings of fluid since they have a plasma expansive effect that is three times greater than crystalloids, thus requiring three times as much volume as crystalloids to achieve the same effect as colloids [32]. As an alternative to synthetic colloids, 15 % albumin solutions can also be used. These unfortunately promote greater formation of edema due to an increase in interstitial oncotic pressure caused by the passage of albumin molecules from the circulation to the interstices. However, since they have a volemic expansive power that is five to six times greater than crystalloids, they may be used in the initial stage of treatment [33].

We have referred to the conservative use of infusions based on exclusive compensation of losses, also by accepting the negative balance, but the greatest problems are in the first phase of treatment, in which the goal is volemic expansion.

Which parameters can be followed to obtain the best results by minimizing the risks?

Let us first say, despite not a few difficulties and uncertainties, that today it is accepted that volemic expansion may be guided with the Fluid Challenge by using at most 3 ml/kg of 6 % HES 130 in 10–15 min and observing the response of SV. It should be remembered that infusions can be continued if SV increases by at least 10–15 % with no significant rise in CVP. Naturally, the restoration of SV does not take long since a moderate dose of the plasma expander administered by the Fluid Challenge and generally around 250 cc is redistributed fairly rapidly and opens the way for new infusions and for the infusion of amines. The absolute CVP value of 8–12 cm H_2O indicated as a target for the Surviving Sepsis Campaign in patients receiving mechanical ventilation is not shared by all. It has, in fact, been demonstrated that in some patients it is necessary to exceed 15 cm H_2O to obtain SV increases and that patients with low CVP may have a negative Fluid Challenge [34].

Even $ScvO_2$, which it is recommended to maintain above 70 %, is not always a good indicator in septic patients, nor are any of the monitoring methods advised to guide the treatment of patients with serious sepsis or septic shock exempt from criticism. This is clearly due to the fact that the commonly used monitoring parameters (CVP, SV, WP) are expressions of macroscopic hemodynamic situations while in sepsis changes to the microcirculation are just as important and are not as easy to monitor.

This reality has led in recent years to microcirculatory control techniques that have been proposed to guide infusions: of these let us refer to the sublingual monitoring of the microcirculation, since it is the easiest to perform. Recently Ospina-Tascon et al., in an interesting study [35], found that it is possible to improve sublingual microcirculation only with infusion in the first 24 h of the diagnosis of sepsis. In later phases it is no longer possible.

This study is further evidence of the importance of correct therapy in the initial phase of sepsis.

A fundamental parameter that cannot be used to guide infusions in the early phase but is extremely important to maintain tissue perfusion is blood pressure. The Surviving Sepsis Campaign of 2008, mentioned above, fixed at 65 mmHg the mean blood pressure to be reached and maintained with infusions and amines. This value, however, may be insufficient in some patients as demonstrated by certain studies, such as that by Jhanji [36], who assessed the effects on the microcirculation of increases in MAP with increasing doses of norepinephrine. Sublingual microcirculation, cutaneous PtO_2 (Clark electrode) and the cutaneous flow of erythrocytes (laser Doppler flowmetry) were analyzed. Therefore, oxygenation and cutaneous microcirculation gradually rose by increasing MAP with norepinephrine from 60 mmHg to 90 mmHg. The authors concluded that in patients with no signs of cardiac compromise, it was possible to have pressure advantages with norepinephrine doses that were even higher than usual without damaging the microcirculation. Similar findings (and in favor of the bolder use of norepinephrine, increasing MAP to 78 mmHg $\pm$ 9 mmHg) were reported in the study by Georger et al. [37]. with NIRS (*Near Infrared Spectroscopy*) on muscular oxygenation in patients with serious septic shock.

From all this it is sufficiently evident that in future we will not always be able to be satisfied only with classic hemodynamic controls to guide the infusion strategy, especially in the early phase of serious sepsis and septic shock, but that we must better focus on controlling the microcirculation.

Fortunately technology seems to be developing. Of particular interest is the possibility of monitoring tissue ΔPCO_2–$PetCO_2$ with a sample of PCO_2 from the ear lobe and a capnograph (maximum value = 26 mmHg) or frequent controls of $\Delta PtCO_2$–$PaCO_2$ ($PtCO_2$ always measured in the ear lobe and $PaCO_2$ with EGA): the maximum value in this case is 16 mmHg [37–39].

The technique is based on the well-known concept that CO_2 accumulates in hypoperfused tissue and therefore the Δ between tissue CO_2 and arterial CO_2 increases.

1.4   Conclusions

In this chapter we have sought to provide an update for resuscitation anesthetists on a vast topic such as fluid therapy but by limiting it to two aspects: one relating to a condition that is the daily bread in our specialization, namely perioperative fluid therapy, and one relating to fluid therapy in septic patients that is still a test bench for all of us.

In particular, fluid therapy in septic patients is a subject that is constantly changing and it is not easy to maneuver between multiple viewpoints that are often contradictory from specialists with doubtful experience. We have sought to provide information that is not linked to any commercial interests, by striving to clarify a highly complex subject.

References

1. Yu M, Chapital A, Ho HC et al (2007) A prospective randomized trial comparing oxygen delivery versus transcutaneous pressure of oxygen values as resuscitative goals. Shock 27:615–622
2. Dyson A, Singer M (2011) Tissue oxygen tension monitoring: will it fill the void? Curr Opin Crit Care 17:281–289
3. Lanke LO, Nilsson GE, Reithner HC (1977) Acta Chir Scand 413:279–284
4. Rehm M, Orth V, Kreimeier U et al (2001) Changes in blood volume during acute normovolemic hemodilution with 5% albumin or 6% HES and intraoperative retransfusion. Anaesthesist 50:569–664
5. Rehm M, Orth V, Kreimeier U et al (2000) Changes in blood volume during acute normovolemic hemodilution and intraoperative retransfusion in patients with radical hysterectomy. Anesthesiology 92:657–664
6. Hecke K, Strunden MS, Reuter DA (2011) Facing the challenge: a rational strategy for fluid and volume management annual update in intensive care and emergency medicine. In: Vincent JL (ed) pp 340–352
7. Chappel D, Jacob M, Hofmann-Kiefer K et al (2008) A rational approach to perioperative fluid management. Anesthesiology 109:723–740
8. Lowell JA, Schifferdecker C, Driscoll DF et al (1990) Postoperative fluid overload: not a benign problem Crit. Care Med 18:728–733
9. Marx G, Ledder S, Smith L et al (2004) Resuscitation from septic shock with capillary leakage: Hydroxyethyl starch (130 kd) but not ringer's solution maintains plasma volume and systemic oxygenation. Shock 21:336–341
10. Cochran Injuries Group (1998) Human albumin administration in critically ill patients: systematic review of randomized controlled trials. Cochrane Injuries Group Albumin Reviewers B.M.G. 317:235–240
11. The Safe Study Investigators (2004) A comparison of albumin and saline for fluid resuscitation in the intensive care unit. NEJM 350:2247–2256
12. Mahmood A, Gosling P, Vohra RK (2007) Randomized clinical trial comparing the effects on renal function of HES or gelatin during aortic aneurysm surgery. Br J Surg 94:427–433
13. Boldt J, Brosch CH, Röhm K et al (2008) Comparison of the effects of gelatin and modern HES solution in renal function and inflammatory response in elderly cardiac surgery patients. Br J Anaesth 100:457–465
14. Neff TA, Doelberg M, Jungheinrich C (2003) Ripetitive large-dose infusion of the novel HES 130/0.4 in patients with severe head injury. Anesth Analg 96:453–459
15. Sakr Y, Payen D, Reinhart K et al (2007) Effects of HES administration on renal function in critically ill patients. Br J Anaesth 98:216–224
16. Michardi F, Teboul JL (2002) Predicting fluid responsiveness in ICU patients: a critical analysis of the evidence. Chest 121:2000–2008
17. Cecconi M, Singer B, Rhodes A (2011) The fluid challenge annual update in intensive care and emergency medicine. In: Vincent JL (ed), Springer pp 332–339

18. Venn R, Steele A, Richardson P et al (2002) Randomized controlled trial to investigate influence of the fluid challenge on duration of hospital stay and perioperative morbidity in patients with hip fractures. Br J Anaesth 88:65–71
19. Vincent GL, Neil MH (2006) Fluid challenge revisited. Crit Care Med 34:1333–1337
20. Isakow W, Shuster DP (2006) Extravascular lung water measurements and hemodynamic monitoring in the critically ill: bedside alternatives to the pulmonary artery catheter. Am J Physiol Lung Cell Med Physiol 291:1118–1131
21. Sakka SG, Klein M, Reinhart K et al (2002) Prognostic value of EVLW in critically ill patients. Chest 122:2080–2086
22. Berkowitz DM, Danai PA, Eaton S et al (2008) Accurate characterization of EVLW in ARDS. Crit Care Med 36:1803–1809
23. Malbrain ML, Cheatham ML, Kirkpatrick A et al (2006) Results from the international conference of experts on intra-abdominal hypertension and abdominal compartment syndrome I definitions. Int Care Med 32:1722–1732
24. Marik PE (2010) Handbook of evidence based critical care. Springer, Verlag, pp 55–77
25. Healey MA, Davis RE, Lin FC et al (1998) Lactated ringer's is superior to normal saline in a model of massive hemorrhage and resuscitation. J Trauma 45:894–899
26. Wilcox CS (1983) Regulation of renal blood flow by plasma chloride. J Clin Invest 71:726–735
27. Dellinger RP, Levy MM, Carlet JH et al (2008) Sepsis campaign: International guidelines for management of severe sepsis and septic shock. Crit Care Med 36:296–327
28. Murphy CV, Schramm GE, Dokerty JA et al (2009) The importance of fluid management in ALI secondary to septic shock. Chest 136:102–109
29. Bruegger D, Jacob M, Rehm M et al (2005) Atrial natriuretic peptide induces shedding of endothelial glycocalyx in coronary vascular bed of guinea pig hearts. Am J Physiol Heart Circ Physiol 289: 1993–1999
30. Lund T, Wiig H, Reed RK et al (1987) A new mechanism for edema generation: strongly negative interstitial fluid pressure causes rapid fluid flow into thermally injured skin. Acta Physiol Scand 129:433–435
31. Hedenstierna G, Lattuada M (2008) Lymphatics and lynph in ALI. Curr Opin Crit Care 14:31–36
32. Trof PJ, Groeneveld ABJ (2011) Cristalloid or colloid fluids: a matter of volumes. In: Annual update in intensive care and emergency medicine, pp 313–321
33. Ernest D, Balzberg AS, Dodek PM (1999) Distribution of normal saline and 5% albumin infusions in septic patients. Crit Care Med 27:46–50
34. Osrnan D, Ridel C, Ray P et al (2007) Cardiac filling pressure are not appropriate to predict hemodynamic response to volume challenge. Crit Care Med 35:64–68
35. Ospina-Tascon G, Neves AP, Occhipinti G et al (2010) Effects of fluids on microvascular perfusion in patients with severe sepsis. Int Care Med 36:949–955
36. Jhanji S, Stirling S, Patel N et al (2009) The effect of increasing doses of norepinephrine on tissue oxygenation and microvascular flow in patients with septic shock. Crit Care Med 37:1961–1966
37. Allée F, Mateo J, Dubreuil G et al (2010) Cutaneous ear lobe PCO2 at 37°t evaluate microperfusion in patients with septic shock. Chest 138:1062–1070
38. Georger JF, Hamzooni O, Chaari A et al (2010) Restoring arterial pressure with norepinephrine improves muscle tissue oxygenation assessed by near infrared spectroscopy in severly hypotensive septic patients. Int Care Med 36:1882–1889
39. Fang X, Tang W, Sun S et al (2006) Comparison of buccal microcirculation between septic and hemorrhagic shock. Crit Care Med 34:S447–S453

Enough has been Written About the Treatment of ALI, but has Enough been Said About how to Prevent It?

Biagio Allaria

Acute Lung Injury (ALI) is a syndrome characterized by the presence of non-cardiogenic pulmonary edema and hypoxemia as a result of various types of disease or condition.

The difference between ALI and ARDS is predominantly linked to the severity of hypoxemia. According to the terminology coined by the NAECC (North American European Consensus Conference) in 1994 [1], and which is still in used, ALI applies to patients with $PaO_2/FiO_2 < 300$ while ARDS applies to patients with $O_2/FiO_2 < 200$. ALI and ARDS are therefore two differing levels of severity of the same phenomenon and a high proportion of ALI leads to ARDS.

As we shall see below, the factors that may lead to the onset of ALI/ARDS are numerous and can mostly be influenced. There are therefore wide margins for the prevention of this syndrome.

Naturally, to implement effective preventive action it is first necessary to identify patients who are at risk, i.e., those who are most likely to develop this syndrome.

We must distinguish between patients with ongoing acute diseases or specific situations known to cause ALI/ARDS, whether pulmonary diseases such as bronchopneumonia (whose severe forms occur in ALI/ARDS in 47 % of cases [2], septic shock (47 %), acute pancreatitis (33 %), massive transfusions (26 %), multiple trauma (16 %) [3]) or patients who simply due to mechanical ventilation,

B. Allaria (✉)
Former Director of the Critical Patient Department of the National Institute
for the Study and Treatment of Tumors, currently Consultant in Clinical Risk Management,
National Institute for the Study and Treatment of Tumors,
Via Venezian 1, 20133, Milan, Italy
e-mail: biagio.allaria@tiscali.it

B. Allaria (ed.), *Practical Issues in Anesthesia and Intensive Care 2013*,
DOI: 10.1007/978-88-470-5529-2_2, © Springer-Verlag Italia 2014

even under general anesthesia, experience changes to their lungs that may lead to ALI/ARDS.

Among the latter, we must include those for whom the incorrect use of fluids may worsen respiratory insufficiency that would have remained moderate without the input of this iatrogenic injury.

In our preventive work, it is necessary not only to try to avoid the onset of ALI/ARDS but also not to provoke deterioration with inappropriate therapeutic action. Thus, it is also important to understand ALI at the onset and therefore useful to spend some time discussing the rapid diagnosis of ALI.

This chapter is therefore divided into 5 sections in which we shall examine in depth the concepts that enable the prevention of ALI with correct mechanical ventilation, appropriate fluid management, a transfusion strategy, correct use of insulin perioperatively and in critical patients, and knowledge of the mechanisms that can prevent organ damage by toxic substances transported from the intestinal lymphatic circulation.

2.1   Can Mechanical Ventilation Alone Cause Lung Damage in Patients with Healthy Lungs? Can this be Optimized?

From controversial data in the literature it seems possible to say that the mechanical ventilation of a healthy lung, as during surgery under general anesthesia, cannot, per se, cause acute pulmonary damage with the characteristics of ALI/ARDS.

It is true that during major abdominal surgery and lung surgery pro-inflammatory cytokines increase. This, however, is linked closely to the degree of surgical trauma and does not seem to be affected by the ventilation technique.

An interesting work in this regard was performed by Wrigge et al. [4], who used different techniques to ventilate patients undergoing thoracotomy or laparotomy for pulmonary or major abdominal interventions, and assessed the extent of pro-inflammatory cytokines in the blood and tracheal aspiration. A group of patients were ventilated with a VT of 12–15 ml/kg ideal weight and 0 PEEP, and another group was managed with "protective" ventilation: VT 6 ml/kg ideal weight and PEEP 10 cm H_2O. All patients had an increased level of cytokines but no significant difference was found between the two groups of patients.

The authors concluded that the method of normal pulmonary ventilation during this type of surgery did not alter the inflammatory response as a consequence of surgery. However, a few years earlier the authors had shown that mechanical ventilation in healthy lungs, with no surgical intervention, did not increase plasma concentrations of inflammatory mediators (TNF, IL6, IL1, IL8, IL10, and IL12).

These observations seem to support the "two-hit model", i.e., the "double damage" model for ALI/ARDS.

The first damage would be pulmonary inflammation, and the second would be ventilation.

In fact, when various methods of ventilation are used on "inflamed" lungs, the differences in the production of cytokines are certainly felt. In these lungs, low VT ventilation with PEEP is certainly less harmful than high VT ventilation with 0 PEEP. This is a reality that has been known for some time and is accepted by all.

There is, however, also evidence that the various means of ventilation influence the inflammatory response, particularly in the case of esophagectomy operations. In an interesting work published in Anesthesiology in 2006 [5], Michelet et al. controlled the inflammatory response (IL1β, IL6, IL8, and TNF) in two groups of patients undergoing esophagectomy who, as was known, were supposed to receive One Lung Ventilation (OLV).

The first group were treated with OLV equal to bi-pulmonary ventilation (VT 9 ml/kg), and the second with VT reduced to 5 ml/kg with the introduction of PEEP 5 cm H_2O. The pattern of the inflammatory response varied greatly: patients with "protective" ventilation had a lower inflammatory response, a better PaO_2/FiO_2 ratio during OLV and 1 h after surgery, and an earlier possibility of extubation.

It would seem to be expected that switching from bi-pulmonary ventilation to OLV would be logical in reducing ventilation. However, many still maintain the same standards of ventilation used for bi-pulmonary ventilation; obviously for fear that a reduction may promote phenomena of alveolar involvement and thus atelectasis.

This means, however, that by beginning trauma ventilation for a lung may promote a greater inflammatory response and an increase in extravascular pulmonary water, which may trigger the onset of ALI.

We are therefore at the point where, in general, different ventilation strategies in patients with healthy lungs do not have different inflammatory responses but there are signs that in any type of surgery involving periods of OLV differing ventilation strategies may be important in affecting patient outcomes.

This applies to the inflammatory response to ventilation. But the ventilation of healthy lungs under general anesthesia is at the basis of other major respiratory dysfunctions that are worth describing since that may be the starting point for postoperative bronchopneumonia complications and therefore ALI.

The point about the effects of anesthesia on the respiratory system was made in length by Hedenstierna and Edmark in 2005 [6]. The authors, starting with the premise that oxygen desaturation is common under general anesthesia and that it is exacerbated immediately after surgery leading to pulmonary complications in 3–10 % of patients, analyzed the possible causes of such changes and later proposed measures required to prevent it.

In patients under general anesthesia the percentage of shunt (alveoli that are perfused by not ventilated) is 8–10 %, while in awake patients it is 1–2 %. The lung, however, does not only contain two populations of alveoli (normal and shunted). There are in fact a certain number of alveoli in which ventilation is not fully abolished but only reduced. In these regions of the lung, there is not a real shunt but only a reduction in the ventilation/perfusion ratio (V/Q), which falls from the normal value of 0.8 to lower levels. In the usual calculation to assess the shunt, both these pulmonary regions are used: those that really are shunted and those with a low V/Q ratio. For this reason it would be more precise to speak of "venous admixture," which therefore includes shunt and reduced V/Q.

Of these two components, V/Q tends to be reduced and transform into shunt if elevated FiO_2 levels are used. In this case, in fact, the reabsorption of oxygen transforms poorly ventilated alveoli into collapsed alveoli. But it is another mechanism with which elevated FiO_2 promotes the shunt: by increasing alveolar PO_2 (PAO_2) it reduces hypoxic vasoconstriction (HPV = hypoxic pulmonary vasoconstriction).

Normally, in poorly ventilated regions HPV diverts blood toward the ventilated regions, thus preserving the shunt; by hyperoxygenating the patient, HPV is inhibited and therefore the shunt is promoted.

But in anesthesia it is another mechanism that inhibits HPV and promotes the shunt: that of halogenated anesthesia. This has been shown to reduce HPV by 50 % [7].

We have therefore seen that in anesthesia there is a tendency to increase the shunt and that this is promoted by using elevated FiO_2 in the case of volatile anesthesia.

But why are there such ventilation problems in anesthesia?

A reduction in respiratory system compliance has been documented with anesthesia (lungs + thoracic walls) from a mean value of 95 ml/cm H_2O to 60 ml/cm H_2O, which occurs in particular due to lung compliance. The phenomenon is linked to a reduction in FRC of approximately 0.5 l, which has also been documented in general anesthesia.

The reduction of FRC and pulmonary compliance is at the basis of atelectasis that occurs very rapidly at the beginning of anesthesia. It has been shown that after the induction of anesthesia and before surgery, 15–20 % of lungs are collapsed at the base and that such atelectatic phenomena may persist for several hours or days after surgery [8].

The phenomenon does not seem to be influenced by the patient's weight, and this is certainly of less importance in those with COPD.

As is to be expected, there is a strict correlation between the degree of atelectasis evaluated by computerized tomography and the degree of shunt.

Finally, Hedenstierna emphasizes that, at least in part, the problems of ventilation in general anesthesia are linked to changes in the volume of closure of the peripheral airways that are responsible for the reduction in ventilation in the regions immediately above those that are atelectatic. In conclusion, a lung under general anesthesia may be divided into three sections: one normal, with a normal V/Q ratio; one with changes to the closure volume (greater than FRC) that inhibits ventilation; and one with collapsed alveoli, where ventilation is completely non-existent.

After this description of respiratory changes that occur under general anesthesia, the similarity between anesthesia and ALI/ARDS stands out, considering that in both cases hypoxemia, atelectasis, shunt, and reduced compliance are observed even if in ALI/ARDS these phenomena are much more serious.

These changes are due to reductions in muscle tone that are confirmed in anesthesia (even without the use of curares) and due to the use of elevated FiO_2 that is still common.

How can we prevent or diminish atelectasis under general anesthesia?

The first strategy that comes to mind is to introduce PEEP, but this is not a good idea.

The introduction of PEEP, by increasing intrathoracic pressure, actually redistributes the flow in favor of lower sections of the lung, where, if dysventilation already exists, shunt increases; moreover, as soon as PEEP is removed, the previously collapsed regions collapse once more immediately. The result is that at the end of anesthesia we still have the same level of atelectasis [9].

The second strategy that can be considered is to maintain respiratory muscle tone but, even without using myorelaxants, all anesthetics reduce muscle tone and therefore it is difficult to follow this route. There is only one anesthetic that does not reduce muscle tone: ketamine, but if a myorelaxant is added the objective is not achieved equally. Therefore, both PEEP and a different use of anesthetics do not constitute appropriate paths for the reduction of atelectasis.

The only clearly useful method for this objective is to use maneuvers capable of reopening all collapsed alveoli simply with insufflation pressure of 40 cm H_2O, which corresponds to the maximum inhalation potential. For this reason, it is called the "vital capacity maneuver" [10]. The recommended duration of this maneuver is 7–8 s and since it may cause hemodynamic imbalance it is advisable to perform it with a careful control of pressure values and heart rate.

A final useful strategy to reduce the incidence of atelectasis is to minimize the reabsorption of alveolar gas that occurs in the reduction of FiO_2. For this reason, the maneuvers described above are not performed with pure O_2, since in this case, the alveoli collapse very soon after the maneuver to the same level as before the maneuver [11]. Even by using the usual mix of gas in anesthesia (N_2O/V_2 60/40) for the maneuver, 40 min after the end of the maneuver atelectasis is only 20 % of the level prior to the maneuver. For these reasons it is advisable never to exceed an FiO_2 of 30–40 % in general anesthesia, unless it is not a situation of emergency hypoxemia.

Even preoxygenation, which is still much used before intubation to have a longer time of acceptable oxygenation in the case of difficult intubations, promotes the formation of atelectasis. According to Hedenstierna, preoxygenation with 100 % FiO_2 causes atelectasis of approximately 7 min and this continues for another 7 min and may persist even longer, possibly exacerbated by other previously described mechanisms, until the end of anesthesia and the postoperative phase.

This long section on the possible implications of the incorrect use of a life-support system during surgical interventions is oriented toward anesthetists with the objective that optimizing ventilation techniques can reduce atelectasis which certainly is a considerable part of the cause of postoperative bronchopneumonia complications.

We have thus far spoken about patients with healthy lungs under general anesthesia, but the concepts described above also apply to patients with mechanically ventilated lungs in ICU for extrapulmonary reasons, who, since they are often deeply sedated, are similar to anesthetized patients. We are furthermore in agreement with the findings of Schultz et al. [12] in their excellent work in Anesthesiology in 2007, namely that protective ventilation with VT of 6 ml/kg and PEEP of 5 cm H_2O is advisable in patients with respiratory insufficiency for the widest range of reasons but that they still are not covered by criteria for the diagnosis of ALI/ARDS. This ventilation strategy reduces, according to Schultz, the possibility that these situations develop into ALI or ARDS.

Finally, regarding the prevention of ALI/ARDS in patients with shock, we should point out that there are few possibilities, but that such possibilities exist and need to be taken into account. We cite the two most important: correct management of fluid treatment, which we shall discuss shortly, and the timeliness of therapeutic intervention.

Iscimen et al. have written about the importance of the timeliness of treatment in the prevention of ALI/ARDS in patients in shock in Critical Care Medicine in 2008 [13]. The authors, aware that at least 50 % of patients with shock experience ALI/ARDS, hypothesized that the delay in treatment in the acute phase may have an important role in causing this. In seeking to confirm the accuracy of the hypothesis, they observed 160 patients in shock who at the onset of symptoms had no picture of ongoing ALI/ARDS. Of these, 71 (equivalent to 44 %) developed ALI, on average 5 h after the onset of shock and in every case within 12 h: two factors emerged as important in causing the respiratory complication: a delay in intensive treatment and inadequate and delayed antibiotic therapy.

2.2   Correct Fluid Management

It has long been discussed whether in patients with ALI it is worth restricting fluids whether or not in addition to diuretic treatment. This strategy emerged because in this disease, characterized by a change in the alveolar/capillary membrane, each increase in hydrostatic pressure leads to an increase in pulmonary edema and thus the worsening of respiratory function.

On the other hand, a restricted infusion accompanied by the use of diuretics exposes the patient to the risk of reduced cardiac output and a resultant fall in organ perfusion. Since patients with ALI/ARDS die most often from multiple organ insufficiency, it is understood how this type of strategy has long been under discussion. However, in 2006 the results of a randomized, multi-center study in a large number of patients appeared in the New England Journal of Medicine was the final word in the debate [14]. There were 500 patients with ALI/ARDS ($PaO_2/FiO_2 < 300$) treated restrictively compared with 500 patients in whom the infusions were conducted liberally. All were monitored with Swan-Ganz catheters for the first 3 days and, if hemodynamic stability was achieved, with CVP from Day 4.

The monitoring of all organ functions continued for 28 days. The conclusions were that conservative treatment improved respiratory function, and reduced the duration of mechanical ventilation and hospitalization in ICU without causing an increase in multiple organ insufficiency.

There is therefore no doubt whatsoever that, if accurate monitoring is possible, a restrictive strategy for fluids is preferable in patients with ALI/ARDS.

This, however, does not necessarily mean that a strategy of this type is also useful for patients who do not have ALI/ARDS but who are simply at risk of contracting it (patients with acute pancreatitis, bronchopneumonia, massive transfusions, multiple trauma, shock, etc.). This is because there is nothing in the literature that convincingly supports a restrictive fluid strategy for all patients who are at risk for ALI and who are admitted to ICU even if a retrospective study of 2,583 mechanically ventilated patients seems to demonstrate that a positive overall fluid balance is a risk factor for the onset of ALI [15].

A potentially more convincing study, albeit in a smaller number of surgical patients admitted to ICU, appeared in Anesthesia Analgesia in 2010 [16]. This study of patients with postoperative respiratory insufficiency seems to show the presence of a statistically significant correlation between the onset of ALI and the positive intraoperative fluid balance.

It nevertheless seems possible to say that cautious use of infusions may be part of the strategy for preventing ALI.

2.3 Use of Blood Derivatives

ALI as a result of transfusion (TRALI = Transfusion-Related Acute Lung Injury) was first described in 1983 by Popovsky [17] and was interpreted as acute respiratory insufficiency caused by antileukocyte antibodies. With the passage of time it was seen that TRALI was essentially linked to the use of whole blood, plasma, and platelets from donors (especially women) with positive antileukocyte antibodies. From the study by Khan in 2007, it was clear that in 841 critical patients the incidence of ALI was greater in those who had received fresh frozen plasma and platelets compared to those who had received only concentrated red blood cells [18].

In accordance with the "double damage" theory for the onset of ALI, it is necessary to point out the importance of the coexistence of a predisposing factor from the patient (pancreatitis, shock, bronchopneumonia, etc.) alongside the presence of antileukocyte antibodies from the donor that interact with antigens in the recipient. The finding of a greater number of TRALI cases due to blood derivatives from female donors has led the UK National Transfusion Service to virtually eliminate plasma and its components from female donors and similar initiatives have been implemented in the USA [19].

The incidence of TRALI is certainly lower in recent years following the decision that was adopted (even though implementation of correct strategies is not uniform) but the fact remains that the use of whole blood, plasma, and platelets should be highly frugal and not liberal. Once again, as with fluid therapy, we should recommend a restrictive approach.

A study by Murphy in 2009 [20] showed that 47 % of patients with ARDS received blood without sufficient reason to justify this and that 67 % were transfused despite Hb being higher than the threshold value of 7 g/dl. In the prevention of ALI, therefore, the frugal use of blood and derivatives plays a role and sensitization to the problem of transfusion centers. This strategy was implemented together with protective ventilation in critical patients by Ylmar et al. In a study published by these authors in Critical Care in 2007, the combination of protective ventilation and the conservative use of blood and derivatives enabled an 18 % reduction in the incidence of ALI [21].

This is one of the first attempts to combine various strategies to prevent ALI and we wish that from this chapter the appropriate messages of the need for simultaneous intervention in all known risk factors are received.

2.4   The Mystery of Diabetes: Risk Factor or Protection Factor?

Diabetes has been and continues to be considered an important risk factor when associated with numerous diseases such as multiple trauma, renal insufficiency, and cardiovascular diseases. In contrast, a protective effect for diabetes in patients with shock has been found with the onset of ALI. In a study by Moss et al., published more than 10 years ago in Critical Care Medicine in patients with shock, it was revealed that non-diabetic shock patients more frequently developed ARDS compared to diabetic patients (47 % vs. 25 %) [22].

Much more recently, in 2008, a study by Iscimen et al. in the same journal, confirmed Moss's findings [23]. Since the presence of diabetes is inevitably accompanied by higher glycemic values and since it has been proven many times that hyperglycemia is associated with higher mortality rates in critical patients, it is difficult to think of hyperglycemia or diabetes as a disease is at the origin of protection in the onset of ALI. Many other studies in animals have shown that hyperglycemia causes oxidative stress which occurs alongside the stress that is present with ALI/ARDS [24].

Moreover, hyperglycemic states induce the formation of advanced glycation end products (AGEs) that promote inflammation and endothelial dysfunction [25].

AGEs have recently been used as markers for type I alveolar cell damage and it has been shown that a higher level of circulating AGEs is associated with the seriousness of ALI and the outcome of patients with ALI/ARDS [26].

Yet metabolic changes in diabetes are not limited to hyperglycemia. For example, it is known that in type 2 diabetes (which is the most common form by a long way) the level of insulin-like growth factor (IGF1) is low and that this low level is at least in part responsible for insulin resistance. IGF1 is nevertheless considered important in causing inflammation in ALI/ARDS. Since in diabetic patients IGF1 is barely represented, its pro-inflammatory effect on the lungs is felt to a lesser extent [27].

But the explanation of the protective effect of diabetes in ALI occurs in particular in drugs that are used to treat it, primarily insulin, which in perioperative phases and in ICU is the most frequently used drug. It is known that insulin is able to modulate inflammation, regulate cell apoptosis, prevent endothelial dysfunction and hypercoagulability, reduce neutrophil chemotaxis, and prevent the excessive production of NO. Practically all these mechanisms are involved in the pathogenesis of ALI.

With the current state of knowledge, it, therefore, appears possible to conclude that careful perioperative insulin therapy and the treatment of critical patients may be considered one of the useful strategies to reduce the incidence of ALI and/or to slow down the development toward ARDS. Especially in perioperative phases, there are still too many departments where instead of using insulin for continuous infusion, as is universally recommended, the hyperglycemic phase is undertaken with an IV insulin bolus or, worse still, a subcutaneous bolus, thus promoting inacceptable and dangerous variability in glycemia.

Even other drugs used to treat diabetes have been found to be useful in the prevention of ALI: we refer to metformin, rosiglitazone, ACE inhibitors, and statins [27].

The latter in particular are capable of contrasting vascular permeability and inflammation [28].

2.5   The Hypothesis of Organ Damage Due to Lymphatic Fluid from the Bowel

Animal studies have repeatedly shown that the bowel, in critical situations (shock, hemorrhage, multiple trauma, etc.) is an important source of toxic mediators that are transported from the bowel to the general circulation of mesenteric lymph nodes. Thus, toxic substances of local origin are distributed throughout the body, causing distant organ damage [29].

It is not entirely clear with which mechanisms these toxic substances are produced, but it is likely that intestinal ischemia, mucosa damage, and bacterial translocation are all factors encountered by the lymphatic fluid once the thoracic duct and subclavian vein are reached, and the possibility of first-line pulmonary damage is evident.

It is interesting to note that the production of toxic substances in shock in animals is confirmed early in fluid resuscitation. This leads to the hypothesis that the mechanism of ischemia–reperfusion is important in causing this pathological situation.

We have mentioned this risk factor, the acquisition of which is fairly recent, because in the literature there are suggestions that contradict it. The most promising strategy is that of early enteral nutrition in septic patients, using immunologically active products such as Impact. In a study by Galaban et al., published in 2003 in Critical Care Medicine, it was shown how immunologically active early enteral nutrition (Impact) may be more effective that the most common method used to date (Nutrodip Protein) in terms of reducing mortality, multiple organ compromise, and episodes of bacteremia [30].

This possibility is still confirmed in the excellent review of ALI prevention possibilities published by Galvin in 2011 [3].

It therefore seems possible to conclude that, especially in septic patients who most often suffer from ALI/ARDS, early enteral nutrition should be considered as one of the ALI prevention strategies.

2.6   Conclusions

In view of the importance of ALI, as a cause of death and in extending the hospitalization either of critical patients in ICU or those with a perioperatively elevated risk requiring more advanced monitoring, implementing, any prevention strategy is a specific duty of anesthetists and resuscitation experts.

Whereas, for years the objective of treating this disease in the best possible way has commendably been pursued, much less has been done in terms of prevention.

What we have said justifies the decision to proceed with greater energy along this path.

References

1. Bernard GR, Artigos A, Brigham Kl et al (1994) The American European consensus conference on ARDS: definitions, mechanism, relevant outcomes and clinical trial coordination. Am J Resp Care Med 149:818–824
2. Ferguson ND, Frutos F, Esteban A et al (2007) Clinical risk conditions for ALI in the intensive care unit and Hospital ward: a prospective observational study. Crit Care 11:R96
3. Galvin I, Ferguson ND (2011) Acute Lung Injury in the ICU: focus on prevention annual update in intensive care and emergency medicine. In: Vincent JL (ed) pp 117–128
4. Wrigge H, Uhlig U, Zinserling J et al (2004) The effects of different ventilator settings on pulmonary and systemic inflammation responses during major surgery. Anesth Analg 98:775–781
5. Michelet P, D'Joumo XP, Roch A et al (2006) Protective ventilation influence systemic inflammation after esophagectomy. Anesthesiology 105:911–919
6. Hedenstierna G, Edmark L (2005) The effects of anesthesia and muscle paralysis on the respiratory system. Intens Care Med 31:1327–1335
7. Marshall BE (1998) Effects of anesthetics on pulmonary gas exchange. In: Stanley TH, Sperry RJ (ed) Anesthesia and the Lung. Kluwer, London, pp 117–125
8. Lindberg P, Gunnarsson L, Tokics L et al (1992) Atelectasis, gas exchange and lung function in the postoperative period. Acta Anaesth Scand 36:546–553

9. Brismar B, Hedenstierna G, Lundquist H et al (1985) Pulmonary densities during anesthesia with muscular relaxation: a proposal of atelectasis. Anesthesiology 62:422–428
10. Rothen HU, Sporre B, Engberg G et al (1993) Reexpansion of atelectasis during general anesthesia: a computed tomography study. Br J Anesth 71:788–795
11. Rothen HU, Sporre B, Engberg G et al (1995) Influence of gas composition on recurrence of atelectasis after a reexpansion maneuver during general anesthesia. Anesthesilogy 82:832–842
12. Schultz MJ, Hitsma JJ, Slutsky AS et al (2007) What TV should be used in patients without ALI? Anesthesiology 106:1226–1231
13. Iscimen R, Cartu R, Ylmer M et al (2008) Risk factors for the development of ALI in patients with septic shock: an observational cohort study. Crit Care Med 36:1518–1522
14. The National Heart (2006) Lung and blood institute ARDS clinical trials network comparison of two fluid-management strategies in ALI. N Engl J Med 354:2564–2576
15. Jia X, Malhorta A, Saeed M et al (2008) Risk factors for ARDS in patients without ARDS. Chest 133:853–861
16. Huges CG, Weavind L, Banerjee A et al (2010) Intraoperative risk factors for ARDS in critically ill patients. Anesth Analg 111:464–467
17. Popovsky MA, Abel MP, Moore SB (1983) Transfusion related acute lung injury associated with passive transfer of antileukocyte antibodies. Am Rev Resp Dis 118:185–189
18. Kahn H, Belshar J, Yilmer M et al (2007) FFP and platelet transfusion are associated with development of ALI in critically ill medical patients. Chest 131:1308–1314
19. Hume HA (2009) TRALI: moving toward prevention. Transfusion 49:402–405
20. Murphy DJ, Howard D, Muriithi A et al (2009) Red blood cell transfusion practices in ALI: what do patient factors contribute? Crit Care Med 36:1935–1940
21. Ylmar M, Keegan MT, Iscimen R et al (2007) Protocol-guided limitation of large TV ventilation and inappropriate transfusion. Crit Care 35:1660–1666
22. Moss M, Guidot DM, Steinberg KP et al (2000) Diabetic patients have a decreased incidence of ARDS. Crit Care Med 28:2187–2192
23. Iscimen R, Cartin-Ceba R, Ylmar M et al (2008) Risk factors for the development of ALI in patients with septic shock: an observational cohort study. Crit Care Med 36:1518–1522
24. HagiwareS, Iwasoka H, Hazegawa a et al (2008) Effects of hyperglycemia and insulin therapy on high mobility group box 1 in endotoxin-induced ALI in a rat model. Crit Care Med 36:2407–2413
25. Ramasamy R, Yan SF, Herold K et al (2008) Receptor for advanced glycation end products: fundamental roles in the inflammatory response: winding the way to the pathogenesis of endothelial disfunction and atherosclerosis. Ann NY Scand Sci 1126:7–18
26. Calfec CS, Ware LB, Eisner MD et al (2008) Plasma receptor for AGE products and clinical outcome in ALI. Thorax 63:1083–1089
27. Schnapp LM, Donhoe S, Chen J et al (2006) Missing ARDS proteome: identification of the insulin-like growth factor (IGF)/IGF binding protein-3 pathway in ALI. Am J Pathol 169:86–95
28. Pirat A, Zeyneloghn P, Aldemir D et al (2006) Pretreatment with simvastin reduces lung injury related to intestinal ischemia reperfusion in rats. Anesth Analg 102:225–232
29. Dietch EA (2001) Role of gut lymphatic in MOF. Curr Opin Crit Care 7:92–98
30. Galban C, Montejo JC, Mesejo A et al (2000) An immune-enhancing enteral diet reduces mortality rate and episodes of bacteremia in septic intensive care unit patients. Crit Care Med 28:643–648
31. Wrigge H, Zinserling J, Stüber F et al (2000) Effects of mechanical ventilation on release of cytokines into systemic circulation in patients with normal pulmonary function. Anesthesiology 93:1413–1417
32. Honiden S, Gong M (2009) Diabetes, insulin, and development of ALI. Crit Care Med 37:2455–2464

Prevention of Perioperative Myocardial Ischemia

3

Biagio Allaria

The prevention of perioperative myocardial ischemia is based in particular on substantial knowledge of the mechanisms that are liable to trigger it. Only by understanding these mechanisms is it possible to block them effectively. Since, however, they are mainly factors that lead to disturbance of the physiology the coronary circulation, it is necessary to take into account both the physiology and pathophysiology of the coronary circulation in order to understand how to prevent myocardial ischemia.

Another useful basis to recall in this preventive work is the identification of patients who are at risk of coronary ischemia, but unfortunately not enough importance has been given to this aspect over the years since, once patients have been identified as being at risk, insufficient attention is usually paid to them to avoid ischemia-inducing mechanisms. In fact, in recent years at-risk patients have carefully been identified but they have been directed toward procedures that are substantially similar to those for patients who are not at risk, whereas they would have needed better monitoring, a more appropriate choice of anesthesia and, above all, operating teams with greater understanding and experience in "protected" postoperative situations.

In the absence of such an effort that would lead to an effective prevention strategy, early diagnosis and early treatment, the proposal of generalized protection of these patients with beta blockers has had considerable success. Beta blockers, as the result of scientific articles by names of great international renown,

B. Allaria (✉)
Former Director of the Critical Patient Department of the National Institute
for the Study and Treatment of Tumors, currently Consultant in Clinical Risk Management,
National Institute for the Study and Treatment of Tumors,
Via Venezian 1, 20133, Milan, Italy
e-mail: biagio.allaria@tiscali.it

B. Allaria (ed.), *Practical Issues in Anesthesia and Intensive Care 2013*,
DOI: 10.1007/978-88-470-5529-2_3, © Springer-Verlag Italia 2014

have been widely welcomed with enthusiasm as they are capable of protecting patients from myocardial ischemic events. Paradoxically, the general protective strategy with beta blockers once again serves to "cover" the insufficiency of control systems and the poor quality of treatment.

Since tachycardia was perhaps the main cause of perioperative ischemia, instead of an early understanding of its causes and preventing it or treating it early, it is preferable to have it at constantly lower levels with a drug. From the time of the first interest in this type of "aspecific protection", the over-simplified nature of the strategy did not escape many of us. Often, in the course of surgery, maintaining satisfactory blood pressure and cardiac output levels is possible thanks to an increase in heart rate, and this phenomenon, albeit moderate, is a sign for the anesthetist that the cause will soon be individualized (too light anesthesia? Absolute or relative hypovolemia?) and corrected just as quickly, preventing tachycardia from becoming an ischemia-inducing factor. It should be restated that the identification of at-risk patients remains an underused strategy during and after surgery, together with updated knowledge of the pathophysiology of the coronary circulation, which is a *sine qua non* condition for preventing ischemic complications, rapidly diagnosing them and correctly adjusting them.

3.1 Pathophysiological Signs in Coronary Circulation

The heart is the only organ that generates its own flow and which influences it with the same activity that generates it: the vast majority of coronary flow (80 %), in fact, occurs in the diastolic phase when the cardiac muscle is relaxed.

Coronary flow at rest is high in proportion to each gram of tissue, as with the brain and kidneys, and gradually tends to diminish with age. The similarity with the brain persists even with high oxygen extraction (which is not characteristic of the kidneys) and for this reason coronary venous blood has a very low oxygen content ($SVO_2 = 20$ %).

The already elevated oxygen extraction at rest cannot later be increased under stress and/or when metabolic demands rise for any reason: in this case, only an increase in flow can therefore counter the rise in oxygen demand.

Normally, therefore, there is a direct relation between oxygen demand in the myocardial tissue and the degree of coronary flow.

This close dependence of myocardial oxygenation of flow, regardless of the impossibility of increasing oxygen extraction in the case of rising metabolic demands, demonstrates the importance of the so-called "coronary reserve".

This "coronary reserve" is an important concept and can be defined in a few words as the difference between flow in baseline conditions and flow at the peak of vasodilatation in a specific condition of mean pressure in arterial perfusion and heart rate. The coronary reserve, in fact, varies with the heart rate and perfusion pressure.

The coronary reserve is decreased when coronary perfusion pressure is lower. When the latter falls below 50 mmHg, a compensatory mechanism is triggered that involves lengthening of the diastolic phase to enable adequate tissue perfusion. This compensatory mechanism appears to be mediated by nitric oxide [1].

This information highlights the danger of certain cases of hypotension in the perioperative phase that are too often accepted unthinkingly, a danger that is obviously propelled if there is simultaneous tachycardia that reduces the duration of diastole and/or if endothelial dysfunction causes insufficient production of nitric oxide.

Endothelial dysfunction is anything but rare and is present even in apparently normal coronary arteries in diabetic patients, hypertensive patients, smokers, and those with a family history of heart disease. If coronary stenosis is present, obviously the coronary reserve later decreases as it does anyway for age alone, in the case of left ventricular hypertrophy, in diabetic patients, and in those with aortic valve disease.

Coronary flow is influenced by pressure from the tissue surrounding the vessels, and therefore, as has been said, it falls during systole, especially in the left ventricle where the contraction force is greater and since intramyocardial pressure is greater at the subendocardial level, flow during systole is redistributed in favor of the subepicardial regions.

Coronary flow of the left ventricle therefore falls considerably during systole and increases at the beginning and in the intermediate phase of diastole and falls again in the final phase of diastole (during which aortic pressure is at minimal values) and stops for practically the entire isometric phase of the following systole.

During diastole perfusion is assured by the pressure gradient between the aortic root (where the coronary arteries emerge) and the right atrium (into which the coronary veins drain). A rough estimate of coronary perfusion pressure (CPP) can be obtained with the following equation:

$$CPP = diastolic\ blood\ pressure - CVP\ (measured\ at\ the\ end\ of\ diastole,$$

$$i.e.\ corresponding\ to\ the\ QRS\ of\ the\ ECG)$$

It is clear that a reduction in this gradient negatively affects flow.

Let us think what may occur in an elderly patient with COPD (with elevated right atrial pressure) and atherosclerotic stenosis of the aortic valve (and therefore very low diastolic pressure at the aortic root). This type of subject is in the most apt conditions for myocardial ischemia, especially if a hypotensive event with tachycardia is confirmed.

In reality the COPD patient is to be considered at high risk for ischemic events in the perioperative phase and the anesthetist, who mostly thinks of the respiratory complications that may arise, would do well to worry about possible ischemic complications too. It should be emphasized that in a patient with COPD characterized by high pulmonary compliance, pulmonary ventilation is particularly felt with venous return, often causing falls in load and pressure. In such conditions, even moderate coronary changes may cause considerable falls in subendocardial perfusion [2]. In order to later refer our attention to the importance of tachycardia (and therefore the reduction in the duration of diastole, which is essential for perfusion), it is sufficient to consider the observation made by Ferro in 1995: a reduction in the duration of diastole from 54 to 45 % of the cardiac cycle has the same effect as coronary stenosis that increases from 40 to 90 % [3].

In determining perfusion of the myocardium, however, not only do the duration of diastole and the right aorta-atrium gradient play a role, but also the aorta-intramyocardial pressure gradient in diastole. We have, in fact, seen how increases in intramyocardial pressure surrounding the vessels cause a reduction in perfusion. A phenomenon of this type is confirmed in chronic heart failure (CHF), where an increase in telediastolic pressure in the left ventricle may reduce this gradient and therefore perfusion, especially in the subendocardial layers.

Even in this case it is useful to recall the attention of anesthetists when they must operate on a patient with precarious cardiac compensation, even for routine surgery. Such a patient, due to increased ventricular diastolic pressure, has a reduced aorta-myocardial gradient and is at risk for ischemia, especially if the duration of diastole is reduced by tachycardia and, in particular, if coronary disease is at the basis of cardiac insufficiency, as is usually the case.

We have repeatedly referred to the particular vulnerability of the subendocardial layers in decreases in perfusion. The phenomenon is clearly understandable if we think that flow is greatly favored in epicardial vessels, which are larger, more superficial, and closer to the aortic root. From the epicardial vessels others branch off that, by detaching themselves perpendicularly, enter the myocardium and thus reach the endocardium. The endocardial vessels, therefore, are further from the origin of flow and more influenced by intramyocardial pressure.

The leveling of ST that we observe on our monitors is the expression of an ischemic condition affecting the subendocardial layers. The phenomenon is greater if accompanied by left ventricular hypertrophy as occurs in hypertension in elderly patients.

It should be noted that if ischemia involves sufficiently wide-ranging parts of the left ventricle, the diastolic release is altered, as is systolic function, resulting in an increase in diastolic pressure on the ventricle, often accompanied by tachycardia that later exacerbates ischemia by creating a vicious circle which, if not interrupted, leads to acute myocardial infarction (AMI).

For this reason a careful observation of the ST tract during surgery in patients with an ischemic risk is fundamental in understanding the phenomenon early and also implementing any possible action to interrupt it.

In conclusion, we should briefly recall the important function that the coronary endothelium plays in vessel motility (vasodilatation and vasoconstriction). Endothelial disease (which, as we have already outlined, is observed not only with atherosclerotic disease but also in smokers, diabetics, those with dyslipidemia and even patients with macroscopically healthy coronary arteries but with considerable family history of coronary disease), characterized by a reduced capacity to produce nitric oxide (NO), reduces the possibility of promoting vasodilatation when necessary, for example to increase myocardial oxygen consumption (MVO_2).

Therefore, when required, flow cannot be sufficient for demand, thus promoting an ischemic event.

Let us consider mild anesthesia with tachycardia, hypertension, and a resulting increase in MVO_2 in a patient with endothelial dysfunction. The adjustment of flow to metabolic requirements does not happen and the precursors are formed for the emergence of ischemia.

But endothelial dysfunction does not impede the adjustment of flow to metabolic needs alone but is also at the basis of enhanced responses or paradoxes that lead to disorders.

For example, acetylcholine, a vagal mediator, which normally causes coronary dilation, may, in the case of endothelial dysfunction, cause coronary constriction.

Amines, which normally have a coronary constrictive effect, enhance this activity. Therefore, in patients with endothelial dysfunction which, as we have seen, is present in many cases, either vagal stimuli or adrenergic stimuli may cause coronary constriction.

We all know how common events of this type are in the perioperative phase; it is worth considering mild anesthesia, visceral traction, awakening with shiver, preoperative emotions, and postoperative pain.

3.2 Identification of Patients at Risk for Ischemia and Early Diagnosis of Ischemia

It should first be said that, even without specific diagnostic measures, we should consider the following as patients with a risk of ischemia: those with a known coronary disease, those with vascular disease in general, diabetics, patients with COPD, those with CHF, and aortic valve disease, and also more simply those with hypertension, especially elderly patients, heavy smokers, and patients with considerable family history of coronary disease. However, it may be useful to assess the coronary reserve of these patients to identify those on whom we should mostly concentrate our monitoring possibilities.

Stress ECG remains a fundamental examination to assess coronary reserve but it is often unusable either because the patient is unable to exert the force or due to difficult interpretation of changes due to the frequent presence of left bundle branch block (LBBB).

If the ECG stress test is impossible, pharmacological stress tests associated with ECG are possible, such as echo-dobutamine and/or echo-dipyridamole. The first reproduces a situation that is similar to that of force due to the increase in heart rate and cardiac output that it produces, and the second, as a result of the coronary dilator effect of the drug used, reproduces a situation of coronary loss.

The advantage in terms of cost and time of an echo-stress in comparison with myocardial scintigraphy is now universally recognized, taking into account the fact that among the two techniques there is no difference in terms of either sensitivity or specificity. The international guidelines establish the absolute interchangeability of these methods [4]. In identifying patients with a particularly high risk, plasma BNP concentrations (brain natriuretic peptide) or pro-BNP concentrations are assuming an increasingly important role or similar significance. BNP is released from the heart chambers under pressure and, considering the importance of the aorta-myocardial gradient in triggering ischemia, its diagnostic value is understood.

All patients at risk for ischemia must be monitored closely, possibly with the automatic analysis of ST with D2, V4, and V5 leads. It has been shown that without an automatic analysis at least 50 % of changes are lost.

Early diagnosis of the ischemic event is naturally possible even with transesophageal echocardiography, since ischemia is accompanied invariably by kinetic changes.

This type of control is thus more effective in ECG since the latter, being highly specific, is less sensitive. Intraoperative echocardiography, however, is not the most available technique in many patients with a high ischemic risk but can be reserved for selected patients such as those with serious known coronary disease and those with post-infarct CHF undergoing complex surgery, especially if large-scale blood loss is expected.

In the case of patients with CHF secondary to significant coronary disease, invasive monitoring with Swan-Ganz catheters may be taken into consideration as it may enable more accurate guiding of infusions since it is the only means to enable the control of Wedge Pressure (WP) that is validly representative of tele-diastolic pressure in the left ventricle and which makes it possible to reduce the risk of overloading and therefore the increase in extravascular lung water (EVLW).

Upon leaving the operating room it is advisable that patients who are at risk for ischemic events undergo 12-lead ECG and that this is repeated at least every day for the first 3–4 days.

In patients with proven changes, even transient, to the ST tract (and, according to some authors, in all patients at risk for ischemia) enzyme control is recommended.

The most commonly used ischemia marker today that is recommended in the postoperative phase is cardiac troponin (cTn). The cTn marker is highly sensitive and specific for myocardial necrosis and certainly more sensitive and specific for CK-MB but, whereas the values to be considered indicative are well known in acute coronary syndromes beyond the surgical environment, there has long been a debate over how to interpret cTn values in the postoperative phase.

A study that clarified the debate was published in 2003 by Landsberg et al. These authors studied 447 patients who underwent vascular surgery with continuous 12-lead ECG in the perioperative phase and cTn and CK-MB controls in the first 3 days following surgery. The cTn marker was more sensitive than CK-MD.

Values for cTnI of 1.5 ng/ml and cTnT values of >0.1 ng/ml are considered positive for the presence of myocardial ischemia [5].

It should, however, be pointed out that cTn values above 0 occur in 0.7 % of the population and are generally associated with cardiac diseases such as left ventricular hypertrophy and either diastolic or systolic disorders of the left ventricle. Such changes, though to a lesser extent than the critical changes highlighted by Landsberg, show that in patients at risk for ischemia baseline cTn controls are performed by observing possible changes in the perioperative period.

The significance of a rise in cTn has long been debated, i.e., whether it is a marker of irreversible damage (i.e., necrosis) or reversible damage. There is much evidence in favor of the fact that cTn elevation may indicate, often briefly, reversible damage alone. Transient increases in cTn observed in triathlon and marathon athletes are indicative of this, as are those observed in patients with pulmonary embolisms [6].

We have already discussed the predictive value of BNP. In particular, the association of cTn and BNP is now considered useful in predicting the ischemic risk [7]. The ischemic risk in patients with COPD has already been outlined. It is also worth noting the observational study in 5,468 patients with COPD by Hjart and Luina [8], who demonstrated that morbidity and mortality in such subjects was twice as high as in the general population.

Patients with COPD are therefore particularly at risk for perioperative ischemic events. It should be noted that, due to their increased pulmonary compliance they in particular "feel" the negative hemodynamic effects of mechanical ventilation, especially if, as is often the case, there is dynamic hyperinflation and intrinsic PEEP. It is therefore not rare that during surgery we face conditions of hypotension and tachycardia that, as we have often said, are the most important predisposing conditions for ischemic events. Correction of ventilation with a Tidal Volume that is not excessive and a sufficiently long expiration time are the most important strategies for preventing decreases in load, hypotension, and tachycardia. However, in such patients it is vital to implement control of the Stroke Volume (SV) with one of the noninvasive measures available today and, as with all patients at risk for ischemia, continuous monitoring of the ST tract on the three recommended leads (D2, V4 and V5) in addition to 12-lead ECG in the first 3 days after surgery, thus controlling ischemia markers as we mentioned a little while ago.

3.3 Prevention of Perioperative Ischemic Events

The first commandment in the strategy for preventing ischemic events is to "AVOID TACHYCARDIA".

We have seen how the reduction in diastolic time corresponds to a reduction in the time available for coronary perfusion and how, in the case of preexisting coronary disease, the final result is equivalent to that of deteriorating stenosis.

In addition there is an increase in MVO_2 which accompanies tachycardia, and the discrepancy that results from its availability and use can lead to an ischemic event.

These simple concepts have been known for years and have led some authors to pursue the short-cut of perioperative beta blockers [9, 10]: considering that tachycardia is a significant cause of ischemia it would seem useful to keep the heart rate constantly low during the perioperative period. Studies like this, even though not large scale, seem to show, especially in patients undergoing vascular surgery especially with a high ischemic risk, that beta blockers enable a reduction in mortality and the incidence of postoperative AMI.

For those who, like us, have worked for many years in vascular surgery, this strategy has barely been accepted.

Patients undergoing vascular surgery often have considerable hemodynamic disturbances, usually due to blood loss, which is often sudden and threatening, due to aortic clamping and de-clamping and even significant changes in body temperature in the intraoperative and postoperative phases. In such situations the mechanisms for compensatory adaptation even include increases in heart rate. Blocking this may trigger falls in output that have repercussions on the intestines, liver, and kidneys.

Beta blockers in all patients may reduce myocardial ischemic events but promote decreases in intestinal, hepatic, renal, and pulmonary perfusion (paralytic ileus, acute renal insufficiency, increased pulmonary dead space, etc.).

Notwithstanding these considerations, which are shared by many and would seem reasonable, the cited works published in prestigious reviews such as the New England Journal of Medicine have little following in the scientific world, in that perioperative beta blockers are still recommended in ACC/AHA guidelines in 2007 and recommended and considered an index of quality in hospital work by the Joint Commission.

Finally, a study published in The Lancet in 2008 and which is clearly reliably for its characteristic large sample and randomized international study—the POISE study (Perioperative Ischemia Evaluation)—has demonstrated the problem of preventing ischemia with a concrete basis [11].

This study has concluded that it is not advisable to carry out indiscriminate perioperative treatment with beta blockers in all patients with an ischemic risk. This type of therapy, in fact, brings about a reduction in perioperative AMI but is associated with an overall increase in mortality. This just corroborates our conviction that beta blocker action is maintained only in patients who have already received beta blocker therapy [12].

In our opinion, these patients may also carry the risk of ischemia with constitutionally increased baseline heart rate or tachycardia due to concomitant diseases such as hyperthyroidism.

We do not, however, use certain beta blockers in patients with tachycardia due to preexisting anemia or hypovolemia, for which we should nevertheless treat the causes of tachycardia rather than reduce it pharmacologically.

From the above it can be understood that our aim is to prevent and quickly correct tachycardia, in particular by maintaining an optimal level of anesthesia and repletion of the circulation by seeking, moreover, to avoid an excessive fall in body temperature during surgery, which often results in shivering upon awakening with substantial consumption of oxygen and associated tachycardia.

The objective of avoiding excessive falls in body temperature will also have the advantage of reducing the incidence of infections from surgical wounds that are tripled in the case of even moderate hypothermia, possibly using the technique of preoperative heating in addition to well known devices to avoid dispersion of temperature and preheating of infusion fluids.

It cannot be forgotten that hypothermia in the operative phase, and particularly immediately after surgery when the vasodilatory effects of anesthesia are not present, produces cutaneous vasoconstriction with centralization of circulation. Consequently, in this phase, possible hypovolemia is masked but later reappears, even dangerously, with an increase in the patient's body temperature a few hours after waking up, when the patient's awareness is often impaired.

Therefore the prevention of ischemic events rests upon certain fundamental cornerstones: careful repletion of the circulation that enables maintenance of a satisfactory SV, a good level of anesthesia, good preoperative sedation, and accurate prevention of falls in body temperature.

Monitoring of circulatory repletion may occur in various ways, even very simply. CVP, which at absolute values is not a good indicator of circulatory repletion, is invaluable if analyzed in its evolution, especially if supported by controls of other parameters such as SPV or PPV.

In practice, if during surgery there is a sudden fall in CVP and an increase in SPV and PPV, it is highly likely that the patient requires circulatory filling.

Even a sudden and rapid fall in $EtCO_2$ with constant ventilation signifies a fall in cardiac output. This change, however, does not point to a fall in SV but in cardiac output. This means that until the heart rate compensates for a fall in SV, $EtCO_2$ is not reduced. The most useful parameter to monitor is SV and therefore, where available, monitoring systems that enable continuous control of SV and SPV or PPV in addition to CVP should be used in patients with a risk of ischemia.

In the case of patients with CHF, the problem of maintaining correct circulatory filling is complicated. Since CHF may be derived from diastolic dysfunction (as often is the case in hypertension with left ventricular hypertrophy) or systolic dysfunction (as with primitive cardiomyopathy or post-infarct cardiomyopathy) or the presence of both, a fall in SV in the perioperative phase is to be interpreted.

In dilated cardiomyopathy (an example of systolic dysfunction), compensation is achieved with greater fiber distension. Therefore, acute blood loss, by reducing the preload, also decreases optimal fiber distension, thus breaking the compensation and provoking a fall in SV. It is therefore not rare that such patients also require a filling test with a fluid bolus to explore the heart's response capacity. A heart like this, if inadequately filled, must inevitably resort to an increase in heart rate to maintain the load, with the implications we have already mentioned.

Yet naturally, in such patients it is also necessary to understand whether the potential for fiber distension has been overcome since, if this level is reached, each subsequent fluid load is destined to affect the pulmonary capillary circulation with the formation of edema.

Furthermore, the increase in ventricular telediastolic pressure reduces the aorta-myocardial gradient, leading to ischemia and later exacerbating ventricular insufficiency.

Controlling the ST tract and pulse-oximetry should be particularly important in situations of this type since, as the administration of fluids should be rapid when required, it is also necessary for prompt loop diuretic and/or nitro-derivative administration when an overload is suspected.

Another problem is the management of cardiac insufficiency caused by diastolic dysfunction. In this case, since the left ventricle has low compliance, even moderately excessive fluid administration may increase ventricular telediastolic pressure, affecting either the coronary circulation or the pulmonary capillary circulation.

From the above it is clear that in cardiac insufficiency, whether systolic or diastolic dysfunction, the key to a correct infusion guide is once again SV, but accompanied by monitoring of left ventricular telediastolic pressure that is more simply represented by WP or, better still, pulmonary capillary pressure, which can both be achieved with Swan-Ganz catheters.

Patients with serious CHF and a positive history of acute pulmonary edema must undergo complex surgery and especially if substantial blood loss is expected, monitoring with a Swan-Ganz catheter is once again the best monitoring method.

An alternative is transesophageal echocardiography (TEE), which is able to provide information on filling or the kinetics of the heart chambers, and which can, in expert hands, enable avoidance of invasive monitoring.

It must be remembered that very often these patients have mitral valve dysfunction with a regurgitation fraction that increased when ventricular chamber distension is excessive and it can therefore be adjusted and affected by correct filling.

It is obvious that an increase in the regurgitation fraction decreases anterograde cardiac output and is therefore a further negative factor.

To assess the development of this phenomenon, TEE is unique.

It is worth mentioning prevention of ischemic events in patients undergoing spinal anesthesia which, as is known, is almost always a cause of reduced cardiac output and resultant hypotension.

The prevention of ischemia is identified with the prevention of a fall in load and pressure. An excellent work in Anesthesia and Analgesia in 2009 compared three strategies in the prevention of these phenomena: crystalloid infusion, hyroxyethyl starch infusion (6 % HES), and 15° Trendelenburg [13].

The study concluded that all three strategies implemented immediately after spinal anesthesia were able to prevent a fall in load but:
- Shortly after crystalloid infusion, if not continued, load begins to fall again;
- The positive effect of Trendelenburg continues only if maintained,

- The efficacy of HES continues for at least 30 min after the end of administration (monitoring of CO, however, lasted only 30 min and the authors state that they do not know the real duration of this effect).

Another interesting work published in the same year and in the same journal concerned elderly patients undergoing transurethral prostate resection under spinal anesthesia. In this work the positive effect of a crystalloid (500 ml) + 6 % HES infusion was shown, compared with crystalloid infusion alone, in preventing a fall in cardiac output. However, the authors' statement that in inhibiting the fall in load, the infusion strategies did not inhibit a fall in pressure, is important.

This is worrying since in patients with critical coronary stenosis in whom the poststenotic dilation mechanisms are already at their maximum, maintenance of the trans-stenotic gradient that ensures flow is preserved only by perfusion pressure. In such situations, cautious administration of amines such as ethylephrine and ephedrine may be useful, taking care not to trigger tachycardia, and always with continuous ST monitoring [14].

It should be emphasized that both these studies were conducted with the same noninvasive monitoring technique: impedance cardiography (ICG), a technique that can easily be applied which is recommended for the control of at-risk patients with spontaneous respiration, in whom parameters such as SPV or PPV cannot be used and catheterization of a central vein is not desired to control CVP.

This monitoring system enables, in addition to controlling SV, the accurate assessment of left ventricular contractility, and continuous monitoring of diastole in its two components: isovolumetric (IVRT) and isotonic (ITRT).

In closing this section, we reiterate the concept already expressed that it is important to avoid, particularly in the postoperative phase, emotional or pain stimuli, since our patients may have endothelial dysfunction of the coronary arteries and may react to either vagal or sympathetic stimuli with vasoconstriction, thus abruptly reducing myocardial perfusion or, worse still, breaking a preexisting condition and therefore causing acute obstruction with resultant AMI.

Proper sedation in the preoperative phase and proper analgesia in the postoperative phase are therefore important steps in the prevention of ischemic events.

3.4 Is There a Pharmacological Possibility of Ischemic Preconditioning and Postconditioning?

Let us begin by briefly explaining ischemic preconditioning: it is basically an adaptive response to a brief ischemic event that tends to slow the process of cell damage connected with a longer ischemic event.

The protective event enabled by ischemic preconditioning may be divided into two phases: early, which begins immediately after the initial ischemic event and enables greater protection but is shorter in time (1–2 h), and late, which begins approximately 24 h after the initial event, is less protective but longer lasting (even up to 3 days). Alongside a protective mechanism of ischemic preconditioning is the possibility of protection from damage resulting from reperfusion of an ischemic territory: this phenomenon, known as ischemic "post-conditioning", is a protective adaptation to reperfusion damage. Reperfusion damage, which accompanies the initial ischemic damage, seems to be due to the opening up of pore in the mitochondrial membrane (normally closed), so-called mitochondrial permeability transition pores (MPTPs).

When the MPTP opening is confirmed, the mitochondria lose their ability to produce ATP, the cytosol is invaded by calcium ions, inorganic phosphate and ROS (reactive oxygen species) [15, 16]. If the MPTP opening is minimal, there is generally full recovery of the cells; if the opening is more generalized it may develop to cell death [17].

Therefore the mechanisms that may be used to restrict perioperative ischemic damage are either ischemic preconditioning or postconditioning. On an experimental level, many drugs have been tested to emphasize these protective processes but none has found a safe position in clinical practice other than halogenated anesthetics.

In a study in which 320 patients undergoing coronary surgery were randomized to receive totally intravenous anesthesia or volatile anesthesia, it emerged that those with halogenated anesthesia had a shorter recovery time in intensive care and in hospital.

The greater duration of recovery for patients treated with intravenous anesthesia was linked to the onset of atrial fibrillation and/or an increase in cTnI > 4 ng/ml. Patients treated with halogenated anesthesia also had better myocardial function in the first hours after surgery [18].

A recent meta-analysis that compared patients treated with the latest-generation halogenated anesthesia (desflurane and sevoflurane) with those receiving totally intravenous anesthesia showed lower levels of postoperative cTn, a better cardiac index, less need for inotropic support, lower AMI rate, shorter duration of mechanical ventilation, shorter hospitalization in ICU and hospital in patients treated with halogenated anesthesia [19].

In the current state of knowledge we can say that, while we do not have any drugs that safely play a protective role in emphasizing either ischemic preconditioning or postconditioning, we may include halogenated anesthesia as a protective strategy in perioperative phases.

3.5 Patients with Recently Implanted Coronary Stents: A New Problem for the Anesthetist

We cannot conclude this chapter without making at least some reference to this subject.

Coronary stent implants are always followed by a treatment period involving the combined use of two platelet antiaggregant drugs: acetylsalicylic acid (ASA) and a thienopyridine, in order to prevent acute thrombosis of the stent, which may be fatal. Combined treatment with these two antiaggregants obviously exposes patients to the danger or hemorrhage in the event of surgery.

The anesthetist is therefore faced with a double risk: acute thrombosis of the stent if treatment is interrupted or hemorrhagic complications if it is continued.

It is nevertheless important to recall that the risk of stent thrombosis from antiaggregant suspensions is a reality for 4–6 weeks from the implant of metal stents (BAR) and for 12 months from the implant of pharmacologically treated stents (DES).

The 2007 ACC/AHA guidelines therefore recommend postponing surgical interventions for 4–6 weeks after implant for BAR and 12 months in the case of DES [20].

In fact there is no evidence that replacement therapy for double antiaggregation, such as low-molecular-weight heparin, warfarin or glycoprotein IIb–IIa, has any success.

Even the suspension of thienopyridine, maintaining only ASA, cannot guarantee a satisfactory antithrombotic effect, especially in the case of DES.

The problem arises when surgery cannot be postponed.

In this case the guidelines, in the knowledge that this pattern cannot guarantee an antithrombotic effect, recommend the suspension of thienopyridine alone, maintaining if possible ASA and restarting thienopyridine as soon as possible.

3.6   Conclusions

Theoretically, to effectively prevent perioperative myocardial ischemia, a certain amount of strategic action is required: identifying patients at risk, monitoring them as best as possible to facilitate the maintenance of normal blood pressure values, heart rate and cardiac output, obtaining a normothermic constant, avoiding postoperative emotions and pain, and carefully choosing the form of anesthesia.

In practice, conducting this strategy is anything but simple, especially if we must manage elderly patients or those with diabetes, hypertension, COPD, vascular disease, cardiac insufficiency, or known coronary disease, especially if surgery involves substantial blood loss.

However, satisfactory results can be achieved if our knowledge is constantly updated, if the patient's attention is always exemplary, and if the available technology is at least acceptable, even if not optimal.

Since, however, patients with such problems are numerous, it is not possible to have optimal advanced technology for everyone. It is therefore essential that the anesthetist knows how to use common forms of monitoring, and understands all the details that often elude an observer who is not very aware.

We hope that this chapter may provide at least a minor contribution to the debate.

References

1. Nichols WN, O' Rourke MF (1995) Mc Donald's blood flow in arteries 1995. The coronary Circ, Hodder Arnold, pp 321–337
2. Allaria B, Dei Poli M (2011) Il monitoraggio delle funzioni vitali nel perioperatorio non cardochirurgico. Springer-Verlag pp 21–39
3. Ferro KE, Muhlmann MH, Bagnet JP et al (1995) Relation between diastolic perfusion time and coronary artery stenosis during stress-induced myocardial ischemia. Circulation 92:342–347
4. Fox K, Garcia MA, Ardinino D et al (2006) Task force on the management of stable angina pectoris of the Eurpean society of cardiology, ESC committee for practice guidelines. Eur Heart J 27:1341–1381
5. Landsberg G, Shatz V et al (2003) Association of cardiac troponin, CK-MB and postoperative myocardial ischemia with long term survival after major vascular surgery. J Am Coll Cardiol 42:1547–1554
6. Shose RC, Atkinson G et al (2007) Exercise reduced cardiac troponin T release: a meta-analysis. Med Sci Sports Exerc 39:2099–2106
7. O'donoghne M, Morrow DA (2008) The future of biomarkers in the management of patients with the acute coronary syndrome. Curr Opin Cardiol 23:309–314
8. Hjart LE, Swissa S (2005) Cardiovascular morbidity and mortality in COPD. Chest 128:2640
9. Mangano DT, Laying FC, Wallace A et al. (1996) Effect of atenolol on mortality and cardiovascular morbidity after non cardiac surgery: multicenter study of perioperative ischemia research group. N Engl J Med 335:1713–1720
10. Poldermans D, Boerome E, Rax JJ et al. (1999) The effect of bisoprolol in perioperative mortality and myocardial infection in high risk patients undergoing vascular surgery. N Engl J Med 341:1789–1794
11. Deveraux PJ, Yang H, Yusuf S et al (2008) Effects of extended release metoprolol succinal in patients undergoing non cardiac surgery (POISE trial). Lancet 371:1839–1847
12. Sear JW, Giles JW, Howard-Alpe G et al. (2008) Perioperative β-blocked: What does POISE tell us, and was our earlier caution justified? Brit J Anesth 101:135–136
13. Zorko N, Kamenik M, Starc U (2009) The effect of Trendelenburg position, lactated Ringer's solution and 6 % HES solution on cardiac output after spinal anesthesia. Anesth Analg 108:655–659
14. Riesmeier A, Schellhaass A, Bildt J et al (2009) Crystalloid/Colloid versus crystalloid intravascular volume administration before spinal anesthesia in elderly patients: the influence on cardiac output and stroke volume. Anesth Analg 108:650–654
15. Halestrap AP, Clarke SJ, Jarvadov SA (2004) Mitochondrial permeability transition pore opening during myocardial reperfusion: a target for cardioprotection. Cardiovasc Res 61:372–385
16. Hansenloy DJ, Ong SP, Yellen DM (2009) The mythocondrial permeability transition pore as a target for preconditioning and postconditioning. Basic Res Cardiol 104:189–202
17. De Hert SG, Wonters PF (2011) Perioperative myocardial ischemia/reperfusion injury: pathophysiology and treatment. Annual update in intensive care and emergency medicine, Springer-Verlag, Berlin, p 471–478
18. De Hert SG, Van der Linden PJ, Cromheeck S et al (2004) Choice of primary anesthetic regimen core influence intensive care unit length of stay after coronary surgery with cardiopulmonary bypass. Anesthesiology 101:9–20
19. Piper HM, Abdallah Y, Shafer C (2004) The first minutes of reperfusion: a window of opportunity for cardioprotection. Cardiovasc Res 61:365–371
20. Fleisher LA, Beckman JA, Brown KA et al (2007) ACC/AHA guidelines on perioperative cardiovascular evaluation and care for noncardiac surgery: executive summary. Circulation 116:1971–1996

Postoperative Respiratory Failure after Major Abdominal Surgery: Definition, Diagnosis and Prevention

4

Davide Chiumello and Cristina Mietto

4.1 Introduction

Postoperative respiratory failure is one of the most important causes of morbidity, mortality, and longer hospital stay in surgical patients, high incidence is comparable only with cardiac complications. However, no univocal and widely accepted definition is available throughout epidemiological studies. Different aspects are involved in the pathogenesis of postoperative respiratory complications, such as the kind of surgery, comorbidities, risk factors, and the population in study. Complications can be related to surgery and anesthesia per se, i.e., general complications, or they can depend upon alterations of the normal physiology of the respiratory system caused by abdominal surgery. Complications may be related to infections, usually fever occurring more than 48 h after surgery is of infective origin, or it can occur in the early postoperative period and usually not due to infections. Beside an etiological classification, we can use temporal limits and subdivide complications in acute, subacute, and late (i.e., pneumonia can be related to surgery if occur within a week from the operation). Therefore, this nonspecific definition can suit different diagnosis: laryngospasm, bronchospasm, hypoxemia, atelectasis, pneumothorax, pleural effusion, pneumonia, aspiration,

D. Chiumello (✉)
Dipartimento di Anestesia, Rianimazione (Intensiva e Subintensiva) E Terapia del Dolore,
Fondazione IRCCS Ca' Granda-Ospedale Maggiore Policlinico, Via Francesco Sforza 35,
20122, Milan, Italy
e-mail: chiumello@libero.it

C. Mietto
Dipartimento di Fisiopatologia Medico-Chirurgica e dei Trapianti, Università degli Studi di
Milano, Via Festa del Perdono, 7, 20122, Milan, Italy
e-mail: Cristina.mietto@gmail.com

B. Allaria (ed.), *Practical Issues in Anesthesia and Intensive Care 2013*,
DOI: 10.1007/978-88-470-5529-2_4, © Springer-Verlag Italia 2014

chronic obstructive pulmonary disease (COPD), acute respiratory failure, thromboembolic disease [1]. Some studies, instead, defined diagnosis as the presence of acute respiratory failure after 48–72 h from surgery [2]. Another approach is to set precise criteria, for example in the study of Brooks-Bunn at least two of the following criteria were to be satisfied during the first six postoperative days: cough or pathological pulmonary auscultation, fever higher than 38 °C, new infiltrate or atelectasis at the chest X-ray, clinical signs of atelectasis, or pneumonia [3]. Traditionally, postoperative respiratory failure incidence is comprised between 2 and 19 % [4], being consistent with what reported for major abdominal surgical patient (3–10 %) [5, 6]; lower values are associated to elective surgery in confront of urgent procedures.

4.2   Pathophysiology of the Respiratory System under Anesthesia

Anesthesia induces changes in the normal physiology of the respiratory system that are involved in the development of postoperative complications.

4.2.1   Respiratory Mechanics

Anesthesia and supine positioning cause a reduction greater than 50 % in lung volumes. In healthy and upright subjects the Functional Residual Capacity (FRC), that is the rest lung volume, is 3.5 l on the average. Supine positioning entails a reduction of FRC of 0.8–1 l even in awake subjects; an additional decrease of 0.4–0.5 l has to be added after the induction of anesthesia, leading to an FRC of nearly 2 l, a value close to Residual Volume (RV) [7, 8]. The effect on lung volumes is common to all anesthetics, except for ketamine [9]. The loss of muscular tone correlates with the reduction in FRC, due to the shift of the equilibrium point of the respiratory system toward lower volumes and to the cephalic displacement of the diaphragm. These changes are not completely reversible at the awakening, in fact a 40 % reduction in Vital Capacity (VC) and a decreased forced expiratory volume in 1 s (FEV1) can persist for more than a week after surgery [10]. Muscular dysfunction can be present even after 7 days from operation, entailing a reduction of tidal volume (Vt) and maximal forced expiratory flow [11]. Simultaneously, the Compliance (Crs) of the respiratory system decreases, mainly for a reduction of lung compliance (Cl) from 200 ml/cm H_2O in awoken subjects to 150 ml/cm H_2O during anesthesia [12]. A proof of the reduction in Crs is the fact that a peak airway pressure of 30 cm H_2O expands the lung to only 70 % of preoperatory total lung capacity (TLC) [13]. This effect and also the increase in respiratory system resistance are caused by the reduction in FRC. Only minor changes are provoked by paralyzing agents, suggesting a more important role of anesthesia than curares [14].

4.2.2 Atelectasis

Atelectasis, defined as the loss of air within pulmonary alveoli causing lung parenchyma collapse (reversible with the application of higher airways pressures), develop quickly during anesthesia and play an important role in the worsening of gas exchange and in the increasing of pulmonary vascular resistances. Moreover, atelectasis predispose to infection. Shunt is consequent to atelectasis and is responsible of hypoxemia. More than 90 % of patients undergoing to general anesthesia develop atelectasis [15]. From early 1980s studies using Computer Tomography (CT) showed how atelectasis distribute preferentially to dependent area near lung basis, while spearing the apical parts; usually the 5–6 % of lung parenchyma is involved, but the percentage can reach more than 15–20 % in some cases [16]. Muscular paralysis promotes this phenomenon, while abdominal surgery has a minor role. Principal determinants are: parenchymal compression due to the weight of lung tissue upon dependent regions, the loss of muscular strength limiting inspiratory effort, and the cephalic displacement of the diaphragm with higher transmission of abdominal pressure and alveolar gas reabsorption, especially when using high FiO_2. It is important to highlight that in healthy spontaneously breathing subjects the use of high FiO_2 does not cause reabsorption atelectasis, suggesting that the loss of muscular strength and the low lung volumes are involved in this process. The total amount of atelectasis is not correlated with age, but it correlates with Body Mass Index (BMI), even if at a lesser extent than what would be imaginable [17]. COPD patients are relatively spared because the high Cl and the dynamic hyperinflation that prevents lung collapse [18]. Anyway, atelectasis per se does not cause fever, while the reason for the rise in temperature has to be searched in an infective process or inflammatory response to tissue injury [19].

4.2.3 Ventilation/Perfusion Ratio

The alteration of ventilation/perfusion (VA/Q) ratio is another mechanism involved in the worsening of oxygenation. The closure of distal airways during expiration causes the appearance of areas with low VA/Q, mainly in the dependent regions upon atelectasis [20]. A low VA/Q means that some lung zones have a greater perfusion than ventilation, the extreme case is the shunt where the VA/Q is equal to zero. On the other side there are zones that are ventilated but not perfused, called alveolar death space (Vd/Vt) and responsible for inadequate clearance of CO_2. Vd/Vt is increased in anesthesia as shown by the higher minute ventilation required to maintain constant partial pressure of CO_2 (PaCO). This can make more difficult the management of ventilation in case of chronic lung diseases, like COPD.

4.3   Preoperative Evaluation and Risk Factors

4.3.1   Risk Factors

The identification of those patients who will develop respiratory failure in the postoperative period is of the greatest importance. Risk factors for pulmonary complications are less studied than those of cardiovascular system and can be related to numerous aspects (Table 4.1). Fundamental factor to consider during preoperative evaluation is the type of surgery: a greater risk is associated with thoracic and high abdomen procedures, with an incidence between 13 and 33 % [21, 22]. The rates are lower (16 %) in case of lower abdomen, or even more considering extra-abdominal surgery [21]. Procedures that last more than 4 h have been shown to be associated to higher risk of complication regardless the kind of surgery [23]. Also physical considerations must be kept in mind, such as the orientation of surgical incision, matter; if the muscular fibers are cut transversally to their main axis, the effects on respiratory function will be more relevant. Diaphragmatic dysfunction is always present in abdominal surgery, grading upon the proximity of surgical insult and the muscle. Regarding the surgical technique, a study on patients undergone to laparoscopic or open cholecystectomy reported that the laparoscopic technique was associated to better FEV1 and forced vital capacity at 24–28 h and to a quicker return to preoperative values [24]. Anyway, laparoscopic surgery seems to grant better postoperative respiratory recovery but evidences are not all consistent about this issue [25]. Anesthetic technique may have great importance but also here the data are not univocal and the studies involved mainly extra-abdominal surgery, like orthopedics [26]. A large meta-analysis found a reduction of mortality, pneumonia, and respiratory failure with regional anesthesia (spinal and epidural) [27]; however this study has several limitations, such as heterogeneity of the included studies, some of those are old and with few patients. Regional anesthesia may be a better option in high-risk patients. Other risk factors are related to the patient: age, smoking, general physical status, obesity, chronic disease (especially pulmonary, COPD, asthma, etc.); moreover alcoholic dependence, weight loss, neurologic deficits, anemia (Hb < 10 g/dl), thrombocytopenia, low plasmatic albumin levels, and renal disease [23, 28]. However, age is not an independent risk factor for respiratory failure probably age-related comorbidities entail a greater role [29]. COPD patients have a risk 4.7-fold higher for postoperative respiratory complications [30] and the optimization of medical therapy is pivotal before surgery, the same about asthma. Recent lung infections, antibiotic use, health-care facility stay, and current infection are associated with higher risk [31]. Different scores and classification are available for preoperative evaluation. Among the others, the American Society of Anesthesiologists (ASA) physical status has been found to correlate with the incidence of postoperative complications (Table 4.2); rates rise from 10 % in ASA II, 28 % in ASA III patients to 46 % in ASA IV [32]. The Goldman cardiac risk can be used for respiratory system risk assessment. This score take into account different factors: medical history, physical status, cardiac diseases and type of surgery (urgent vs nonurgent) [33]. Epstein et al.

Table 4.1 Preoperative risk factors

Patient	Surgery	Anesthesia
Pulmonary disease (COPD, asthma, current infections)	High abdomen > low abdomen	Anesthetic technique (spinal/epidural vs. general)
Smoke	Procedure time > 4 h	Postoperative analgesia
Age	Surgical technique (laparotomy vs. laparoscopic)	
Obesity	Type of incision	
Physical status/nutritioning		
EtOH abuse		
Neurology		
Anemia, trombhocytopenia		
Ipoalbuminemia		
Kidney disease		

Table 4.2 ASA physical status (American Society of Anesthesiologists)

Class	
ASA I	Good health status
ASA II	Mild systemic disease without functional limitations
ASA III	Severe systemic disease and mild function limitation
ASA IV	Severe life threatening disease
ASA V	Survival is not assured for more than 24 h, with or without surgery
ASA VI	Cerebral death
ASA I–V E	Emergency

developed, from the Goldman score, another index including also specific respiratory variables: obesity, smoke, purulent sputum and cough, pathological chest auscultation, FEV1/FVC lower than 70 % and arterial carbon dioxide partial pressure ($PaCO_2$) higher than 45 mmHg (Table 4.3) [34]. Unlikely this index is not validated for abdominal surgery. A similar approach has been used to develop the Respiratory Failure Risk Index (Table 4.4), using logistic regression model seven variables has been associated to the risk of pulmonary complications (type of surgery, emergency, serum albumin level, BUN, general physical status, COPD, age); patients are then assigned to one of five classes and higher scores characterized progressively higher risks [35]. Expressely on abdominal surgical patients the risk factors are, listed in decreasing importance: pathological findings on chest X-ray, high Goldman cardiac risk score, and a high Charlson comorbidity index (a score designed to predict the 10-year mortality) [36, 37].

Table 4.3 Cardiopulmonary risk index [34]

Cardiac risk index (CRI)		Pulmonary risk index (PRI)	
Variable	Score	Variable	Score
Chronic heart failure	11	Obesity (BMI > 27 kg/m^2)	1
Recent IMA	10	Smoke	1
More than 5 BEVs/min	7	Cough	1
Arrhythmia	7	Crackles rales	1
Svere aortic stenosis	3	FEV1/FVC < 70 %	1
Poor general status	3	PaCO$_2$ > 45 mmHg	1
CRI = 0–41		PRI = 0–6	
Cardio-pulmonary risk index (CPRI) = CRI + PRI			

Table 4.4 Respiratory failure risk index [35]

Variable	Score	
Type of surgery		
■ Abdominal aneurism repair	27	
■ Thoracic	21	
■ High abdomen, neurosurgery, peripheral vascular	14	
■ Neck	11	
Urgency	11	
Albuminemia (< 3 mg/dl)	9	
BUN (> 30 mg/dl)	8	
Partial or total disability	7	
COPD	6	
Age		
■ ≥ 70	6	
■ 60–69	4	
Total score = 0–84		
Class	Score	Risk (%)
I	≤ 10	0.5
II	11–19	2.2
III	20–27	5.0
IV	28–40	11.6

4.3.2 Preoperative Evaluation

A correct preoperative evaluation is a key moment to detect those patients who have the highest risk to develop postoperative complications. Careful medical history recording and physical assessment are pivotal to detect signs and symptoms of any known or unknown lung disease. Symptoms of pulmonary compromise must be evaluated, like cough, exercise intolerance, shortness of breath, or chest pain. A proper and careful preoperative exam is more important than any laboratory result [38]. A complete evaluation of the respiratory system must include: 1—respiratory mechanics through pulmonary function testing (spirometry); 2—gas exchange and CO diffusibility (DLCO); 3—heart–lung interaction and maximum oxygen consumption (VO_2); 4—chest imaging, X-ray, or other technique. Pulmonary function tests are necessary for diagnosis and monitoring the response to therapies, but they have no utility for preoperative risk assessment [39]. Traditionally, pulmonary function tests are used in thoracic surgery, where a FEV1 < 2 l or 50 % of predicted value, FVC < 50 % or DLCO < 60 % of predicted usually define a significant higher risk of death after pneumonectomy [40]. Spirometry is not a routine test in patients undergoing extrathoracic surgery, but it can play a role (together with emogasanalysis—ABG) in case of chronic lung diseases. In patients with COPD or asthma, spirometry defines the severity and the response to therapy prior to surgery. It is also recommended in smokers or in patients with respiratory symptoms scheduled for high abdomen surgery. Cases of new dyspnea is an indication even in case of lower abdomen surgery [38]. Different targets have been proposed: a FEV1 lower than 1.2 l is associated to an incidence of 37 % of complications and to a mortality of 47 % [41]. Otherwise, FEV1 < 50 % of predicted value or FEV1/FVC < 70 % have been proposed as indexes of higer risk [30]. In a study on heavy smokers scheduled for abdominal surgery, a FEV1 < 40 % of predicted value was associated to only 5 % of risk [42], but the modification of therapy done upon the spirometry test may be the reason for such a low incidence. However, it is important to keep in mind that no spirometric value avoids surgery [23]. Gas exchange are studied with ABG and, as previously stated for pulmonary function tests, it have to be used in patients with history of lung disease or new symptoms. Hypercapnia ($PaCO_2 > 45$ mmHg) is associated with higher mortality and complication rates, being a sign of the severity of the underling disease. A $PaCO_2/PaO_2$ ratio < 0.72 is associated with increased risk of postoperative complications [43]. The cardiopulmonary tests are rarely necessary in abdominal surgery and maximum oxygen consumption can be easily estimated by daily physical activity of the patient: the inability to climb one flight of stairs correspond to a $VO_2 < 10$ ml/kg/min, while if the patient can climb five flights the VO_2 is > 20 ml/kg/min. Patients with very low physical capability ($VO_2 < 10$ ml/kg/min) may have very high surgical risk. Lastly, the routine use of chest X-ray is not advisable, because it is a bad screening test for pulmonary compromise. Indeed, unexpected findings modify the treatment only in 0.2–1 % of cases [44]. Moreover, the biological risk and the costs are to be taken into account.

Patients with known or suspected cardiopulmonary disease can benefit from chest X-ray, and it has been proposed for subjects with ASA III, older than 65 years, smoking, native of regions endemic for tuberculosis, malign neoplasm, immuno-compromised, progress radio-therapy or undergoing to major surgery (National Institute for Clinical Excellence—National Health Service > 3) [44].

4.4 Preventive Measures

Preventive strategies are always to be implemented, regardless the preoperative risk (Table 4.5).

4.4.1 Smoking

Smokers have an increased risk of postoperative respiratory complications, with direct correlation between the time and number of packages/year. Smoking causes an increase of carboxyhemoglobin and decrease in oxygen arterial saturation; the half-life of carboxyhemoglobin is about six hours and so avoiding smoking can be useful even if only 24 h before the procedure (no evidences are available in this regard). Only one study showed that smoking cessation 8 weeks before surgery decreases the need of postoperative mechanical ventilation [45]. This time lapse is required for mucocyliar and small airways function to recovering. Shorter period of time may determine a paradoxical increase in secretions and mucus production. Numerous studies have not found any difference between patients who quit smoking or not before surgery [46]. A recent meta-analysis, including only studies in which the smoking cessation was within 8 weeks from surgery, did not find any increased risk even if smoking was stop before the classical time limits (Relative Risk—RR, 0.78, IC95 % 0.57–1.07) [47].

Table 4.5 Preventive strategies

Preoperative	Intra-operative	Post-operative
Smoking cessation	Spinal/Epidural anesthesia	Epidural analgesia
Optimization of therapy if pulmonary disease	Laparoscopy	Recruitment maneuvers
Delay surgery or start antibiotics if current infection	Surgical time < 4 h	CPAP and NIMV
Weight loss	No long lasting paralyzing agent	Physiotherapy
Teaching of physiotherapy exercises	Nasogastric tube only if aspiration risk	

4.4.2 Nutritional Status

Despite obesity is associated with shorter life expectance and higher perioperative mortality, no clear and precise evidence is available to correlate BMI and postoperative respiratory failure risk [23]. On the opposite, debilitated patients need to be recovered to optimize their nutritional status and protein requirement before surgery. Nasogastric tube use should be limited to patients with nausea, vomiting, or abdominal distention because its routine use has been associated to higher incidence of pulmonary complications, without benefit on adverse outcomes [48].

4.4.3 Pulmonary Diseases

In patients affected by chronic obstructive diseases (COPD, asthma) the preoperative introduction of an effective therapy is pivotal for risk reduction [49]. First line drugs are bronchodilatators like beta2-adrenergic and anticholinergic (other drugs, like theophylline, are to be considered only as second line in patients with not responding bronchospasm) plus steroids. Steroids must be administered at lest 12 h prior surgery, because of their long onset time and no increased in infective risk with short cycles [50]. Patients with hyper-reactivity of the respiratory system, treated with inhalation albuterol and methylprednisolone for 5 days before surgery, showed a reduced incidence of bronchospasm at intubation [51]. No evidence is available in support to the prophylactic use of antibiotics, antimicrobials should be restricted to patients with current infections. In case of elective surgery, the operation should be postponed until the resolution of the infectious disease.

4.4.4 Pain Management

Bad pain control can impair the inspiratory effort and cough, thus contributing to the development of atelectasis in the postoperative period. Epidural analgesia provides better pain control in confront to intravascular route and is associated to lower occurrence of respiratory failure, duration of mechanical ventilation, and necessity of reintubation [52]. Beside in thoracic surgery, the positioning of an epidural catheter is recommended also in patients at risk of pulmonary complications undergoing major abdominal surgery in which can reduce adverse events of one-third [53]. A meta-analysis on 20,000 patients found better pain relief with epidural than intravenous (patient controlled analgesia—PCA) or intramuscular opioid analgesia: analgesia was inadequate in 7.8 % of cases treated with epidural, 20.9 % for PCA and 20.1 % for intramuscular analgesia [54]. Usually a combination of opioid and local anesthetic is used to guarantee a better pain control at rest and during movements (i.e., cough, physiotherapy, walking, …). The rationale is the synergic effect of the two drugs, thus allowing lower dosages and risks of overdose/toxicity with better results. In abdominal surgical patients, pain was better controlled even with only the infusion of fentanyl trough an epidural catheter in confront to morphine or fentanyl i.v. [55, 56]. A common concern about epidural analgesia is respiratory depression. However, a study on 2696 patients showed that epidural infusion with bupivacaine and morphine was associated to lower incidence of respiratory depression than with intravascular morphine (0.04 % vs. 1.2 %, respectively) [57]. In case adverse events occur earlier in the immediate postoperative period, rather than with i.v. opioids when respiratory depression is maximal during the first postoperative day [57]. The effects on respiratory drive is strictly connected with the use of opioids, in addition to local anesthetics; more hydrophilic drugs like morphine can spread more easily though the central nervous system (CNS) and cause a late depression. Morphine dosages < 0.2 mg/h are not associated to higher risks. A meta-analysis found that epidural extended release morphine (EREM), which guarantee a prolong effect without the necessity of a catheter in place, is associated to a higher risk of respiratory depression (Odds ratio 5.80; IC95 % 1.05–31.93, $p = 0.004$) compared to PCA, requiring in case a close monitoring [58].

4.4.5 Anesthetic and Surgical Technique

A wide meta-analysis showed that locoregional anesthesia (spinal or epidural) provides better results [27]. One hundred and fourty one randomized and controlled studies have been included in the analysis: neuroaxial analgesia did not show same results about postoperative pneumonia (Odds ratio 0.61; IC95 % 0.48–0.76) or respiratory failure (Odds ratio 0.41; IC95 % 0.23–0.73). Short acting curare may be helpful because they reduce the occurrence of residual paralysis [59]. About the surgical technique, no definite data is available in favor of laparoscopy, however in bariatric surgery the open approach is associated to an almost double risk compared to laparoscopy [60].

4.4.6 Respiratory Physiotherapy

Respiratory physiotherapy is recommended for all patients after major abdominal surgery, while during the preoperative period it is to limit for high-risk subjects [23]. Numerous techniques are available but no clear evidence showed the superiority of one over the others [61]. The correct use of devices and exercises is essential and these skills have to be reached before surgery so to be used effectively during the postoperative period. However, opposite evidences are reported, and a recent meta-analysis failed in showing a beneficial effects in terms of reduction of complications or outcome [62].

4.4.7 Ventilatory Strategies

Postoperative respiratory failure has been defined as the impossibility to extubate or the necessity of reintubate the patient within 48 h after surgery. Clinical signs of respiratory failure are gas exchange (hypoxemia and hypercapnia) and respiratory mechanics alterations (tachypnea, dyspnea, use of accessory muscles). Considering that atelectasis is the main cause of hypoxemia and infection susceptibility, it is important to ensure lung expansion during the postoperative period. Anyway, intubation and mechanical ventilation require sedation with increased hemodynamic compromise, longer ICU, and hospital stay. First, it is essential to exclude mechanical obstruction for atelectasis development, like the presence of bronchial secretions. In this case a bronchoscopy is useful to remove secretions, especially when proximal bronchial obstructions cause lobar dysventilation. Noninvasive ventilation is widely used for prevention of postoperative respiratory failure. Noninvasive ventilation comprises all those techniques that do not require intubation to deliver positive airway pressure. The two main modalities are continuous positive airway pressure (CPAP) in which a constant positive pressure is maintained during the whole respiratory cycle, and noninvasive intermittent positive pressure ventilation (NIPPV) in which two pressures levels are delivered: one is inspiratory (pressure support—PS) and patient's inspiratory effort triggers the ventilator to deliver a positive pressure, while during expiration a positive pressure (positive end-expiratory pressure (PEEP) is maintained in all the system. CPAP causes an increase in intrathoracic pressure and FRC, with better gas exchanges due to changes in VA/Q ratio, reduce work of breathing in case or intrinsic PEEP (i.e., COPD patients) and the afterload of the left ventricle. NIPPV allows for a higher support to respiratory muscles, an increase in minute ventilation with consequent better CO_2 clearance and dyspnea relief. The rationale for NIV use is based upon better lung inflation and ventilation, better gas exchanges and lower degree of atelectasis, together with decreased work of breathing. A great advantage is that NIV does not require intubation, so avoiding sedation and infection risk (VAP—ventilator associated pneumonia) and higher patient comfort. Both modalities (CPAP and NIPPV) can be delivered with the helmet or the mask, but better results have been reported with the helmet (80 %) than the face mask (52 %) [63, 64]. Patients with higher risk are those who may have greatest benefit from NIV use: elder, COPD and obese patients. Contraindications are a reduced level of alertness and consciousness, hemodynamic instability, impaired airway protection, cardiac or respiratory arrest, trauma or facial surgery, hematemesis, and hemoptysis (Table 4.6). Numerous meta-analysis evaluated NIV in the postoperative period. Ferreyra et al. showed that CPAP can be helpful in decreasing the incidence of postoperative complications after abdominal surgery (RR 0.66; CI95 % 0.52–0.85), corresponding to a number of patients to treat (NNT) of 14.2 (IC95 % 9.9–32.4); moreover NIV reduced the risk of pneumonia (RR 0.33; IC95 % 0.14–0.75) and atelectasis (RR 0.75; IC95 % 0.58–0.97) [65]. NIV can be an option not only for prevention but also for ventilatory support of postoperative respiratory complications [66]. Studies found NIV useful after extubation in order to

Table 4.6 Contraindications for noninvasive ventilation (NIV)

Absolute	Relative
Cardiac or respiratory arrest	Mild alteration of consciousness
Coma, encephalopathia, agitation	Evolving respiratory failure
Impaired airway protection	Oppositional patients
Vomiting	
Recent trauma o facial surgery	
Hematemesis or hemoptysis	
Abundant secretions	
Hemodynamic instability	
Severe comorbidities	

prevent the onset of respiratory distress, reduction of atelectasis, and improved oxygenation [67]. Joris et al. showed beneficial effects of NIV during the first 24 h after surgery in obese patients, regarding gas exchange, FEV1 and FVC [68]. The improvements of respiratory function were confirmed even after 48 h and the return to baseline values was quickest. In another study the use of CPAP 10 cmH_2O for 12–24 h was associated to shorter ICU stay [69]. Consistent results have been published in case of treatment for respiratory failure. Jaber et al. reported a successful rate of 66 % in avoid intubation for postoperative respiratory failure in 72 patients scheduled for abdominal surgery [70]. Worst hypoxemia and no improvement in PaO_2 are predictors of failure. Similar results have been shown after liver transplant in a study in which NIV was compared to only oxygen supplement. Authors found lower reintubation (20 % vs. 70 %, $p = 0.02$) and ICU mortality (20 % vs. 50 %, $p = 0.05$) in the NIV group, even if hospital outcome was not different [71]. In a randomized multicenter study, 209 patients with $PaO_2/FiO_2 < 300$ have been enrolled to one CPAP (7.5 cm H_2O) cycle of 6 h or to control group (only oxygen supplement). Results reported lower incidence of pneumonia, reintubation, and sepsis in the interventional group, parallel to a trend in shorter ICU stay [6]. The study was stopped earlier for significant benefit in the CPAP group (reintubation 1 % vs. 10 %, $p = 0.005$). A common concern for CPAP use in abdominal surgery is the risk of air leakage through enteric anastomosis, but no study found evidences in support [72]. Indeed, in a post-esophagectomy study, NIV was associated to lower risks of air leakage, reintubation, ARDS (Acute Respiratory Distress Syndrome) and shorter ICU stay [73]. Finally, NIV can be a role both in the preoperative period for better preoxygenation (especially in obese and hypoxemic patients) before intubation or as physiotherapy: NIV delivered at home for a week before surgery provided higher oxygenation and lung volumes (atelectasis 14 vs. 49 %) [74]. Instead in case of required intubation and invasive mechanical ventilation, a lung protective ventilation showed to be preferable also in patients without acute respiratory distress syndrome (ARDS). In a study enrolling surgical patients (except for neuro- and cardiac surgery) authors found that a tidal volume of 6 ml/kgIBW versus 12 ml/kgIDW was associated to a reduction in the length of mechanical ventilation, ICU stay and incidence of lung infections [75]. Gajic et al. reported that 24 % of 332 patients, ventilated for more than 48 h, satisfied the criteria of ARDS at the fifth day of intubation. ARDS incidence was higher in females (29 % vs. 20 %, $p = 0.68$) with a parallel trend in higher tidal volume (11.4 ml/kgIBW vs. 10.4 ml/kgIBW, $p < 0.0001$). Risk factors were high Vt, lung restrictive disease, academia, and massive blood products transfusion [76]. Alteration of inflammatory markers in response to mechanical ventilation can be detected as early as in the intra-operative period: in elective abdominal procedures lasting more than 5 h, the use of 6 ml/kgIBW and 10 cm H_2O PEEP compared to 12 ml/kgIBW and 0 PEEP was associated to lower inflammatory activation and local procaogulatory effects [77]. In the bronchoalveolar lavage liquid of patients with higher Vt could be detected higher levels of thombin–antithrombin complex, soluble tissue factor, and factor VIIa, that is, a usual pattern associated to alveolar damage. In another study, Michelet et al. found lower concentration of Interlukine-1 (IL-1), IL-6, and IL.8 in patients with protective ventilation during surgery and for 18 h after the procedure [78]. Conversely, some studies did not find any difference [79, 80]. Lastly, anesthesia and surgery promote alterations of normal physiology of the respiratory system that lead to lung collapse. Recruiting maneuvers (defined as an increase in transpulmonary pressure) are required to reexpand lung tissue, improving ventilation and oxygenation. Different modalities of recruitment has been proposed, manual vs in mechanical ventilation, but no evidence of superiority of one over the others are available [81, 82]. Once the lung is open, then it is essential to maintain alveolar recruitment with the correct PEEP level. A recent meta-analysis did not find any influence on outcome, despite better oxygenation and lower number of atelectasis at computer tomography scanning (CT) [83]. The response of the individual patient to the rise of ventilatory pressure is usually based upon changes in respiratory system mechanics (total respiratory system compliance, or divided in lung and chest wall parts), gas exchange (PaO_2, $PaCO_2$), functional indexes (shunt, dead space), and lung volumes (FRC, EELV—end expiratory lung volume), or with imaging techniques (CT). Recently lung ultrasound is becoming widespread and allows evaluating lung ventilation and inflation [84]. Recruitment maneuvers guided by direct lung ultrasound visualization of areas closed that regain aeration can be useful to evaluate at bed side and in real time the response and the correct pressure required (limiting the risk of over distention and not reaching correct pressure necessary to reopen the lung).

References

1. Johnson DC, Kaplan LJ (2011) Perioperative pulmonary complications. Curr Opin Crit Care 17(4):362–369
2. Svensson LG, Hess KR, Coselli JS, Safi HJ, Crawford ES (1991) A prospective study of respiratory failure after high-risk surgery on the thoracoabdominal aorta. J Vasc Surg 14(3):271–282
3. Brooks-Brunn JA (1997) Predictors of postoperative pulmonary complications following abdominal surgery. Chest 111(3):564–571

4. Fisher BW, Majumdar SR, McAlister FA (2002) Predicting pulmonary complications after nonthoracic surgery: a systematic review of blinded studies. Am J Med 112(3):219–225
5. McAlister FA, Bertsch K, Man J, Bradley J, Jacka M (2005) Incidence of and risk factors for pulmonary complications after nonthoracic surgery. Am J Respir Crit Care Med 171(5):514–517
6. Squadrone V, Coha M, Cerutti E, Schellino MM, Biolino P, Occella P et al (2005) Continuous positive airway pressure for treatment of postoperative hypoxemia: a randomized controlled trial. JAMA 293(5):589–595
7. Lumb AB, Nunn JF (1991) Respiratory function and ribcage contribution to ventilation in body positions commonly used during anesthesia. Anesth Analg 73(4):422–426
8. Wahba RW (1991) Perioperative functional residual capacity. Can J Anaesth 38(3):384–400
9. Chawla G, Drummond GB (2008) Fentanyl decreases end-expiratory lung volume in patients anaesthetized with sevoflurane. Br J Anaesth 100(3):411–414
10. Westerdahl E, Lindmark B, Eriksson T, Friberg O, Hedenstierna G, Tenling A (2005) Deep-breathing exercises reduce atelectasis and improve pulmonary function after coronary artery bypass surgery. Chest 128(5):3482–3488
11. Chuter TA, Weissman C, Mathews DM, Starker PM (1990) Diaphragmatic breathing maneuvers and movement of the diaphragm after cholecystectomy. Chest 97(5):1110–1114
12. Don H (1977) The mechanical properties of the respiratory system during anesthesia. Int Anesthesiol Clin 15(2):113–136
13. Lumb AB, Nunn JF (2005) Nunn's applied respiratory physiology. Elsevier, Boston
14. Hedenstierna G, Jarnberg PO, Gottlieb I (1981) Thoracic gas volume measured by body plethysmography during anesthesia and muscle paralysis: description and validation of a method. Anesthesiology 55(4):439–443
15. Gunnarsson L, Tokics L, Gustavsson H, Hedenstierna G (1991) Influence of age on atelectasis formation and gas exchange impairment during general anaesthesia. Br J Anaesth 66(4):423–432
16. Brismar B, Hedenstierna G, Lundquist H, Strandberg A, Svensson L, Tokics L (1985) Pulmonary densities during anesthesia with muscular relaxation–a proposal of atelectasis. Anesthesiology 62(4):422–428
17. Strandberg A, Tokics L, Brismar B, Lundquist H, Hedenstierna G (1987) Constitutional factors promoting development of atelectasis during anaesthesia. Acta Anaesthesiol Scand 31(1):21–24
18. Gunnarsson L, Tokics L, Lundquist H, Brismar B, Strandberg A, Berg B et al (1991) Chronic obstructive pulmonary disease and anaesthesia: formation of atelectasis and gas exchange impairment. Eur Respir J 4(9):1106–1116
19. Mavros MN, Velmahos GC, Falagas ME (2011) Atelectasis as a cause of postoperative fever: where is the clinical evidence? Chest 140(2):418–424
20. Rothen HU, Sporre B, Engberg G, Wegenius G, Hedenstierna G (1998) Airway closure, atelectasis and gas exchange during general anaesthesia. Br J Anaesth 81(5):681–686
21. Pedersen T, Eliasen K, Henriksen E (1990) A prospective study of risk factors and cardiopulmonary complications associated with anaesthesia and surgery: risk indicators of cardiopulmonary morbidity. Acta Anaesthesiol Scand 34(2):144–155
22. Tarhan S, Moffitt EA, Sessler AD, Douglas WW, Taylor WF (1973) Risk of anesthesia and surgery in patients with chronic bronchitis and chronic obstructive pulmonary disease. Surgery 74(5):720–726
23. Qaseem A, Snow V, Fitterman N, Hornbake ER, Lawrence VA, Smetana GW et al (2006) Risk assessment for and strategies to reduce perioperative pulmonary complications for patients undergoing noncardiothoracic surgery: a guideline from the American College of Physicians. Ann Intern Med 144(8):575–580
24. Widdison AL (1996) A systematic review of the effectiveness and safety of laparoscopic cholecystectomy. Ann R Coll Surg Engl 78(5):476

25. Guller U, Jain N, Hervey S, Purves H, Pietrobon R (2003) Laparoscopic vs open colectomy: outcomes comparison based on large nationwide databases. Arch Surg 138(11):1179–1186
26. Urwin SC, Parker MJ, Griffiths R (2000) General versus regional anaesthesia for hip fracture surgery: a meta-analysis of randomized trials. Br J Anaesth 84(4):450–455
27. Rodgers A, Walker N, Schug S, McKee A, Kehlet H, van Zundert A et al (2000) Reduction of postoperative mortality and morbidity with epidural or spinal anaesthesia: results from overview of randomised trials. BMJ 321(7275):1493
28. Canet J, Gallart L, Gomar C, Paluzie G, Valles J, Castillo J et al (2010) Prediction of postoperative pulmonary complications in a population-based surgical cohort. Anesthesiology 113(6):1338–1350
29. Mohr DN (1983) Estimation of surgical risk in the elderly: a correlative review. J Am Geriatr Soc 31(2):99–102
30. Kroenke K, Lawrence VA, Theroux JF, Tuley MR, Hilsenbeck S (1993) Postoperative complications after thoracic and major abdominal surgery in patients with and without obstructive lung disease. Chest 104(5):1445–1451
31. Bochicchio GV, Joshi M, Scalea T (2000) Community-acquired infections in the geriatric trauma population. Shock 14(3):338–342
32. Kroenke K, Lawrence VA, Theroux JF, Tuley MR (1992) Operative risk in patients with severe obstructive pulmonary disease. Arch Intern Med 152(5):967–971
33. Goldman L, Caldera DL, Nussbaum SR, Southwick FS, Krogstad D, Murray B et al (1977) Multifactorial index of cardiac risk in noncardiac surgical procedures. N Engl J Med 297(16):845–850
34. Epstein SK, Faling LJ, Daly BD, Celli BR (1993) Predicting complications after pulmonary resection. Preoperative exercise testing versus a multifactorial cardiopulmonary risk index. Chest 104(3):694–700
35. Arozullah AM, Daley J, Henderson WG, Khuri SF (2000) Multifactorial risk index for predicting postoperative respiratory failure in men after major noncardiac surgery. The National Veterans Administration Surgical Quality Improvement Program. Ann Surg 232(2):242–253
36. Charlson ME, Pompei P, Ales KL, MacKenzie CR (1987) A new method of classifying prognostic comorbidity in longitudinal studies: development and validation. J Chronic Dis 40(5):373–383
37. Smetana GW, Lawrence VA, Cornell JE (2006) Preoperative pulmonary risk stratification for noncardiothoracic surgery: systematic review for the American College of Physicians. Ann Intern Med 144(8):581–595
38. Smetana GW (1999) Preoperative pulmonary evaluation. N Engl J Med 340(12):937–944
39. De Nino LA, Lawrence VA, Averyt EC, Hilsenbeck SG, Dhanda R, Page CP (1997) Preoperative spirometry and laparotomy: blowing away dollars. Chest 111(6):1536–1541
40. Celli BR, MacNee W (2004) Standards for the diagnosis and treatment of patients with COPD: a summary of the ATS/ERS position paper. Eur Respir J 23(6):932–946
41. Wong DH, Weber EC, Schell MJ, Wong AB, Anderson CT, Barker SJ (1995) Factors associated with postoperative pulmonary complications in patients with severe chronic obstructive pulmonary disease. Anesth Analg 80(2):276–284
42. Warner DO, Warner MA, Offord KP, Schroeder DR, Maxson P, Scanlon PD (1999) Airway obstruction and perioperative complications in smokers undergoing abdominal surgery. Anesthesiology 90(2):372–379
43. Carrillo G, Estrada A, Pedroza J, Aragon B, Mejia M, Navarro C et al (2005) Preoperative risk factors associated with mortality in lung biopsy patients with interstitial lung disease. J Invest Surg 18(1):39–45
44. Calderini E, Adrario E, Petrini F, Salvo I, Solca M, Bonomo L et al (2004) Indications to chest radiograph in preoperative adult assessment: recommendations of the SIAARTI-SIRM commission. Minerva Anestesiol 70(6):443–451

45. Moller AM, Villebro N, Pedersen T, Tonnesen H (2002) Effect of preoperative smoking intervention on postoperative complications: a randomised clinical trial. Lancet 359(9301):114–117
46. Bluman LG, Mosca L, Newman N, Simon DG (1998) Preoperative smoking habits and postoperative pulmonary complications. Chest 113(4):883–889
47. Myers K, Hajek P, Hinds C, McRobbie H (2011) Stopping smoking shortly before surgery and postoperative complications: a systematic review and meta-analysis. Arch Intern Med 171(11):983–989
48. Nelson R, Edwards S, Tse B (2007) Prophylactic nasogastric decompression after abdominal surgery. Cochrane Database Syst Rev (3):CD004929
49. Liccardi G, Salzillo A, De Blasio F, D'Amato G (2009) Control of asthma for reducing the risk of bronchospasm in asthmatics undergoing general anesthesia and/or intravascular administration of radiographic contrast media. Curr Med Res Opin 25(7):1621–1630
50. Kabalin CS, Yarnold PR, Grammer LC (1995) Low complication rate of corticosteroid-treated asthmatics undergoing surgical procedures. Arch Intern Med 155(13):1379–1384
51. Silvanus MT, Groeben H, Peters J (2004) Corticosteroids and inhaled salbutamol in patients with reversible airway obstruction markedly decrease the incidence of bronchospasm after tracheal intubation. Anesthesiology 100(5):1052–1057
52. Popping DM, Elia N, Marret E, Remy C, Tramer MR (2008) Protective effects of epidural analgesia on pulmonary complications after abdominal and thoracic surgery: a meta-analysis. Arch Surg 143(10):990–999
53. Liu SS, Wu CL (2007) The effect of analgesic technique on postoperative patient-reported outcomes including analgesia: a systematic review. Anesth Analg 105(3):789–808
54. Dolin SJ, Cashman JN, Bland JM (2002) Effectiveness of acute postoperative pain management: I. Evidence from published data. Br J Anaesth 89(3):409–423
55. Mann C, Pouzeratte Y, Boccara G, Peccoux C, Vergne C, Brunat G et al (2000) Comparison of intravenous or epidural patient-controlled analgesia in the elderly after major abdominal surgery. Anesthesiology 92(2):433–441
56. Cooper DW, Saleh U, Taylor M, Whyte S, Ryall D, Kokri MS et al (1999) Patient-controlled analgesia: epidural fentanyl and i.v. morphine compared after caesarean section. Br J Anaesth 82(3):366–370
57. Flisberg P, Rudin A, Linner R, Lundberg CJ (2003) Pain relief and safety after major surgery. A prospective study of epidural and intravenous analgesia in 2696 patients. Acta Anaesthesiol Scand 47(4):457–465
58. Sumida S, Lesley MR, Hanna MN, Murphy JD, Kumar K, Wu CL (2009) Meta-analysis of the effect of extended-release epidural morphine versus intravenous patient-controlled analgesia on respiratory depression. J Opioid Manag 5(5):301–305
59. Berg H, Roed J, Viby-Mogensen J, Mortensen CR, Engbaek J, Skovgaard LT et al (1997) Residual neuromuscular block is a risk factor for postoperative pulmonary complications. A prospective, randomised, and blinded study of postoperative pulmonary complications after atracurium, vecuronium and pancuronium. Acta Anaesthesiol Scand 41(9):1095–1103
60. Weller WE, Rosati C (2008) Comparing outcomes of laparoscopic versus open bariatric surgery. Ann Surg 248(1):10–15
61. Ambrosino N, Gabbrielli L (2010) Physiotherapy in the perioperative period. Best Pract Res Clin Anaesthesiol 24(2):283–289
62. Guimaraes MM, El Dib R, Smith AF, Matos D (2009) Incentive spirometry for prevention of postoperative pulmonary complications in upper abdominal surgery. Cochrane Database Syst Rev (3):CD006058
63. Conti G, Cavaliere F, Costa R, Craba A, Catarci S, Festa V et al (2007) Noninvasive positive-pressure ventilation with different interfaces in patients with respiratory failure after abdominal surgery: a matched-control study. Respir Care 52(11):1463–1471

64. Chiumello D, Pelosi P, Carlesso E, Severgnini P, Aspesi M, Gamberoni C et al (2003) Noninvasive positive pressure ventilation delivered by helmet vs. standard face mask. Intensive Care Med 29(10):1671–1679
65. Ferreyra GP, Baussano I, Squadrone V, Richiardi L, Marchiaro G, Del Sorbo L et al (2008) Continuous positive airway pressure for treatment of respiratory complications after abdominal surgery: a systematic review and meta-analysis. Ann Surg 247(4):617–626
66. Chiumello D, Chevallard G, Gregoretti C (2011) Non-invasive ventilation in postoperative patients: a systematic review. Intensive Care Med 37(6):918–929
67. Stock MC, Downs JB, Gauer PK, Alster JM, Imrey PB (1985) Prevention of postoperative pulmonary complications with CPAP, incentive spirometry, and conservative therapy. Chest 87(2):151–157
68. Joris JL, Sottiaux TM, Chiche JD, Desaive CJ, Lamy ML (1997) Effect of bi-level positive airway pressure (BiPAP) nasal ventilation on the postoperative pulmonary restrictive syndrome in obese patients undergoing gastroplasty. Chest 111(3):665–670
69. Kindgen-Milles D, Muller E, Buhl R, Bohner H, Ritter D, Sandmann W et al (2005) Nasal-continuous positive airway pressure reduces pulmonary morbidity and length of hospital stay following thoracoabdominal aortic surgery. Chest 128(2):821–828
70. Jaber S, Delay JM, Chanques G, Sebbane M, Jacquet E, Souche B et al (2005) Outcomes of patients with acute respiratory failure after abdominal surgery treated with noninvasive positive pressure ventilation. Chest 128(4):2688–2695
71. Antonelli M, Conti G, Bufi M, Costa MG, Lappa A, Rocco M et al (2000) Noninvasive ventilation for treatment of acute respiratory failure in patients undergoing solid organ transplantation: a randomized trial. JAMA 283(2):235–241
72. Huerta S, DeShields S, Shpiner R, Li Z, Liu C, Sawicki M et al (2002) Safety and efficacy of postoperative continuous positive airway pressure to prevent pulmonary complications after Roux-en-Y gastric bypass. J Gastrointest Surg 6(3):354–358
73. Michelet P, D'Journo XB, Seinaye F, Forel JM, Papazian L, Thomas P (2009) Non-invasive ventilation for treatment of postoperative respiratory failure after oesophagectomy. Br J Surg 96(1):54–60
74. Perrin C, Jullien V, Venissac N, Berthier F, Padovani B, Guillot F et al (2007) Prophylactic use of noninvasive ventilation in patients undergoing lung resectional surgery. Respir Med 101(7):1572–1578
75. Lee PC, Helsmoortel CM, Cohn SM, Fink MP (1990) Are low tidal volumes safe? Chest 97(2):430–434
76. Gajic O, Dara SI, Mendez JL, Adesanya AO, Festic E, Caples SM et al (2004) Ventilator-associated lung injury in patients without acute lung injury at the onset of mechanical ventilation. Crit Care Med 32(9):1817–1824
77. Choi G, Wolthuis EK, Bresser P, Levi M, van der PT, Dzoljic M et al (2006) Mechanical ventilation with lower tidal volumes and positive end-expiratory pressure prevents alveolar coagulation in patients without lung injury. Anesthesiology 105(4):689–695
78. Michelet P, D'Journo XB, Roch A, Doddoli C, Marin V, Papazian L et al (2006) Protective ventilation influences systemic inflammation after esophagectomy: a randomized controlled study. Anesthesiology 105(5):911–919
79. Wrigge H, Zinserling J, Stuber F, von Spiegel T, Hering R, Wetegrove S et al (2000) Effects of mechanical ventilation on release of cytokines into systemic circulation in patients with normal pulmonary function. Anesthesiology 93(6):1413–1417
80. Wrigge H, Uhlig U, Zinserling J, Behrends-Callsen E, Ottersbach G, Fischer M et al (2004) The effects of different ventilatory settings on pulmonary and systemic inflammatory responses during major surgery. Anesth Analg 98(3):775–781 (Table)
81. Malbouisson LM, Humberto F, Rodrigues RR, Carmona MJ, Auler JO (2008) Atelectasis during anesthesia: pathophysiology and treatment. Rev Bras Anestesiol 58(1):73–83

82. Maa SH, Hung TJ, Hsu KH, Hsieh YI, Wang KY, Wang CH et al (2005) Manual hyperinflation improves alveolar recruitment in difficult-to-wean patients. Chest 128(4):2714–2721

83. Imberger G, McIlroy D, Pace NL, Wetterslev J, Brok J, Moller AM (2010) Positive end-expiratory pressure (PEEP) during anaesthesia for the prevention of mortality and postoperative pulmonary complications. Cochrane Database Syst Rev (9):CD007922

84. Bouhemad B, Brisson H, Le Guen M, Arbelot C, Lu Q, Rouby JJ (2011) Bedside ultrasound assessment of positive end-expiratory pressure-induced lung recruitment. Am J Respir Crit Care Med 183(3):341–347

85. Chetta A, Tzani P, Marangio E, Carbognani P, Bobbio A, Olivieri D (2006) Respiratory effects of surgery and pulmonary function testing in the preoperative evaluation. Acta Biomed 77(2):69–74

86. Delay JM, Sebbane M, Jung B, Nocca D, Verzilli D, Pouzeratte Y et al (2008) The effectiveness of noninvasive positive pressure ventilation to enhance preoxygenation in morbidly obese patients: a randomized controlled study. Anesth Analg 107(5):1707–1713

87. Cavaliere F, Biasucci D, Costa R, Soave M, Addabbo G, Proietti R (2011) Chest ultrasounds to guide manual reexpansion of a postoperative pulmonary atelectasis: a case report. Minerva Anestesiol 77(7):750–753

Lights and Shadows on Aerosol Therapy in Mechanically Ventilated Patients

5

Davide Chiumello and Silvia Coppola

The term aerosol refers to the fine dispersion in a gas, suitable to be breathed in, (dispersing phase) of liquid or solid particles (dispersed phase). It can be considered as the means of transport of a drug to the airways in the form of small liquid or solid particles (with a diameter from 2 to 100 μ).

The deposition of the aerosol in the airways depends from several parameters, some dependent on the drug itself, such as the physicochemical properties of the particles, some dependent on the anatomical and physiological characteristics of the patient, such as the anatomy of the respiratory tree and the inhalation pattern [1].

The administration of drugs by aerosol is commonly implemented by three types of devices:

- pressurized metered-dose inhalers (pressurized metered dose inhaler—pMDI)
- providers of dry powder (dry powder inhaler—DPI)
- nebulizers.

The advantages that lead to prefer drugs for topical use in the treatment of respiratory diseases are manifold. In the first place, the possibility of obtaining important therapeutic effects at significantly lower doses than those required by the systemic route, and second, the lower incidence of systemic side effects, and third, the better bioavailability of the drug that is released in an active form directly on 'target organ' with reduced first pass effect and overall catabolism, and fourth, the

D. Chiumello (✉) · S. Coppola
Dipartimento di Anestesia, Rianimazione (Intensiva E Subintensiva) e Terapia Del Dolore, Fondazione IRCCS Ca' Granda-Ospedale Maggiore Policlinico, Via Francesco Sforza 35, 20122, Milan, Italy
e-mail: chiumello@libero.it

S. Coppola
e-mail: silvia_coppola@libero.it

B. Allaria (ed.), *Practical Issues in Anesthesia and Intensive Care 2013*,
DOI: 10.1007/978-88-470-5529-2_5, © Springer-Verlag Italia 2014

rapid availability of drugs into the systemic circulation. This latter effect exploits the easily accesible exchange surface, of great absorption and the minimum distance from the vascular bed that characterizes the respiratory tract avoiding the enterohepatic metabolism of the first phase [2].

However, the administration of drugs by aerosol is not without disadvantages. These include the fact that a relatively small fraction of aerosol administered actually reaches the lungs, the lack of a titratable and reliable dose, the lack of a standardized technical information on inhalers for clinicians, all variables that affect the deposit, the lungs, and the reproducibility of the administered dose.

Furthermore, the risks associated with drug therapy taken via aerosol may occur due to the type of inhaled medication, the type of generator used, the technique of administration. Most of the risks associated with aerosol therapy are attributed to adverse reactions to administred drugs. Other potential risks are: bronchospasm following the administration of a cold aerosol and with high density in patients suffering from asthma or from other respiratory diseases, exposure to high doses of inhaled medication subsequently to the modifications of the drug concentration caused by evaporation, heating, or inability of the device to spray efficiently suspension and finally the increased risk of infection due to the fact that the aerosol may be contaminated with bacteria.

By aerosol, several drugs can be administered such as $\beta2$ agonists, steroids, anticholinergics, antibiotics, antivirals, and rhDNase [3].

The possible clinical applications relate to all respiratory diseases characterized by airway obstruction, both acute and chronic, recurrent bronchospasm during infections, especially viral, all respiratory infections that occur with a component asthmatiform and infections of upper and lower airways.

For many years, aerosol therapy has been reserved for spontaneously breathing patients able to cooperate and synchronize with the delivery of the drug. Moreover, the lack of a reliable and titratable dose has limited the use of aerosol therapies in patients on mechanical ventilation to the empirical administration of bronchodilators, also given the availability in these patients of a venous access that can be readily used to infuse drugs [4].

5.1 Basic Aerosol Physics

The ability of particles to remain suspended in a gas can be predicted from their size, shape and density, and the density and viscosity of the gas – known as Stokes law [5]. The properties of an aerosol are commonly expressed by two variables, the mass median aerosol diameter (MMAD), a measure of the average particle size, and the geometric standard deviation (GSD), a measure of the distribution or heterogeneity of particle sizes. Both can be calculated from the cumulative particle size distribution curve [6]. Reliable estimates of likely deposition site within the respiratory tree/ventilator circuit can be made based upon particle size.

Fig. 5.1 Effect of aerosol particle according to their size along the airway tree [7]

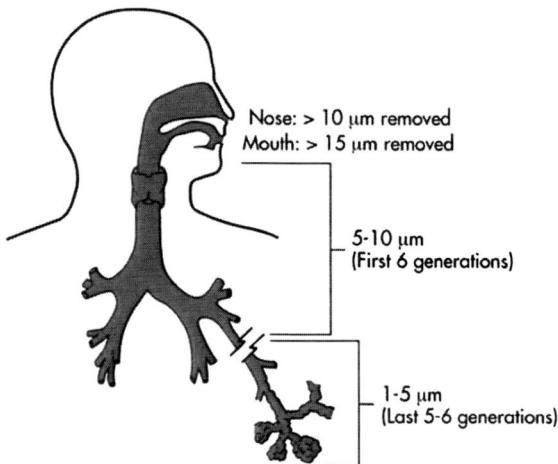

Nose: > 10 μm removed
Mouth: > 15 μm removed

5-10 μm
(First 6 generations)

1-5 μm
(Last 5-6 generations)

Generally, the deposition site in the respiratory tract is the upper airways or the ventilator circuit for the particle with a diamater >5 μ, the tracheobronchial tree for particles with a diameter of 2–10 μ; the small particles with a diameter of 0.5–5 μ have an alveolar deposition, the smaller particles with a diameter <0.5 μ stay suspended in gas and are exhaled [4] (Fig. 5.1).

In order to assess the efficiency of an aerosol generator, it is necessary to determine both the distribution of particle sizes and the rate at which they are produced.

5.2 Pharmacodynamics and Pharmacokinetics of Aerosol Therapy

Although the concept of topical therapy may sound simple, its application in practice has needed the design and construction of complex and sophisticated tools, still evolving. In respect of the specific characteristics of each drug (mechanism of action, pharmacokinetics, and pharmacodynamics) devices should provide the drug to predefined constant dose over time. Under this light the physical and chemical characteristics of the substance to be nebulized represent a key factor.

The water solubility, in particular, is crucial to obtain a good respirable particles in these conditions; the drug is uniformly distributed, more soluble in the bronchial secretion, and therefore more readily available to be absorbed. Some inhaled corticosteroids, such as beclomethasone dipropionate, fluticasone propionate, and budesonide, being lipophilic molecules have a lower solubility with the most commonly used diluents (saline solutions), compared to other molecules such as flunisolide. These characteristics have practical influence on the final size of the generated particles. The drug should reach that particular sector of the respiratory system where there are the anatomical conditions (receptors) that allow it to fully express its specific action.

Bronchodilators, both $\beta2$-stimulants that anticholinergics, for example, have to arrive on the surface of small bronchi and bronchioles to interact with receptors capable of mediating the bronchodilator effect. The amount of drug that is distributed on the main bronchi or at the level of the alveoli has not pharmacological effects. Therefore, from this point of view, *the size of the particles* that are emitted from the aerosol generator represents a critical element; an average diameter should optimally be between 2.5 and 6 μ and ideally all emitted particles should have the same characteristics (but this happens only in theory).

Another important factor to take into consideration is represented by the flow with which the aerosol is inhaled and also by the *breathing pattern* of the patient: if the patient is tachypneic the deposition of a greater amount of drug will be on the oropharynx, while if the subject has a slow breathing pattern (bradypnea), perhaps interspersed with phases of apnea, the drug reaches more easily the distal areas of the bronchial tree.

Moving from these considerations it is easy to comprehend which important role plays the behavior of the patient in this type of treatment, and especially the ventilatory setting in a patient on mechanical ventilation to be subjected to aerosol therapy [8].

To study the complex problem of pharmacokinetics aerosol therapy in the intubated patient, Palmer and colleagues studied a method to measure the deposition of particles in the lung; aerosol particles were captured from the ventilator circuit at the level of a inspiratory filter placed before the endotracheal tube, subsequently in a separate experiment another dose of antibiotic was nebulized and inhaled by the patient, the amount captured by a expiratory filter represented the mass exhaled [9]. The difference between the inhaled and exhaled amount indicated the portion deposited in the lungs.

Summarizing the aerosol deposition in the airways depends on characteristics of the aerosol particles, such as size, density and hygroscopicity, and also on anatomical and clinical factors, such as morphology of the airways, current pathologies, age and physiological factors such as tidal volume, functional residual capacity, and respiratory rate.

5.3   Methods of Aerosol Delivery

5.3.1   Pressurized Metered Dose Inhalers

These devices contain a pressurized mixture of propellants, surfactants, preservatives, flavoring agents, and active drug, the latter comprising approximately 1 % of the total contents.

Pressurized Metered Dose Inhalers (MDI) (Fig. 5.2a) are formed by a pressurized canister in which the active ingredient is in suspension with surfactants and

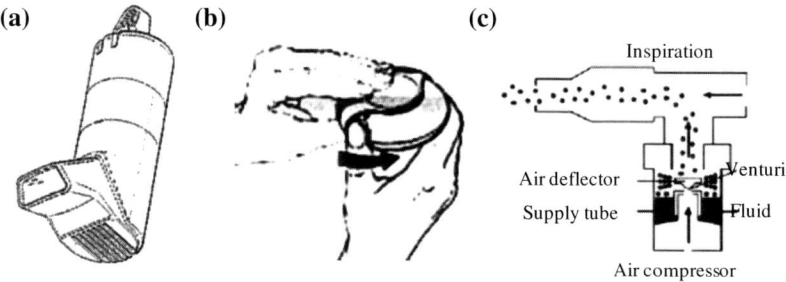

Fig. 5.2 **a** pressurized *MDI* metered dose inhaler, **b** *DPI* dry powder inhalers, **c** air jet nebulizer

gaseous propellants. Exerting pressure on the bottom of the canister, a predetermined amount of medication is released in aerosol form with particle size between 1 and 2 μ. As the mixture is released, the propellant evaporates. The extent to which evaporation occurs is dependent on the ambient temperature and the physical properties of the mixture. Patient-device synchrony is difficult to achieve, but it is essential to ensure the effective delivery of active ingredient.

This can be largely overcome by deploying the drug dose into a holding chamber or spacer both in spontaneous breathing patients and in mechanically ventilated patients, attaching the device to the endotracheal tube or to the inspiratory arm of the ventilatory circuit [2]. A variety of such chambers that interface with mechanical ventilator circuits have been developed [10]. However, the reliable delivery of an aerosol via these devices still requires a complex number of steps: heat the can up to body temperature, shake the inhaler well, wait a minute for subsequent doses [4].

Given the comparative simplicity of nebulizers and the limited number of available drugs, pressurized MDI used in mechanically ventilated patients is employed in only a minority of ICUs.

5.3.2 Dry Powder Inhalers

These devices produce reliable aerosols by placing a fixed volume of loosely aggregated, or carrier particle bound, micronized powder at the end of a shaped tube.

The aerosolization of the powder requires energy, supplied by the patient; thanks to the inspiratory flow produced during inhalation. They consist of a tank, a body, and a mouthpiece (Fig. 5.2b). The patient should take an inspiration that drives the dose along the suction channels up to the mouthpiece and produces a turbulence that breaks the aggregates of dust in respirable particles. The optimal inspiratory maneuver for pulmonary deposition of the particles is given by the force of inhalation (peak inspiratory flow), from the total time of inhalation, and the speed with which the flow increases.

Unlike pressurized MDIs, no patient device synchronization is required. However, the aerosolization process tends to produce a comparatively higher percentage of charged particles which results in a higher proportion of early/upper airway particle deposition [5].

Although interface devices that integrate DPIs into mechanical ventilator circuits have been developed [4], none is currently in widespread use [10].

5.3.3 Nebulizers

There are three principal designs of nebulizer: Jet, ultrasonic, and vibrating mesh. The performance of these devices varies widely [5].

5.3.3.1 Jet Nebulizers

The jet nebulizers (Fig. 5.2c) are powered by compressed air or oxygen in order to nebulize liquid drugs. They push the liquid contained in a chamber reservoir by a jet of compressed air at a rate of 5–10 L/min. The gas is accelerated through a narrow orifice placed at 90° of the free end of a second nozzle which fish inside the liquid drug. For the Bernoulli law, in the second nozzle there is a negative pressure gradient that pushes the liquid to rise in the tube where the jet of compressed air shatters and turns it into aerosol. The particle size varies greatly, but the majority of the particles except the smallest collides on the walls and return to the reservoir. In the ventilatory circuit, the aerosol is transported through the flow of gas to a point close to the patient. These air jet devices cool the solution and tend to concentrate the solution. Furthermore, they develop tangential forces that can degrade larger molecules as well as the microstructures of the protein complexes.

5.3.3.2 Ultrasonic Nebulizers

These devices are based on a high frequency vibrating piezoelectric crystal. The crystal emits ultrasonic vibrations, classically at 3 MHz, which are transmitted via one of various designs to a liquid reservoir. The transmitted energy disrupts the liquid surface tension causing cavitation and aerosolization. As a rule, the higher the frequency, the smaller the particle generated.

Ultrasonic nebulizers heat solutions, the effect being proportional to the frequency and, hence, the smaller are generated particles, the more marked is the effect.

Their use is limited by the cost of the necessary equipment.

5.3.3.3 Vibrating Mesh Nebulizers

These devices are also based on a high frequency vibrating piezoelectric crystal.

The crystal is used to vibrate a precision engineered micron mesh at very high frequency. A micro pump delivers a small volume of liquid from a reservoir onto the vibrating mesh resulting in a precise aerosol. These devices neither cool nor heat the solution. Then, they inflict significant sheer stresses and they are consequently recommended for use with complex microstructures and large molecules [11].

5.4   Comparison of the Different Types of Nebulizer

There are no outcome studies comparing different types of nebulizer in mechanically ventilated patients. Jet nebulizers are simple and cheap in comparison to ultrasonic or vibrating mesh devices and hence are by far the commonest technology employed. Because of the heterogeneity of the performance of different jet nebulizer, and of their technologies, it seems unlikely that any comparative outcome studies are feasible. The most important disadvantage of jet nebulizers is the need to entrain an additional 5–10 l/min of gas into the ventilator circuit, which inevitably affects tidal volume and potentially the dynamic compliance of the patient's ventilatory profile.

Regarding the percentage of administered therapy in the correct site, this depends much more from the ventilator circuit and the ventilatory setting rather than the type of nebulizer. The dose of delivered bronchodilator by the nebulizer is much greater than the delivered dose by MDI, but the response to bronchodilators is often the same with the two systems. Despite the difference of nearly 10 times of the total dose of drug (example: 5 mg with a nebulizer versus 0.7 mg with MDI if the patient is breathing spontaneously) bronchodilator response is the same [12].

The discrepancy in the dose of the drug is partially explained by the great loss of drug inside the nebulizer. The response to the administration by MDI is better when you use the spacers; the spacer must be connected to the inspiratory limb of the ventilator through a Y-connector and puff provided into the spacer will be inhaled into the inspiratory phase of ventilation [13].

In general, the administration with MDI has the advantage of a more simple use without the risk of bacterial contamination and without the need for correction of the flow velocity.

In conclusion, the most commonly used methods in the ventilated patient are the pneumatic nebulizers and metered dose inhalers without a clear evidence of superiority of one device versus the other.

5.5   Problems with Aerosol Administration in Patients on Mechanical Ventilation

The administration of aerosol particles up to the distal airways or alveoli in mechanically ventilated patients can be a challenge. Compared to aerosol administration in spontaneously breathing patients, there are some peculiarities. The humidification of the inhaled gas is an issue to be taken into consideration as it reduces the deposition of the aerosol particles of approximately 40 % by increasing the deposition of the particles themselves in the ventilator circuit. The aerosol therapy during mechanical ventilation therefore requires an increase of the doses to achieve the desired therapeutic effect [14].

Only nebulizers and pressurized metered dose inhalers can be used as aerosol dispensing devices; dry powder inhalers cannot be used as the humidification of the circuit, prevents the formation of particles. Factors that can influence the proportion of the drug administered with success are inspiratory flow profile, respiratory rate, tidal volume and the modality of administration, continuous or synchronized with inspiration. Both the ventilatory set and the type of the used device affect on the efficacy of the drug in situ [15].

To allow an adequate peripheral deposition of the drug, the ventilatory setting should include:

- a low inspiratory flow that facilitates the mixture of the aerosol and its transport to the lower airways;
- a tidal volume greater than 500 ml which should ensure a wider distribution;
- a long slow continuous inspiratory profile to reduce the turbulent flow and the deposition of the particles in the proximal airways;
- a long inspiratory pause to maximize particle deposition in the periphery;
- a minimum level of positive end-expiratory pressure [16].

Generally, the ventilator setting is never changed or optimized when spraying.

However, it has been widely demonstrated that the use of a constant flow in the ventilator circuit during all phases of ventilation may increase the losses of aerosol while the aerosol administration synchronized with the inhalation significantly increases the levels of antibiotics deposited in sputum.

In addition to the variables of ventilatory pattern, also humidification and the type of device are relevant.

Humidification is achieved using active humidifiers in the inspiratory arm, or by means of heat and moisture exchangers (HME). There is no evidence to suggest that one method is superior to the other [17]. While the performance of active humidifiers is almost uniform, the performance of heat and moisture exchangers varies considerably [18].

When the aerosol is exposed to gas saturated with water vapor, the particles hydrate and become bigger and consequently the availability of peripheral aerosol particles decrease. In the same way, the humidification of the ventilator circuit increases the size of the particles [19, 20]. In contrast, the aerosol, when exposed to dry gas, is dehydrated and this causes crystallization of drugs or additives and the reduction of the availability of drug. The entity of this phenomenon depends on the exposure time and the position of the nebulizer in the circuit [13, 19]. Results of in vitro experiments suggest that a fresh gas without water vapor is a better aerosol carrier than a gas saturated with water vapor and that the better position of the device should be approximately 15–30 cm before the Y of ventilator circuit. It was also shown that the ratio of inhaled particles in non-humidified gas versus inhaled particles in humidified gas was 2:1, indicating a double availability of the drug when the humidifier was turned off [20]. However, if you use HME as a filter, the nebulizer should be placed distal to the filter between this one and the corrugated tubing.

Numerous studies have been performed in vitro regarding systems of administration of aerosol therapy in mechanical ventilators; they have proved less useful in the clinical application. In vivo studies are very limited and often have been performed with not accurate methods.

As regards the type of device, metered dose inhalers require an adapter and a spacer to ensure an efficient administration of the drug, if properly used is able to provide drug doses more consistent of those of nebulizers [21].

Although the optimal method for administering aerosol therapy by nebulizers is yet to be established, the use of an inspiratory pause, a slow inspiratory flow and an adequate tidal volume much more influence the effectiveness of therapy with nebulizers rather that with MDI [19, 22].

The disadvantages of nebulizers in mechanical ventilation consist in a contamination of the ventilator circuit, the reduced ability to "trigger" from the patient and in the increased tidal volume and medium airways pressure due to the aerosol flow. In general, the nebulizer is perhaps less efficient than MDI during mechanical ventilation, but it can deliver a higher cumulative dose to the distal airways. Therefore, nebulizers and MDI produce similar therapeutic effects in ventilated patients, but the pressurized metered dose inhalers are easier to use, require less attention from the nursing staff, are able to release more predictable doses of drug and do not increase the risk of contamination bacterial.

Also, when MDI are used with a spacer, the ventilator circuit should not be disconnected during the aerosol treatment to reduce the risk of ventilator-associated pneumonia and prevent the loss of positive end-expiratory pressure in patients with severe respiratory failure [23, 24]. Despite the optimal nebulizer has to be identified, there is consensus that the aerosol administration synchronized with the inspiration, the humidified circuit, the correct position of the device in the circuit are conditions that promote an efficient aerosol therapy (Table 5.1).

5.6   Clinical Use

5.6.1   Bronchodilators

The drug administered by inhalatory route most commonly prescribed in patients on mechanical ventilation is the racemic salbutamol (albuterol). This $\beta2$ agonist has an important role in the treatment of acute asthma and chronic obstructive pulmonary disease (COPD). In addition to the bronchodilator action, racemic salbutamol seems to have a function in the clearance of alveolar fluid as demonstrated in experimental studies and in some small trials [25] and seems to promote the mucociliary clearance [26].

As already known, there is a distinct difference between the administered dose and the dose of drug that actually reaches the airways, in fact most of the drug remains on the walls of the endotracheal tube. As above discussed, the airways'

Table 5.1 Advantages and disadvantages of different aerosol devices

Device	Advantages	Disadvantages
Pressurized meter dose inhaler MDI	Dose and diameter of the particles are independent of inhalation maneuvers Fast delivery Reproducible delivered doses Difficult contamination Cheap	Possible reactions to propellants High oropharyngeal deposition Need for coordination with inspiration. Limited availability of drugs, Difficult to administer high doses
Dry powder inhaler DPI	Less need for coordination between inhalation and drug delivery. Not need to propellant Cheap	Need for high inspiratory flow between 30 and 60 L/min. Limited availability of drugs Effect of humidity on the drug Difficult to administer high doses
Nebulizers Air jet nebulizers	Coordination between inspiration and delivery is not required Possibility to administer high doses	Expensive Need for an energy source Slow delivery time Risk of contamination Unpredictable effective dose.
Ultrasonic nebulizers	Coordination between inspiration and delivery is not required Possibility to administer high doses Fast delivery	Expensive Risk of contamination Different performance among devices Slow delivery time
Vibrating mesh nebulizers	Coordination between inspiration and delivery is not required Possibility to administer high doses Fast delivery Tidal volume is sufficient for a good efficacy Accuracy in the drug delivery	Expensive Risk of contamination Limited availability of drugs

patient anatomy, the ventilator parameters and the type of device greatly affect the effectiveness of the administered aerosol therapy.

Therefore, in mechanically ventilated patients, bronchodilators $\beta2$ agonists should be administered according to their pharmacological effect or their toxicity, rather than prescribing an arbitrary number of puffs. Manthous and colleagues recommended to start with 5–10 puffs of albuterol administered by MDI with spacer or 2.5 mg of albuterol administered with a nebulizer [27]. If the airway resistance, defined as the difference between the peak pressure and plateau pressure remained above 15 cm H_2O L/s and there were no toxic reactions, the treatment had to be repeated at a higher dose. Once the effective dose was determined on the basis of a reduction of the resistive component, this dose could be repeated every 2–6 h depending on the severity of bronchospasm and half-life of the drug. In patients who did not respond to high doses of $\beta2$ agonist (20 puffs by MDI with spacer or a triple dose of nebulizer) inhaled anticholinergics should be always administered, and in case of therapeutic failure, systemic corticosteroids should be the following step [28].

The use of bronchodilator is also described in patients on mechanical ventilation even in the absence of a proven or suspected reversible obstruction of the airways, although no clinical trial has demonstrated that albuterol or any other $\beta2$ agonist has a beneficial effect in these patients [29]. To date, two large multicenter randomized trials in patients with acute respiratory failure were abandoned after an interim analysis due to lack of efficacy [29, 30]. It should also be remembered that the toxicity of salbutamol is not completely clarified [31], there is instead a well-documented propensity to induce lactic acidosis. [32] The literature regarding a possible clinical deterioration in patients with acute heart failure is anecdotal [33].

In general, therapy with high-dose inhaled $\beta2$ agonists can have side effects such as tachycardia, tremor, hyperglycemia, and decreased levels of serum potassium, magnesium, and phosphate. The decrease in serum potassium is the result of the shift mediated by receptors β, of the potassium into the cells and the effect is remarkable, if one considers that high doses of inhaled $\beta2$ agonists can be used for the acute treatment of hyperkalemia [34].

The second most commonly prescribed bronchodilator as aerosol therapy in ventilated patients is the anticholinergic ipratropium bromide. Systemic absorption is minimal then the side effects of anticholinergics (tachycardia, dry mouth, blurred vision, urinary retention) are minimal. Ipratropium is not a bronchodilator of first choice for asthma and is recommended in combination with $\beta2$ agonists. Magnesium sulfate is widely used and recommended as an additional bronchodilator in the treatment of life threatening acute asthmatic attack [35, 36]. It is usually administered intravenously, but can be equally effective when nebulized [37].

Although no longer used, the nebulized adrenaline had its rational for the acute airway obstruction secondary to inflammation, corticosteroids, and surfactant [2], as well as there could be a biological and pharmacological rational, despite of the little evidence, on the clinical use of lidocaine spray [38, 39].

In summary, although the bronchodilators have a well-established role in the acute or chronic treatment of asthma and COPD, there is a lack of evidence regarding the effectiveness of the empiric bronchodilator therapy in mechanically ventilated patients without these particular conditions.

5.6.2   Corticosteroids

As well as bronchodilators, inhaled corticosteroids have a well-established role in the treatment of chronic asthma and COPD. In exacerbations and in the acute events, it is recommended the systemic steroid therapy while the role of inhalation therapy is not clear [40]. It is known that corticosteroids have an important effect on the physiological down regulation of $\beta2$ receptors. This role is so important that all major guidelines recommend the use of corticosteroids in all patients requiring chronic therapy with $\beta2$ agonists. So, if the nebulized albuterol is used in an empirical way or actually tested in acute, you should consider to administer simultaneously, inhaled or systemic steroid therapy, in particular to reduce the incidence of relapse in the medium/long term [41]. However, currently there are no clear indications on the use of inhaled corticosteroids.

5.6.3 Mucolytics

The main components of the normal respiratory secretions are glycoproteins that form a mucous gel of large oligomeric structures. The sputum or the pathological mucus contains additional components including deoxyribonucleic acid derived from necrotic neutrophils together with actin filaments, cellular debris, bacteria. Consequently, sputum tends to have a higher viscosity than the normal secretions [42]. This increased viscosity on the one hand favors the cough, on the other hinders the mucociliary clearance [43]. Because mechanically ventilated patients do not have cough and have a reduced mucusciliary clearance, therapy to reduce the viscosity of sputum has an important rational.

N-acetylcysteine (NAC), administered both per os and by aerosol is perhaps the most widely recommended mucolytic. However, there is no evidence to support its effectiveness in any pathological condition [42, 44].

The NAC administered by aerosol, breaks the disulfide bonds of the structure of the glycoprotein mucin and is associated with an improved clearance of mucus. Because of the increased risk of bronchospasm, its use is limited. It can be used together with a bronchodilator administered by inhalation.

There is also good evidence to support the efficacy of nebulized hypertonic saline (3–14 %) [42, 45]. An alternative therapy is nebulized mannitol [46, 47].

Patients with cystic fibrosis produce few mucin and their secretions have a high viscosity due to the highly polymerized DNA. The human recombinant DNase (rhDNase, dornase alpha) seems to improve lung function in the chronic treatment of patients affected by cystic fibrosis, but it does not provide any significant effect in acute exacerbations of cystic fibrosis.

Up to now, there have been two trials in pediatric patients and both suggest that it could be a promising therapy [48, 49]. It was not demonstrated no efficacy of rhDNase in the bronchiectasis in patients not affected by cystic fibrosis.

5.6.4 Aerosolized Antibiotics

Ventilator-acquired pneumonia (VAP) is a serious complication of mechanical ventilation; its impact can be minimized following the guidelines for infections control [50]. VAP is a syndrome that evolves in a series of stages from the colonization of the respiratory tract, passing through the tracheobronchitis (VAT) and finally pneumonia [51]. The role of the nebulized antibiotic therapy in the prevention and treatment of both VAT and VAP begins to be studied but there are many unanswered questions.

The topical aerosol therapy administered to patients affected with tracheo-bronchitis seems to prevent infection of the lower airways. Although desirable, the aerosol antibiotic therapy is not commonly used, for many reasons including the lack of a clear indication about the correct timing, the risk to increase bacterial resistance, the technical difficulty to administer aerosol to intubated patients, the lack of specific formulations for many antibiotics and because of problems related to the choice of therapeutic end points in critically ill patients.

To minimize the systemic toxicity aerosol therapy should achieve therapeutic levels in the airways but reduce the exposure of the drug to the rest of the organism [52].

Experimental studies have shown pharmacological concentrations in tracheal aspirates up to 100 times higher than the in vitro minimum inhibitory concentration (MIC) for a particular microorganism, that corresponds to 10–50 times normally obtained with the systemic therapy. There are many doubts about the actual availability of the drug especially in the lung consolidation. The penetration of the drug in the thick secretions or areas of lung consolidation can be very limited as demonstrated by detection of antibiotics concentrations below the MIC, favoring the emergence of resistant strains [53]. Systemic therapy and inhalation therapy have many limitations. This opened to the possibility to associate nebulised antibiotics for systemic therapy that seems to show promising results [54]. This approach can be useful in case of VAP/VAT caused by multi-resistant bacteria and by polymicrobial flora.

Although definitive trials on the use of nebulised antibiotics do not exist, there are some results that justify its use: the detection of elevated levels of antibiotic in the sputum, the reduction of the volume of secretions, the reduction of bacterial growth and of cytokines in models of tracheobronchitis. Further advantages of this antibiotic therapy are the reduction of systemic toxicity and the maintenance of an unchanged flora.

Although these studies have found a dose–response phenomenon in the trachea, the significance of this phenomenon remains unclear. To identify clinical end points remains the greatest challenge to prevent or treat VAP [52].

It has been demonstrated that in critically ill patients with ventilator-associated tracheobronchitis, aerosol therapy with antibiotics can reduce the incidence of VAP and the signs and symptoms of respiratory infection, can facilitate weaning and reduces bacterial resistance and the use of systemic antibiotics, thus providing a clinical benefit in the long term outcomes. On the contrary it does not seem to have any additional benefits in the short outcome after an acute infection compared to systemic antibiotic therapy [55].

There is a particular interest versus the aminoglycosides, broad-spectrum antibiotics directed toward the main Gram-negative pathogens responsible for VAP, hospital, and community-acquired pneumonia, whose use is limited because of the systemic toxicity and the poor penetration into lung tissue. The aerosol therapy offers advantage, theoretically, to achieve high pharmacological concentrations in situ with few systemic effects. Although a lot of data already exist regarding the aerosolized antibiotic therapy in patients affected with cystic fibrosis in spontaneous breathing, there are few data in patients on mechanical ventilation. In 2008, it was performed a multicenter trial to evaluate the alveolar penetration of amikacin in mechanically ventilated patients with Gram-negative nosocomial pneumonia. This trial found that the antibiotic concentrations were much higher than the MIC of the microorganisms responsible in the areas involved by the lung infection, with very low serum concentrations. The clinical efficacy in terms of outcomes of aerosol therapy in combination with systemic therapy, however, still to be established [56].

Among the antibiotics, colistin is currently administered by inhalation in patients with cystic fibrosis. It is active against Gram-negative bacteria, already used as a topical therapy in the decontamination of the digestive tract and has several systemic side effects when administered endovenously, such as nephrotoxicity and neurotoxicity. The liquid formulation to inhale by means of a nebulizer is not approved by the FDA because the degradation products of the drug may damage the lung epithelium and cause serious side effects. Therefore, the colistin should be diluted before administration (50–75 mg in 3–4 ml of normal saline for 3–4 times per day).

There are few antibiotic formulations suitable for the administration such as inhaled tobramycin and colistin. The use of intravenous preparations to aerosol therapy exposes the respiratory tract to preservatives, hypertonic solutions, and irritants that can provoke bronchospasm, although in patients on mechanical ventilation it has never been reported as a problem.

It is becoming common the use of inhaled pentamidine for prevention and more rarely as a treatment for Pneumocystis carinii pneumonia, or in immunocompromised patients who have developed an allergy to sulfamidics drugs or resistance to cotrimoxazole.

Currently, the role of antibiotics by aerosol or instillation into the endotracheal tube as adjuvants for the prevention or treatment of pulmonary infections in ICU remains to be further investigated in clinical studies.

5.6.5 Pulmonary Vasodilatators

Mechanically ventilated patients with acute lung injury may develop acute or acute on chronic pulmonary hypertension. It is characterized by refractory hypoxemia and right heart failure. Inhaled prostacyclin and sildenafil represent a good therapeutic opportunity. Currently, aerosolized iloprost, which is a synthetic analog of prostacyclin is approved for the treatment of pulmonary hypertension of stage III and IV [57, 58]. Smaldone and colleagues, that studied the pharmacokinetics and pharmacodynamics of inhaled antibiotic therapy in mechanically ventilated patients, have developed a device for the administration of iloprost in critically ill patients and found that clinically effective doses of iloprost may be administered in patients who require high concentrations of oxygen or mechanical ventilation, following the already known evidences about the nebulization, the ventilatory set, and the ventilator type [59].

5.6.6 Heparin, Antithrombin, Activated Protein C, and Sodium Bicarbonate

The inhalation of smoke or chemicals may cause airway damage and in particular local bleeding and fibrin thrombi. There are plausible arguments to support the use of a combination of unfractionated heparin with antithrombin or activated protein C to break up blood clots and facilitate the removal, but there are few studies that support this approach [60]. The nebulized sodium bicarbonate may have a role in airway hyperactivity syndrome after the exposure to hydrochloric gas.

Table 5.2 Aerosol drug preparations available in Italy

Drug	Device
Bronchodilatators	
Albuterol	Nebulizer/MDI
Salmeterol	DPI
Arformoterol	DPI
Tiotropium	DPI
Ipratropium/albuterol	MDI
Corticosteroids	
Beclomethasone dipropionate	MDI
Fluticasone propionate	MDI
Fluticasone/salmeterolo	DPI
Budesonide	DPI
Mometasone	DPI
Mucolytics	
Dornase α	Nebulizer
Acetylcysteine	Nebulizer
Antibiotics	
Tobramycin	Nebulizer
Pentamidine	Nebulizer
Ribavirin	Nebulizer
Other	
Iloprost	Nebulizer

5.7   Conclusions

The new frontiers of aerosol therapy concern the spread of new devices and the administration of new drug compounds. Among the new devices, there might be an intratracheal catheter currently under study, to place inside the endotracheal tube or a bronchoscope ideal to administer aerosol therapy directly in the lungs. About drug formulations, there is a renewed interest in the use of surfactant therapy in patients with acute respiratory failure and new studies are developing on the use of GM-CSF (granulocyte–macrophage colony stimulating factor) in patients with pulmonary alveolar proteinosis or metastatic tumors because of antitumoral effect toward the lung metastases.

In conclusion, aerosol therapy in ventilated patients has its intuitive utility, but the clinical application continues to be restricted by the limited variability of the pharmacological formulations and the inability to administer a reliable and titratable drug dose.

The new technologies in particular vibrating mesh nebulizers together with a specific ventilator management can solve many problems and many doubts about the effectiveness of aerosol transport in the ventilated patient. The use of inhaled bronchodilators and NAC is already part of the clinical practice in intensive care although sometimes in an empirical modality. The aerosolized antibiotic therapy, that can provide many benefits, is still under study and currently is under-used in patients on mechanical ventilation (Table 5.2).

References

1. Dolovich MB, Ahrens RC, Hess DR, Anderson P et al (2005) Device selection and outcomes of aerosol therapy: evidence-based guidelines American college of chest physicians/ American college of asthma allergy, and immunology. Chest 127:335–371
2. Manocha S, Walley KR (2005) Respiratory therapy. In: Fink MP, Abraham E (eds) Terapia intensiva, Elsevier, Masson, pp 526–531
3. Newman SP (1985) Aerosol deposition considerations in inhalation therapy. Chest 88:152S–160S
4. Ruickbie S, Hall A, Ball J (2011) Therapeutic aerosols in mechanically ventilated patients. In: Vincent J-L (ed) Annual update in intensive care and emergency medicine, Springer, Berlin
5. Crowder TM, Rosati JA, Schroeter JD, Hickey AJ, Martonen TB (2002) Fundamental effects of particle morphology on lung delivery: predictions of Stokes law and the particular relevance to dry powder inhaler formulation and development. Pharm Res 19:239–245
6. Reay CA, Bousfield DR, Colchin ES, Menes JA, Sims AJ (2009) Buyers' guide: Nebulizers. In: NHS purchasing and supply agency centre for evidence-based purchasing, London
7. Rau JL Jr (2002) Respiratory care pharmacology, 6th edn. Mosby, St. Louis
8. Newhouse MT (1982) Principles of aerosol therapy. Chest 82:39S–41S
9. Palmer LB, Smaldone GC, Chen JJ, Baram D, Duan T et al (2008) Aerosolized antibiotics and ventilator-associated tracheobronchitis in the intensive care unit. Crit Care Med 36(7):2008–2013
10. Dhand R (2005) Inhalation therapy with metered-dose inhalers and dry powder inhalers in mechanically ventilated patients. Respir Care 30:1331–1334

11. Hess DR, Myers TR, Rau JL (2005) A guide to aerosol delivery devices for respiratory therapists. American Association for Respiratory Care, Dallas
12. Idris AH, McDermott MF, Raucci JC et al (1993) Emergency department treatment of severe asthma: metered-dose inhaler plus holding chamber is equivalent in effectiveness to nebulizer. Chest 103:665–672
13. AARC (1992) Clinical Practice guidelness. Selection of device, administration of Bronchodilatator and evaluation of response to therapy in mechanically ventilated patients. Respir Care 44:105–113
14. Georgopoulos D, Mouloudi E, Kondili E, Klimathianaki M (2000) Bronchodilator delivery with metered-dose inhaler during mechanical ventilation. Crit Care 4:227–235
15. Lin HL, Fink JB, Zhou Y, Cheng YS (2009) Influence of moisture accumulation in inline spacer on delivery of aerosol using metered-dose inhaler during mechanical ventilation. Respir Care 54:1336–1345
16. Dhand R (2004) Basic techniques for aerosol delivery during mechanical ventilation. Respir Care 49:611–620
17. Kelly M, Gillies D, Todd David A, Lockwood C (2010) Heated humidification versus heat and moisture exchangers for ventilated adults and children. Cochrane Database Syst Rev 2010:CD004711
18. Demers RR (2001) Bacterial/viral filtration. Chest 120:1377–1389
19. Ari A, Areabi H, Fink JB (2010) Evaluation of aerosol generator devices at 3 locations in humidified and non-humidified circuits during adult mechanical ventilation. Respir Care 55:837–844
20. Miller DD, Amin MM, Palmer LB, Shah A. R, and Smaldone GC (2003) Aerosol delivery and modern mechanical ventilation in vitro/in vivo evaluation. Am J Respir Crit Care Med 168:1205–1209
21. Dhand R, Guntur VP (2008) How best to deliver aerosol medications to mechanically ventilated patients. Clin Chest Med 29:277–289
22. Ari A, Atalay OT, Harwood R et al (2010) Influence of nebulizer type, position, and bias flow on aerosol drug delivery in simulated pediatric and adult lung models during mechanical ventilation. Respir Care 55:845–855
23. Hess D (2002) Aerosol delivery during mechanical ventilation. Minerva Anestesiol 68:321–328
24. Dhand R (2008) Aerosol delivery during mechanical ventilation: from basic techniques to new devices. J Aerosol Med Pulm Drug Deliv 21:45
25. Mutlu GM, Factor P (2008) Alveolar epithelial 2-adrenergic receptors. Am J Respir Cell Mol Biol 38:127–134
26. Restrepo RD (2007) Inhaled adrenergics and anticholinergics in obstructive lung disease: do they enhance mucociliary clearance? Respir Care 52:1159–1173
27. Manthous CA, Chatila W, Schmidt GA, Hall JR (1995) Treatment of bronchospasm by metered-dose inhaler albuterol in mechanically ventilated patients. Chest 107:210–213
28. MacIntyre NR, Silver RM, Miller CW, Schuler F, Coleman E (1985) Aerosol delivery in intubated, mechanically ventilated patients. Crit Care Med 13:81–84
29. National Heart, Lung and Blood Institute (NHLBI) (2008) Drug study of Albuterol to treat Acute Lung Injury (ALTA). http://clinaltrials.gov/ct2/show/NCT00434993 Accessed 11 Oct 2010
30. The Beta-2 Agonist Lung Injury Trial 2 UK Clinical Research Network (2010) Balti-2 (Beta Agonist Lung injury Trial-2). http://www2.warwick.ac.uk/fac/med7research/ctu/trials/ecr/balti2 Accessed 11 oct 2010
31. Ameredes BT, Calhoun WJ (2006) (R)-albuterol for asthma:pro [a.k.a (S)-albuterol for asthma:con]. Am J Resp Crit Care Med 174:965–969
32. Creagh-Brown BC, Ball J (2008) An under-recognized complication of treatment of acute severe asthma. Am J Emerg Med 26:514,e 1–3

33. Adam JS, Charles E, Douglas MC et al (2008) bronchodilatator therapy in acute decompensated heart failure patients without a history of chronic obstructive pulmonary disease. Ann Emerg Med 51:25–34
34. Truwit JD (1991) Toxic effects of bronchodilatators. Crit Care Clin 7:1337–1342
35. Camargo CA Jr, Rachelefsky G, Schatz M (2009) Managing asthma exacerbations in the emergency department: summary of the national asthma education and prevention program expert panel report 3 guidelines for the management of asthma exacerbations. Proc Am Thorac Soc 6:357–366
36. British thoracic Society and the Scottish Intercollegiate Guidelines Network (2009) British guidelines on the management of asthma. www.britthoracic.org.uk/Portals/Clinical/ Information/Asthma/guidelines/20 June2009
37. Mohammed S, Goodacre S (2007) Intravenous and nebulised magnesium sulphate for acute asthma: systematic review and meta-analysis. Emer Med J 24:823–830
38. Chong CF, Chen CC, Ma HP, Wu YC, Chen YC, Wang TL (2005) Comparison of lidocaine and bronchodilatator inhalation treatment for cough suppression in patients with chronic obstructive pulmonary disease. Emerg Med J 22:429–432
39. Hunt LW, Friga E, Butterfield JH et al (2004) Treatment of asthma with nebulised lidocaine: A randomized, placebo-controlled study. J Allergy Clin Immunol 113:853–859
40. Mannam P, Siegel MD (2010) Analytic review: management of life-threatening asthma in adults. J Intensive care Med 25:3–15
41. Kay AB (1991) Asthma and inflammation. J Allergy Clin Immunol 87:893–945
42. Rogers DF (2007) Mucoactive agents for airway mucus hypersecretory diseases. Respir Care 52:1176–1193
43. Voynow JA, Rubin BK (2009) Mucins, mucus and sputum. Chest 135:505–512
44. Nash EF, Stephenson A, Ratjen F, Tullis E (2009) Nebulized and oral thiol derivatives for pulmonary disease in cystic fibrosis. Cochrane Database Syst Rev 168:CD007168
45. Wark P, McDonald VM (2009) Nebulised hypertonic saline for cystic fibrosis. Cochrane Database Syst Rev 168:CD001506
46. Jacques A, Daviskas E, Turton JA et al (2008) Inhaled mannitol improves lung function in cystic fibrosis. Chest 133:1338–1396
47. Willis PJ, Greenstone M (2006) Inhaled hyperosmolar agents for bronchiectasis. Cochrane Database Syst Rev 168:CD002996
48. Prodhan P, Greenberg B, Bhutta AT et al (2009) Recombinant human deoxyribonuclease improves atelectsis in mechanically ventilated children with cardiac disease. Congenit Heart Dis 4:166–173
49. Riethmueller J, Kumpf M, Borth- Bruhns T et al (2009) Clinical and in vitro effect for dornase alfa in mechanically ventilated pediatric non cystic fibrosis patients with atelectases. Cell Physiol Biochem 23:205–210
50. Torres A, Ewig S, Lode H, Carlet J (2009) Defining, treating and preventing hospital acquired pneumonia: European perspective. Intensive Care Med 35:9–29
51. Craven DE, Chroneou A, Zias N, Hjalmarson KI (2009) Ventilator associated tracheobronchitis. Chest 135:521–528
52. Smaldone GC (2004) Aerosolized antibiotics in mechanically ventilated patients. Respir Care 49(6):635–639
53. Dhand R (2007) The role of aerosolized antimicrobials in the treatment of ventilator-associated pneumonia. Respir Care 52:866–884
54. Palmer LB (2009) Aerosilized antibiotics in critically ill ventilated patients. Curr Opin Crit Care 15:413–418
55. Palmer L, Smaldone G, Chen JJ et al (2008) Aerosolized antibiotics and ventilator-associated tracheobronchitis in the intensive care unit. Crit Care Med 36:2008–2013
56. Luyt C E et al (2009) Pharmacokinetics and lung delivery of PDDS-aerosolized amikacin (NKTR-061) in intubated and mechanically ventilated patients with nosocomial pneumonia. Critical Care 13(6):R200

57. Afshari A, Brock J, Moller AM, Wetterslev J (2010) Aeosolized prostacyclin for acute lung injury (ALI) and acute respiratory distress syndrome (ARDSS). Cochrane Database Syst Rev 168:CD007733
58. Gomberg- Maitland M, Olshewski H (2008) Prostacyclin therapies for the treatment of pulmonary arterial hypertension. Eur Respir J 31:891–901
59. Harris KW, O'Riordan TG, and Smaldone GC (2007) Aerosolized iloprost customized for the critically ill. Respir Care 52(11):1507–1509
60. Toon MH, Maybauers MO, Greenwood JE, Maybauer DM, Fraser JF (2010) Management of acute smoke inhalation injury. Crit Care Resusc 12:53–61

Update on Lung Imaging to Select Ventilatory Management in ARDS Patients

6

Davide Chiumello, Sara Froio and Silvia Coppola

6.1   Introduction

The lung imaging techniques have always been a crucial component for the pathophysiological knowledge and management of the acute respiratory distress syndrome (ARDS). Recently, the current ARDS definition has been update also clarifying the role of lung imaging in order to optimize the agreement between intensivists and radiologists and to make the clinical use of the definition easier [1–3].

In this chapter, we will focus on the diagnostic assessment, clinical management, technical and clinical limitations of chest X-ray, computed tomography, lung ultrasound (LUS), positron emission tomography, electrical impedance tomography, and finally magnetic resonance for ARDS management.

In Tables 6.1 and 6.2, we summarized some of the original articles that we identified from the recent literature to study the role of Lung Imaging in ARDS patients.

D. Chiumello (✉) · S. Froio · S. Coppola
Dipartimento di Anestesia, Rianimazione (Intensiva E Subintensiva) e Terapia del Dolore,
Fondazione IRCCS Ca' Granda-Ospedale Maggiore Policlinico, Via Francesco Sforza 35,
20122, Milan, Italy
e-mail: chiumello@libero.it

S. Froio
e-mail: sara.froio@hotmail.it

S. Coppola
e-mail: silvia_coppola@libero.it

B. Allaria (ed.), *Practical Issues in Anesthesia and Intensive Care 2013*,
DOI: 10.1007/978-88-470-5529-2_6, © Springer-Verlag Italia 2014

Table 6.1 Original articles identified from the recent literature about the role of lung imaging in ARDS patients

Author	N° pt	Technique	Topic	Results
Pirilla [88]	104	X-ray	Lung assessment	Initial chest X-ray abnormalities were associated with a higher risk of requiring ICU admission
Endo [89]	240	X-ray/CT	Lung assessment	Radiologic techniques might be insufficient to detect lung alteration in the initial stage of deterioration of pulmonary oxygenation in patients with mild symptoms
Wang [90]	60	CT	Lung assessment	In blunt chest trauma patients, the pulmonary contusion volume measured by CT-scan, is useful in predicting ARDS development
Strumwasser [91]	106	CT	Lung assessment	In politrauma patients a critical pulmonary contusion volume was identified as the maximally sensitive and specific screening value for ARDS development and correlated with prolonged ICU stay
Copetti [26]	58	LUS	Lung assessment	A specific LUS pattern of ARDS is strongly predictive, in an early phase, of a non-cardiogenic pulmonary edema
Canchi [92]	12	LUS	Lung assessment	In ECMO patients LUS is a safe and reliable method to follow the pathology evolution/recovery of lung and can limit the number of CT-scan and chest X-ray
Bellani [48]	16	PET/CT	Lung assessment	In ARDS patients the metabolic activity is increased across the entire lung density spectrum, but the intensity of this activation and its regional distribution vary within and between subjects
Rodrigues [1-9]	8	PET	Lung assessment	In thoracic trauma patients diffuse lung uptake of FDG was detected by PET 1-3 days before clinically determined ARDS
Chung [18]	28	CT	Outcome	Specific CT pattern predict mortality in ARDS patients
Masclans [93]	38	CT	Outcome	In ARDS survivors after 6 months CT morphologic alterations are limited to less than 25 % of lung parenchyma
Grieser [94]	23	CT	Outcome	In patients with severe ARDS a score on CT findings has a prognostic value in the prediction of mortality

ICU Intensive Care Unit; *CT* Computed Tomography; *LUS* Lung Ultrasound; *PET* Positron Emission Tomography; *ARDS* Acute Respiratory Distress syndrome; *ECMO* Extra Corporeal Membrane Oxygenation; *FDG* fluoride-2-deoxy-D-glucose

Table 6.2 Original articles identified from the recent literature about the role of lung imaging in ARDS patients

Author	N° pt	Technique	Topic	Results
Yoshida [95]	18	CT	Recruitment	CT quantitative analysis demonstrated that APRV is more efficient than PSV in decreasing atelectasis in ARDS patients
Lu [96]	20	CT	Recruitment	CT quantitative analysis demonstrated that intratracheal surfactant replacement induces a significant lung reareation of poorly or nonaerated lung region
Caironi [97]	68	CT	Recruitment	CT quantitative analysis at three different airway pressures demonstrated that the application of high PEEP in patients with high lung recruitability significantly reduce the amount of opening and closing lung tissue
Mentzekopoulos [98]	15	CT	Recruitment	CT quantitative analysis demonstrated that the percentage of nonaerated lung tissue is lower in patients treated with HFO and tracheal gas insufflation vs HFO or CMV
Brhun [99]	9	CT	Recruitment	Dynamic CT during uninterrupted mechanical ventilation demonstrated that a high tidal volume is a major factor responsible for cycling recruitment and derecruitment in ARDS patients
Chiumello [19]	50	CT	Recruitment	The diagnostic accuracy of visual anatomical analysis compared with quantitative lung CT scan analysis in assessing lung recruitability is acceptable
Bouhemad [37]	40	LUS	Recruitment	Bedside LUS is equivalent to the PV curve method for quantitative assessment of PEEP-induced lung recruitment
Stefanidis [36]	10	LUS	Recruitment	LUS can detect the nonaerated lung area changes during a PEEP trial
Lowaghen [72]	16	EIT	Recruitment	By analysis of intratidal and EELV regional distribution before and after a PEEP trial, EIT could be useful to identify recruitability and optimal PEEP
Lowaghen [73]	16	EIT	Recruitment	Using EIT it is possible to assess potentially recruitable lung volume using a recruitment maneuver and alveolar PV curve
Dakin [100]	14	CT	Lung perfusion	Dynamic CT can quantify the proportion of perfusion applied to consolidated areas (shunt). This data correlated whit the severity of hypoxemia.

CT Computed Tomography; *LUS* Lung Ultrasound; *EIT* Electrical Impedance Tomography; *PEEP* Positive End-Expiratory Airway Pressure; *ARDS* Acute Respiratory Distress Syndrome; *EELV* End Expiratory Lung Volume; *PV* Pressure–Volume; *HFO* High Frequency Oscillation; *APRV* Airway Pressure Release Ventilation; *PSV* Pressure Support Ventilation; *CMV* Controlled Mechanical Ventilation

6.2 Chest X-Ray

6.2.1 Diagnostic Assessment

Radiography is based on electromagnetic radiation partially absorbed by the tissues they traverse. Medical images derived from the different degree of attenuation of X-rays by tissues with radiological density varying from bone to air.

Since the first definition of ARDS in 1967 the presence of bilateral infiltrates on chest X-ray has been one of the diagnostic criteria to define the syndrome. For almost 20 years, the evaluation of extension and distribution of lung opacities in ARDS patients has been limited to only chest X-rays.

Radiographic appearances in ARDS vary depending on stage disease, although a considerable overlap may exist.

In the first 24 h following insult, when there is little alveolar edema, the chest X-ray is generally normal, however when ARDS has followed a severe pneumonia the chest X-ray may be abnormal at the onset. When ARDS evolves, widespread ground-glass opacification becomes apparent and during the following 2 or 3 days chest X-ray shows bilateral homogenous air space opacifications due to exudation of inflammatory fluid into the interstitium and air spaces [4]. After this acute-exudative phase (1–7 days), radiographic appearances usually stabilize during the intermediate-proliferative phase and reticular opacities can develop. In the late phase chest X-ray can appear normal or show reticular opacities of an irreversible fibrosis [5].

The radiographic criterion is made more explicit in the Berlin definition specifying that it should include bilateral opacities, consistent with pulmonary edema that are not fully explained by effusions, lobar/lung collapse or nodules. In fact, when the radiological criteria of the previous ARDS definition were strictly applied (bilateral chest-X-ray infiltrates) the sensitivity was good but specificity was low.

6.2.2 Clinical Management and Limitations

Chest X-ray in clinical practice is a routineous tool:
- to support a diagnosis of ARDS in patients fulfilling clinical criteria
- to detect or confirm a suspected subclinical complication
- to monitor progression or regression of prior findings
- to assess the position of invasive devices.

Chest X-ray, however, cannot discriminate whether opacities are broncopneumonia foci or areas of atelectasis typical of ARDS appearance. In fact when alveolar consolidation is assessed using bedside frontal chest radiography, the correlation with the extent of lung injury is low [6].

Recently, Xirouchaki et al. [7] demonstrated that bedside chest X-ray had lower diagnostic accuracy for pleural effusions (69 %), pneumothorax (89 %) and alveolar consolidation (49 %) when compared to LUS and computed tomography. In this light radiographic information should be taken into consideration together with other clinical data, especially in critically ill patients. The overall clinical picture is also important to interpretate the radiographic changes caused by ARDS therapy. For example, when PEEP is increased, lung opacities may improve; while if PEEP is reduced, the opacities may appear to worsen, despite clinical signs are stable.

Several reports have shown that undergoing critically ill patients to daily chest X-ray is an unuseful practice and has been currently abandoned in most Intensive Care Units (ICUs) [8, 9]. In fact, chest X-ray in ICU is useful to readily identify the position of devices, to monitor the progression and regression of disease. However, it is clinically insufficient to detect and to differentiate clinical events such as pneumonia, pulmonary edema, atelectasis, and lung recruitability. Consequently, this could frequently result in erroneous evaluation of the distribution of gas and tissue within the injured lung parenchyma. In fact distinction between hydrostatic pulmonary edema and changes representative of ARDS *per se*, two patterns that can coexist in critically ill patients, is frequently impossible.

6.2.3 Technical Limitations

Chest X-ray is an ubiquitous and relatively inexpensive imaging technique. However, the intensive care environment and the poor contrast diagnostic resolution can affect the quality of the radiographic film.

Furthermore bedside chest X-ray is often of inferior quality due to the difficulty to control scattered radiations the inability of critically ill patient to cooperate and the anterior posterior view.

6.3   Computed Tomography

6.3.1   Diagnostic Assessment

Computer tomography (CT) scan measures the linear attenuation of radiation intensity upon passage through matter in a given volume of tissue or "voxel" (the CT unit of volume). The X-ray attenuation of tissue is expressed by CT number or Hunsfield unit (HU) [10].

Lung parenchyma, which includes different anatomic entities, is a mixture of air and tissue, its physical density is very close to the one of water in fact its range of density is included between 0 and -1000 HU. The strict correlation between CT density and the lung physical density allows quantification of lung compartments with different degrees of aeration [11]. Due to correlation between CT number and density for any given lung region of interest it is possible to compute for any given voxel of lung CT image the percentage of air and the percentage of lung tissue.

CT has been utilized to study the inhomogenous pattern of the lung ARDS lesion since 1980s. The application of CT provided the morphological and functional characterization of the injured lung and opened a new era in understanding pathophysiological aspects of ARDS.

CT scan abnormalities were not included in the previous ARDS definition, because of concerns regarding cost, safety, lack of widespread availability and poor feasibility of CT scan. Currently, in the diagnostic criteria of Berlin definition, bilateral opacities seen on CT scan, if available, could substitute chest X-ray opacities [3].

All the ARDS definitions have included the presence of bilateral pulmonary infiltrates by chest X-ray; unfortunately, as discussed above, chest radiographic infiltrates may be the morphological sign of many clinical conditions. CT may be a much better tool to detect ARDS "white lungs," characterized by patchy infiltrates interspersed with normally aerated regions.

The ARDS morphological description of the CT scan includes the recognition of normally aerated lung, poorly inflated areas, characterized by increased density, with steel recognizable vessels (ground-glass opacifications) and not inflated areas with increased density and no recognizable vessels (consolidation) [12]. CT scan revealed a typical sterno-vertebral gradient of increasing parenchymal density from non dependent (ventral in supine position) to dependent regions (dorsal in supine position). This gradient of aeration causes the lung to collapse under its own weight in dependent regions [13]. The dependent loss of aeration is the rationale of the "sponge model" developed by Gattinoni et al. [10] by CT scan studies.

The radiological course of ARDS presents in the acute phase of the disease normal regions, frequently located in non dependent areas, ground-glass opacification in the middle lung and consolidation in the most dependent lung. After the acute phase, CT appearances are variable. In the late stage, CT density of lungs decreases and the architecture undergoes extensive modifications: ground-glass opacities representing areas of fine fibrosis, diffuse parenchymal fibrosis, with the distortion of bronchovascular markings and pulmonary cysts of varying sizes and bullae, usually correlated with prolonged ventilation [14].

6.3.2 Clinical Management

Nowadays information from CT scan often influences clinical management of ARDS patients. In fact CT scanning is an effective tool to confirm the diagnosis, to identify complications, to direct ventilation and finally to determine prognosis.

First, CT scanning is a problem solving technique in patients with no clear radiographic evidence of ARDS. In fact thanks to its cross sectional images it provides better tissue discrimination eliminating the superimposition of structures.

Second, in ARDS patients who are deteriorating or not improving as expected, CT can detect occult complications that may not be apparent on the antero-posterior, supine chest X-ray [10, 14] for example pleural effusions, abscess, pneumothorax, sequelae of barotrauma and tube malposition.

Third, CT scan has a relevant role in the life saving treatment of ARDS, allowing a rationale setting of mechanical ventilation. In ARDS the proportion of lung which can be ventilated can be reduced to almost 20–30 % of a normal lung and in fact this aerated lung is not stiff but small, the "baby lung" [15].

The most relevant information to set ventilator strategy has been understood from the quantitative analysis of X-ray density of lung tissue. This method permits to quantify the lung parenchyma as normally aerated, hyperinflated, poorly inflated and not aerated.

By CT quantification of lung compartments, we can study the amount of the lung available for ventilation [16]. It is clear that CT scan quantitative analysis gives the opportunity to target tidal volume to the actual open portion of the lung by preventing the development of ventilator induced lung injury.

CT scan allows also a precise definition of lung recruitability, that should be a prerequisite for a rationale setting of positive end-expiratory pressure (PEEP). We can quantify lung recruitment by measuring how much nonaerated tissue becomes aerated under different ventilatory conditions [17], which implies the use of two CT scans at different airway pressure.

Lung recruitability affects the response to the levels of PEEP in ARDS patients: the higher is the lung recruitability, the higher will be the collapsed lung tissue that PEEP can maintain recruited. High levels of PEEP in patients with high lung recruitability can be beneficial by preventing intratidal opening and closing and the consequent regional excessive stress and strain. Differently, the application of high levels of PEEP in patients with low lung recruitability can lead to overdistention of regions that are already aerated without opening the collapsed tissue [16]. In this context, CT scan is a unique tool to differentiate between recruitment and hyperinflation.

Quantitative analysis on CT provides the possibility to quantify at each level of the lung the pressure (weight) transmitted to the dependent parenchyma along with the sterno-vertebral axis. This "superimposed pressure" depends on the height of tissue above the level and on the density and determines alveolar collapse in most dependent regions. The setting of PEEP should be tailored to counteract this superimposed pressure in order to keep the lung open and to obtain a homogenous distribution of ventilation [12].

Finally, CT characteristics detected in early ARDS can predict long-term prognosis: findings of early fibrosis are a strong independent predictor of mortality, as a contrary a pure consolidation pattern in early phase of disease is associated to better survival [18].

6.3.3 Technical and Clinical Limitations

The benefits of CT scan imaging in the clinical setting have to be weighed against the risks associated with transporting a patient from the ICU to the radiology department, the additional costs and the radiation exposure.

Quantitative CT scan analysis is not a routine tool despite of its role as the reference method for computing PEEP-induced lung recruitment because it needs a dedicated software and a manual delineation of the lung that takes up to 6 h.

However, recently Chiumello et al. [19] demonstrated how the simple visual analysis of lung CT image can be useful in ARDS patients. They showed the accuracy of visual anatomic analysis in detecting patients with high or low recruitability although the interobserver variability and the inability of estimating the hyperinflation are limitations of this simple analysis.

Although these limitations CT scan remains the gold standard technique for the management of ARDS patients. In addition dose reduction strategies, that have been already employed in other clinical settings, might represent an interesting research field.

6.4   Lung Ultrasound

6.4.1   Diagnostic Assessment

Transthoracic LUS is noninvasive, easily repeatable, and reproducible and does not require the transportation of patients outside the ICU. It allows the diagnosis of alveolar-interstitial syndrome, lung consolidation, pleural effusion, and pneumothorax more accurately than auscultation and bedside chest radiography in ICU patients [6, 20, 21]. Recently, evidence-based and expert consensus recommendations for LUS with focus on emergency and ICU settings were provided [22]. LUS appears as an attractive alternative method for bedside assessment of lung aeration during ARDS and effects of therapeutic aiming at improve it.

Ultrasound is an imaging modality which relies upon the use of sound waves which are transmitted into the body and then reflected back again from the structures being examined. The creation of ultrasound image is based on the physical properties of ultrasound pulse formation, the propagation of sound in matter, the interaction of sound with reflective interfaces [21]. Normally, lung parenchyma is not visible beyond the pleura. Thus, the ability to generate real images of lung parenchyma always indicates pathology [23].

6.4.1.1 Ultrasound Patterns of Aeration
A lines, B lines (comet tails), and consolidation are the elementary LUS signs [22]. To summarize, four patterns corresponding to various degree of lung aeration can be described [22].
(1) The presence of artifactual horizontal A lines beyond the pleural line characterizes normal pulmonary aeration.
(2) The presence of multiple and well separated vertical B lines corresponds to moderate decrease in lung aeration resulting from interstitial syndrome
(3) The presence of coalescent B lines less than 3 mm apart corresponds to more severe decrease in lung aeration resulting from partial filling of alveolar spaces by pulmonary edema or confluent bronchopneumonia [24]

(4) The presence of lung consolidation containing white points characterized by an inspiratory reinforcement—dynamic bronchograms—corresponds to complete loss of lung aeration with persisting aeration of distal bronchioles.

To be comprehensive, LUS examination should cover six regions by lung, delineated by anterior and posterior axillary lines: upper and lower parts of anterior, lateral and posterior chest wall [21]. In each region of interest, systematic examination of adjacent intercostal space allows assessment of ultrasound patterns of aeration.

6.4.1.2 Early Diagnosis of ARDS

LUS could be used for early diagnosis of ALI/ARDS. The heterogenous distribution of LUS patterns including well separated or coalescent B lines, spared areas and presence of posterior lung consolidations with dynamic bronchograms is typical of ARDS [16, 25] and allows its early distinction from acute cardiogenic pulmonary edema [26]. Moreover, B lines detected extravascular lung water accumulation early in the course of the oleic acid lung injury in pigs, before change in PaO_2/FiO_2 ratio [27].

6.4.2 Clinical Management

6.4.2.1 LUS to Quantify Lung Reareation

Several studies have showed that an improvement in lung aeration may be accurately detected by corresponding changes in LUS patterns. If the whole lung is examined, LUS using scores based on number of B lines can monitor extension of pulmonary edema, the amount of extravascular lung water, and the corresponding decrease in lung aeration. LUS was used to monitor lung aeration changes during community-acquired or ventilator-associated pneumonia [24, 28], experimental ARDS [27], high altitude pulmonary edema and cardiogenic pulmonary edema [29–31]. Therefore, ultrasound scores exclusively based on the number of B lines are linearly correlated to decrease in lung aeration.

6.4.2.2 LUS for Bedside Assessment of Alveolar Recruitment

The value of LUS for assessing PEEP-induced reareation of lung consolidation has been firstly reported in a case report [32] or using transesophageal echocardiography [33–35]. In the latter studies, based on the examination of the left lower lobe during transesophageal echocardiography, LUS pattern characteristic of lung consolidation was replaced by coalescent B lines after PEEP, indicating partial re aeration of the left lower lobe [34]. Using the same method in patients with ALI/ ARDS, this group monitored daily time-dependent lung reareation by measuring the decrease in the area of consolidated regions within left lower lobe [33]; and detected increase in lung aeration resulting from prone positioning [35]. Although these studies were limited to left dependent lung regions, significant correlations were found between decrease in consolidated areas and improvement of oxygenation [33–35]. Transthoracic LUS was also used to assess reduction of nonaerated areas in the dependent right lung regions during PEEP trials [36].

Indeed the whole lung should be examined in order to estimate the PEEP-induced lung recruitment [37]. In this study, 40 ARDS/ALI patients were prospectively enrolled and PEEP-induced lung recruitment was assessed using the pressure–volume curve method and compared to LUS. Study showed that PEEP-induced lung recruitment can be adequately estimated with LUS using a reareation score. Interestingly in this study, the essential of recruitment results from the reareation of poorly aerated lung regions. It means that coalescent B lines are transformed into separated B or A lines, and separated B lines are transformed into A lines. The reareation of nonaerated lung regions remains marginal: ultrasound consolidations transformed into coalescent or separated B lines, or A lines is a rarely observed event, occurring mostly in the lower parts of anterior, lateral, and posterior lung regions. Only one study assessed accuracy of LUS for measuring lung reareation using CT of the whole lung as gold standard [24]. In this study including patients with ventilator-associated pneumonia, lung reareation resulted from 7 days of antimicrobial therapy was measured by CT scan and compared to LUS score reareation score. A high correlation was found between LUS reareation score and CT reareation. However, studies using CT of the whole lung as gold standard are required to evaluate ability of LUS to reliably estimate PEEP-induced lung recruitment.

6.4.3   Technical and Clinical Limitations

Some of LUS limitations are patient-dependent. Obese patients are frequently difficult to examine using LUS because of the thickness of subcutaneous tissue around the rib cage. The presence of subcutaneous emphysema or large thoracic dressings precludes the propagation of ultrasound beams to the lung periphery and makes LUS examination difficult.

Performing and interpreting LUS requires a training period aimed at acquiring the necessary skills and knowledge.

Finally, LUS cannot detect PEEP-induced lung hyperinflation. CT data of the whole lung have shown that PEEP produces not only end–expiratory reareation of nonaerated parts of the lung (recruitment) but also simultaneous end-expiratory hyperinflation of aerated pulmonary areas in patients with focal ARDS [16, 25].

6.5   Positron Emission Tomography

6.5.1   Diagnostic Assessment

PET is a functional imaging technique based on the administration of a molecule labeled with a radioactive isotope, which decays with the emission of a positron.

PET scanners are often combined with CT scanners, a practice that increases PET usefulness allowing a precise anatomical localization of the physiologic process.

PET provides information about lung function imaging in asthma [38], cystic fibrosis [39], sarcoidosis [40], lung transplant rejection [41], and cancer [42].

Depending on which tracer is used (11-carbon, 13-nitrogen, 15-oxygen, 18-fluoride, which can be used as a substitute for hydrogen) we can study the in vivo imaging of several organic functions. Any molecule virtually can be labeled without altering its properties so that PET scan can be useful to investigate any physiological process characterized by the kinetics of a given molecule.

In recent decades, hundreds of tracers have developed and applied. PET with 18-fluoride-2-deoxy-D-glucose (18-FDG) has been used to monitor cellular metabolic activity, that is believed to reflect the presence and activity of inflammatory cellsin the setting of lung inflammation [43, 44].

The administration of 18-FDG permits the in vivo monitoring of cellular glycolytic activity, because this molecule is an analogue of glucose that is taken up by cells at the same rate of the glucose [43]. In this way, the accumulation of 18-FDG detected by PET is proportional to the intensity of the glycolytic metabolism of the cells. The uptake of 18-FDG is principally related to the activation of neutrophils, whose metabolism is tightly dependent on anaerobic glycolysis and requires an elevated uptake of glucose [45, 46].

There are different methods of quantifying 18-FDG uptake in the lung: the simplest are based on static indices such as the standardized uptake value, defined as the tissue concentration of tracer as measured by PET scanner divided by the activity injected divided by body weight [43]. There are also dynamic indices derived from the kinetics of 18-FDG typically over a period of 60–75 min starting from the endovenous injection of the radio-tracer [47]. These dynamic indices, based on lung specific compartmental models, account for the presence of the extracellular compartment and are influenced by the number of metabolically active cells and the diffusion of radio-tracer into edematous tissue.

During ARDS, PET imaging revealed that the lung metabolic activity is increased, supporting the evidence that no lung region is spared by the inflammatory process. Bellani et al. [48] showed that in a cohort of ten mechanically ventilated patients with ARDS the inflammation was not confined to the regions with density abnormalities on the CT scan (nonaerated, or poorly aerated regions), but also involved normally aerated regions. Previously, Rodrigues et al. [49] observed that in patients who did not developed ARDS, just only a moderate 18-FDG uptake is demonstrated in nonaerated and poorly aerated regions, while in subjects who subsequently developed ARDS, a diffuse 18-FDG uptake was identified 1–3 days before the clinical manifestation of disease.

Early diffuse 18-FDG uptake prior clinical signs of ARDS could signify an accelerated rate of glucose concentration by activated inflammatory cells or nonspecific leaking of the tracer in the alveolar spaces due to increased vascular permeability [49].

In the setting of pulmonary edema, Schuster et al. [50] studied pulmonary vascular permeability by 68-Ga transferrin PET to quantify the severity of pulmonary vascular leak but they could not distinguish between cardiogenic and non cardiogenic pulmonary edema.

The role of PET in the diagnostic assessment should be further investigated especially in the early phase before the development of the overt clinical and radiographic manifestations of ARDS syndrome.

6.5.2   Clinical Management

There is considerable interest in the application of FDG PET to ARDS because noninvasive and accurate quantification of pulmonary inflammation improves understanding of the disease mechanism and assessment of therapeutic strategies. In fact open lung biopsy, the current reference standard, is invasive and restricted to the sampled region, and bronchoalveolar lavage, the less invasive alternative, also is topographically limited [51].

FDG PET may provide molecular and cellular information in the progression of ARDS. This is particularly interesting in a phase of the syndrome for which very little information is available, the early events, prior to development of consensus clinical manifestations of ARDS [49].

FDG PET has been used also to measure the effect of anti-inflammatory interventions suggesting its applicability in the testing of novel drugs [52].

6.5.3   Technical and Clinical Limitations

The use of PET technique involves clinical and technical difficulties: clinical impossibility of patient's transport according to the attending physician, kidney injury, and logistic reason including length of the study procedure and the clinical care of critically ill patients throughout the permanence in the PET facility.

Results of animal studies suggest that the use of lung compartmental models may improve quantification of FDG signal in ARDS patient. Further research is needed to explore the biologic correlates of FDG uptake. Better understanding of such mechanisms is required before FDG PET can be used as a decision-making tool in the treatment of patients with ARDS [47].

6.6   Electrical Impedance Tomography

6.6.1   Diagnostic Assessment

Electrical Impedance Tomography (EIT) is a non-invasive, bedside monitoring technique that provides semi-continuous, real-time information about the regional distribution of the changes in electrical resistivity of the lung tissue due to variations in ventilation (or blood flow—perfusion) in relation to a reference state [53–55].

Information is gained by repeatedly injecting small alternating electric currents (usually 5 mA) at high frequency of 50–80 kHz through a system of skin electrodes (usually 16) applied circumferentially around the thorax in a single plane between the 4th and 6th intercostal space. While an adjacent pair of electrodes "injects" the current ("adjacent drive configuration"), all the remaining adjacent passive electrode pairs measure the differences in electric potential. A resistivity (impedance) image is reconstructed from this data by a mathematical algorithm using a two-dimensional model and a simplified shape to represent the thoracic cross-section.

The resulting images possessed a high temporal and functional resolution making it possible to monitor dynamic physiological phenomena (e.g., delay in regional inflation or recruitment) on a breath by breath basis.

It is important to realize that the EIT images are based on image reconstruction techniques that require at least one measurement on a well-defined reference state. All quantitative data are related to this reference and can only indirectly quantify (relative) changes in local lung impedance (but not absolute).

From this, it is obvious that only functionally active lung structures are displayed, whereas structures—whether normal or pathological (e.g., stable pneumothoraces or pleural effusions)—that do no change over time are functionally mute and cannot be represented as an image. In fact EIT has been evaluated in the detection of pneumothorax and pleural effusions. In an animal study, EIT has shown a sensitivity of 100 % in detecting small pneumothoraces [53, 56]. This could make EIT useful in situations where there is a high likelihood of pneumothorax such as during the insertion of central venous catheters or during a recruitment maneuver.

6.6.2 Clinical Management

In clinical practice EIT can provides a continuous, non-invasive bedside monitoring of functional changes [53, 57] such as regional distribution of ventilation, lung overdistention and collapse, lung recruitability, and lung perfusion [53, 58–63].

6.6.2.1 Assessment of Distribution of Ventilation

Mechanical ventilation can exert injurious effects on the lung tissue through the generation of excessive mechanical forces (lung strain and stress). These are amplified within the injured lung in proportion to the degree of mechanical homogeneity [58, 64, 65].

Studies in recent years have described various methods of analyzing EIT images to derive information about the regional lung mechanics and alveolar behavior [53, 58–63]. With EIT, it has been shown possible to derive regional lung pressure volume (pressure-impedance) curves that demonstrate how opening lung pressures vary significantly in the different lung regions, with the highest pressures found in the dorsal lung regions in accordance with gravitational forces previously described using CT scan.

Analysis of pressure-impedance curves has allowed the representation of the regional distribution of lower and upper inflection points in different parts of the lung [65–68] and more recently, the distribution and quantification of opening and closing alveolar pressures [69].

6.6.2.2 Assessment of Overdistention and Lung Collapse

Furthermore, the analysis of the pressure impedance curve during a decremental PEEP trial can allow the quantification of regional overdistention and collapse [70, 71] by calculating changes in regional compliance (change in impedance divided by the driving pressure). EIT images obtained during stepwise changes of mean airway pressure can be analyzed using a fuzzy logic-based algorithm to identify alveolar opening of collapsed regions, overdistention of previously functional areas, collapse of previously opened alveolar regions and the recovery of previously overdistended alveoli [66].

6.6.2.3 Lung Recruitability

Analysis of regional compliance may be useful in identifying changes in gas distribution and lung recruitability, thereby allowing the titration of PEEP based on the degree of recruitability [72]. EIT can also be used in local compliance estimation and assessment of the intratidal gas distribution—analyzed by dividing the regional tidal impedance signal into eight isovolume parts—of mechanically ventilated patients with ARDS [73]. Optimal PEEP may also be identified by the "global inhomogeneity index," calculated as the normalized sum of differences between the median value of regional impedance changes from the tidal image and the value of every pixel [74, 75]. The high temporal resolution of EIT allows the analysis of the dynamic behaviors of the lung during a slow inflation maneuver. By calculating the delay time needed for the regional impedance to reach a certain threshold value of the maximal local impedance change it has been possible to construct maps of regional delays in ventilation that correlate with the amount of recruited lung and lung inhomogeneity [76, 77].

The overall concept underlying these homogeneity indices is that a PEEP titration strategy aimed at a reduction in regional ventilation inhomogeneity improves lung protection with the assumption that this strategy leads to better ventilation distribution, thus minimizing tidal collapse and hyperinflation.

6.6.2.4 Lung Perfusion

An important objective in the setting of mechanical ventilation is to optimally match ventilation with lung perfusion in order to optimize gas exchange.

As the perfusion-related changes in thoracic impedance are about one order of magnitude smaller than the changes induced by ventilation, it is much more difficult to extract information on lung perfusion.

A promising method to quantify lung perfusion (pulsatile and nonpulsatile components) is by the injection of a contrast agent that possesses much higher electrical conductivity than lung tissues (e.g., hypertonic saline). The hypertonic saline causes a decrease in the impedance signal as it travels though the right heart and the lungs to the left heart during a 10 s breath-hold. Through mathematical calculations of first-pass kinetics of the impedance-time dilution curve, it has been possible to estimate pulmonary perfusion in a way that correlated with single-photon emission computed tomography (SPECT) [78]. However, this technique is limited because assessment of perfusion cannot happen continuously but only as a bolus and the frequency of the measurement is restricted by the potential side effects caused by the use of saline at high concentration (10–20 %).

6.6.3   Technical and Clinical Limitations

Several studies have validated EIT against other methods that measure global (e.g., nitrogen washout-washin) or regional lung volume (e.g., PET, SPECT, and CT) [58–63] and changes in end-expiratory lung impedance seem to correlate with changes in end-expiratory lung volume (EELV) [58, 67, 79, 80]. However, this linear correlation is crucially dependent on electrode position, the conformational changes of the chest wall and diaphragm and the proportion of tidal ventilation distributed in the lung areas falling inside and outside the EIT image during tidal breathing [81].

6.7   Magnetic Resonance Imaging

6.7.1   Diagnostic Assessment

Magnetic resonance is a functional lung imaging technique that can offer the possibility to investigate the pathophysiology of pulmonary disease.

Research in functional magnetic resonance imaging (MRI) of the lung provides an understanding of the relationship between regional pulmonary structure and function.

Although conventional lung MRI offers poor signal intensity due to low proton density and the short T2* relaxation time of lung tissue, hyperpolarized noble gas MRI (HP MRI), can give information about ventilation-perfusion heterogeneity, pulmonary end-capillary diffusion of oxygen and lung microstructure with high spatial resolution [82, 83].

Noble gases such as ^{3}-Helium (3-He) and ^{129}-Xenon (129-Xe) can act as contrast agents diffusing rapidly into the airspaces allowing the visualization and quantification of the ventilated airways and alveolar spaces [84].

3-He has negligible solubility in tissues and remains in the airways and alveolar spaces and it can be used to measure the properties of the pulmonary gas spaces.

In contrast, hyperpolarized ^{129}-Xenon follows the same pathway as oxygen, diffusing from the alveolar gas spaces to the septal tissue and blood, and therefore allows the calculation of gas exchange parameters including alveolar surface area, septal thickness and vascular transit time [85, 86].

Lung MRI has been employed to study lung microstructure, quantify ventilation and lung function, indirectly estimate alveolar oxygen concentration, and measure lung perfusion [68, 84, 87].

6.7.1.1 Lung Microstructure

Diffusion weighted MRI exploits the calculation of the atomic Brownian random motion to measure the diffusion coefficient of the hyperpolarized gas within the lung airspaces. In particular, the motion of the ^{3}He atoms is restricted by the walls of the alveoli and terminal bronchioles. The measured value of diffusion is termed the apparent diffusion coefficient (ADC), which quantifies regional restriction in airway gas diffusivity in proportion to the size of ventilated airspaces. As alveolar space increase (e.g., emphysema) the gas is less restricted and can diffuse over greater lengths resulting in greater signal loss and increase in the value of ADC [82–84]. Alternatively, when gaseous molecules experience diffusion restriction, such as alveolar wall boundaries, ADC is reduced. ADC measurements as a surrogate of changes in alveolar size have been used to assess the effects of atelectasis and alveolar recruitment manoeuvres on alveolar size [82].

6.7.1.2 Assessment of Lung Function

Visualization of ventilation is also possible using oxygen-enhanced MR imaging [82–84]. Molecular oxygen increases MRI signal by causing a concentration dependent shortening of the longitudinal relaxation (T1) of the protons of the capillary blood of the lung. Oxygen-based signal enhancement MRI provides an estimation of lung function by providing combined information about ventilation, perfusion and oxygen diffusion. Oxygen-enhanced MRI has the advantage of greater availability and safety compared to other contrast agents, but the disadvantage of relatively low signal enhancement, and the complex contrast mechanism which results from the combination of effects of ventilation, perfusion, and oxygen diffusion properties of the lung.

The interactions between molecular oxygen and hyperpolarized gas can also quantify alveolar oxygen pressure. The paramagnetic effect of oxygen causes a gradual loss of polarization in the HP gas, and the rate at which this depolarization occurs depends on the concentration of alveolar PO_2 in the gas mixture. It is therefore possible to derive alveolar partial pressure of oxygen (PAO_2) and rate of oxygen uptake into the bloodstream. As oxygen uptake is dependent on lung perfusion, it is possible to noninvasively construct high resolution maps of regional ventilation perfusion distribution.

Newer techniques [82, 83] based on nonenhanced dynamic MR acquisitions and other contrast agents such as aerosolized gadolinium or infusion of water-in-perfluorocarbon emulsions into the lung appear to be a promising although not fully tested in humans.

6.7.2 Technical and Clinical Limitations in the Clinical Management

Studies have used MRI in animal models and in healthy humans to study the structure and the function of lung parenchyma [82, 85]. However, this imaging modality is not currently applied in ARDS patients. Despite the reliability of the HP MRI, there are some significant drawbacks. It is time consuming and it can be technically difficult to perform because it requires multiple arterial blood analysis, the sampling of mixed expired gases and an independent measurement of cardiac output.

Certainly, the possibility to match information about regional capillary blood flow and alveolar ventilation is the great potential of this technique. This makes MRI an exciting new tool to resolve unanswered questions.

6.8 Conclusions

In addition to chest X-ray and CT which remain the most frequent used imaging techniques for daily patient's management, several other techniques such as LUS, positron emission tomography, electrical impedance tomography, and magnetic resonance have significantly contributed to advances in the physiological knowledge of the ARDS in the recent years.

References

1. Ranieri VM, Rubenfeld GD, Thompson BT, Ferguson ND, Caldwell E, Fan E, Camporota L, Slutsky AS (2012) Acute respiratory distress syndrome: the Berlin definition. JAMA 307:2526–2533
2. Camporota L, Ranieri VM (2012) What's new in the "Berlin" definition of acute respiratory distress syndrome? Minerva Anestesiol 78:1162–1166
3. Ferguson ND, Fan E, Camporota L, Antonelli M, Anzueto A, Beale R, Brochard L, Brower R, Esteban A, Gattinoni L, Rhodes A, Slutsky AS, Vincent JL, Rubenfeld GD, Thompson BT, Ranieri VM (2012) The Berlin definition of ARDS: an expanded rationale, justification, and supplementary material. Intensive Care Med 38:1573–1582
4. Aberle DR, Brown K (1990) Radiologic considerations in the adult respiratory distress syndrome. Clin Chest Med 11:737–754
5. Desai SR (2002) Acute respiratory distress syndrome: imaging of the injured lung. Clin Radiol 57:8–17
6. Lichtenstein D, Goldstein I, Mourgeon E, Cluzel P, Grenier P, Rouby JJ (2004) Comparative diagnostic performances of auscultation, chest radiography, and lung ultrasonography in acute respiratory distress syndrome. Anesthesiology 100:9–15
7. Xirouchaki N, Magkanas E, Vaporidi K, Kondili E, Plataki M, Patrianakos A, Akoumianaki E, Georgopoulos D (2011) Lung ultrasound in critically ill patients: comparison with bedside chest radiography. Intensive Care Med 37:1488–1493
8. Graat ME, Choi G, Wolthuis EK, Korevaar JC, Spronk PE, Stoker J, Vroom MB, Schultz MJ (2006) The clinical value of daily routine chest radiographs in a mixed medical-surgical intensive care unit is low. Crit Care 10:R11

9. Hendrikse KA, Gratama JW, Hove W, Rommes JH, Schultz MJ, Spronk PE (2007) Low value of routine chest radiographs in a mixed medical-surgical ICU. Chest 132:823–828
10. Gattinoni L, Caironi P, Pelosi P, Goodman LR (2001) What has computed tomography taught us about the acute respiratory distress syndrome? Am J Respir Crit Care Med 164:1701–1711
11. Caironi P, Carlesso E, Gattinoni L (2006) Radiological imaging in acute lung injury and acute respiratory distress syndrome. Semin Respir Crit Care Med 27:404–415
12. Pelosi P, D'Andrea L, Vitale G, Pesenti A, Gattinoni L (1994) Vertical gradient of regional lung inflation in adult respiratory distress syndrome. Am J Respir Crit Care Med 149:8–13
13. Gattinoni L, Mascheroni D, Torresin A, Marcolin R, Fumagalli R, Vesconi S, Rossi GP, Rossi F, Baglioni S, Bassi F (1986) Morphological response to positive end expiratory pressure in acute respiratory failure. Computerized tomography study. Intensive Care Med 12:137–142
14. Sheard S, Rao P, Devaraj A (2012) Imaging of acute respiratory distress syndrome. Respir Care 57:607–612
15. Gattinoni L, Pesenti A (2005) The concept of "baby lung". Intensive Care Med 31:776–784
16. Gattinoni L, Caironi P, Cressoni M, Chiumello D, Ranieri VM, Quintel M, Russo S, Patroniti N, Cornejo R, Bugedo G (2006) Lung recruitment in patients with the acute respiratory distress syndrome. N Engl J Med 354:1775–1786
17. Gattinoni L, Pesenti A, Avalli L, Rossi F, Bombino M (1987) Pressure-volume curve of total respiratory system in acute respiratory failure. Computed tomographic scan study. Am Rev Respir Dis 136:730–736
18. Chung JH, Kradin RL, Greene RE, Shepard JA, Digumarthy SR (2011) CT predictors of mortality in pathology confirmed ARDS. Eur Radiol 21:730–737
19. Chiumello D, Marino A, Brioni M, Menga F, Cigada I, Lazzerini M, Andrisani MC, Biondetti P, Cesana B, Gattinoni L (2012) Visual anatomical lung CT scan assessment of lung recruitability. Intensive Care Med 39(1):66–73
20. Agricola E, Arbelot C, Blaivas M, Bouhemad B, Copetti R, Dean A, Dulchavsky S, Elbarbary M, Gargani L, Hoppmann R, Kirkpatrick AW, Lichtenstein D, Liteplo A, Mathis G, Melniker L, Neri L, Noble VE, Petrovic T, Reissig A, Rouby JJ, Seibel A, Soldati G, Storti E, Tsung JW, Via G, Volpicelli G (2011) Ultrasound performs better than radiographs. Thorax 66:828–829
21. Bouhemad B, Zhang M, Lu Q, Rouby JJ (2007) Clinical review: Bedside lung ultrasound in critical care practice. Crit Care 11:205
22. Volpicelli G, Elbarbary M, Blaivas M, Lichtenstein DA, Mathis G, Kirkpatrick AW, Melniker L, Gargani L, Noble VE, Via G, Dean A, Tsung JW, Soldati G, Copetti R, Bouhemad B, Reissig A, Agricola E, Rouby JJ, Arbelot C, Liteplo A, Sargsyan A, Silva F, Hoppmann R, Breitkreutz R, Seibel A, Neri L, Storti E, Petrovic T (2012) International evidence-based recommendations for point-of-care lung ultrasound. Intensive Care Med 38:577–591
23. Via G, Storti E, Gulati G, Neri L, Mojoli F, Braschi A (2012) Lung ultrasound in the ICU: from diagnostic instrument to respiratory monitoring tool. Minerva Anestesiol 78:1282–1296
24. Bouhemad B, Liu ZH, Arbelot C, Zhang M, Ferarri F, Le Guen M, Girard M, Lu Q, Rouby JJ (2010) Ultrasound assessment of antibiotic-induced pulmonary reaeration in ventilator-associated pneumonia. Crit Care Med 38:84–92
25. Vieira SR, Puybasset L, Richecoeur J, Lu Q, Cluzel P, Gusman PB, Coriat P, Rouby JJ (1998) A lung computed tomographic assessment of positive end-expiratory pressure-induced lung overdistension. Am J Respir Crit Care Med 158:1571–1577
26. Copetti R, Soldati G, Copetti P (2008) Chest sonography: a useful tool to differentiate acute cardiogenic pulmonary edema from acute respiratory distress syndrome. Cardiovasc Ultrasound 6:16

27. Gargani L, Lionetti V, Di Cristofano C, Bevilacqua G, Recchia FA, Picano E (2007) Early detection of acute lung injury uncoupled to hypoxemia in pigs using ultrasound lung comets. Crit Care Med 35:2769–2774
28. Reissig A, Kroegel C (2007) Sonographic diagnosis and follow-up of pneumonia: a prospective study. Respiration 74:537–547
29. Agricola E, Bove T, Oppizzi M, Marino G, Zangrillo A, Margonato A, Picano E (2005) "Ultrasound comet-tail images": a marker of pulmonary edema: a comparative study with wedge pressure and extravascular lung water. Chest 127:1690–1695
30. Agricola E, Picano E, Oppizzi M, Pisani M, Meris A, Fragasso G, Margonato A (2006) Assessment of stress-induced pulmonary interstitial edema by chest ultrasound during exercise echocardiography and its correlation with left ventricular function. J Am Soc Echocardiogr 19:457–463
31. Volpicelli G, Caramello V, Cardinale L, Mussa A, Bar F, Frascisco MF (2008) Bedside ultrasound of the lung for the monitoring of acute decompensated heart failure. Am J Emerg Med 26:585–591
32. Gardelli G, Feletti F, Gamberini E, Bonarelli S, Nanni A, Mughetti M (2009) Using sonography to assess lung recruitment in patients with acute respiratory distress syndrome. Emerg Radiol 16:219–221
33. Tsubo T, Yatsu Y, Suzuki A, Iwakawa T, Okawa H, Ishihara H, Matsuki A (2001) Daily changes of the area of density in the dependent lung region—evaluation using transesophageal echocardiography. Intensive Care Med 27:1881–1886
34. Tsubo T, Sakai I, Suzuki A, Okawa H, Ishihara H, Matsuki A (2001) Density detection in dependent left lung region using transesophageal echocardiography. Anesthesiology 94:793–798
35. Tsubo T, Yatsu Y, Tanabe T, Okawa H, Ishihara H, Matsuki A (2004) Evaluation of density area in dorsal lung region during prone position using transesophageal echocardiography. Crit Care Med 32:83–87
36. Stefanidis K, Dimopoulos S, Tripodaki ES, Vitzilaios K, Politis P, Piperopoulos P, Nanas S (2011) Lung sonography and recruitment in patients with early acute respiratory distress syndrome: a pilot study. Crit Care 15:R185
37. Bouhemad B, Brisson H, Le Guen M, Arbelot C, Lu Q, Rouby JJ (2011) Bedside ultrasound assessment of positive end-expiratory pressure-induced lung recruitment. Am J Respir Crit Care Med 183:341–347
38. Taylor IK, Hill AA, Hayes M, Rhodes CG, O'Shaughnessy KM, O'Connor BJ, Jones HA, Hughes JM, Jones T, Pride NB, Fuller RW (1996) Imaging allergen-invoked airway inflammation in atopic asthma with [18F]-fluorodeoxyglucose and positron emission tomography. Lancet 347:937–940
39. Chen DL, Ferkol TW, Mintun MA, Pittman JE, Rosenbluth DB, Schuster DP (2006) Quantifying pulmonary inflammation in cystic fibrosis with positron emission tomography. Am J Respir Crit Care Med 173:1363–1369
40. Brudin LH, Valind SO, Rhodes CG, Pantin CF, Sweatman M, Jones T, Hughes JM (1994) Fluorine-18 deoxyglucose uptake in sarcoidosis measured with positron emission tomography. Eur J Nucl Med 21:297–305
41. Jones HA, Donovan T, Goddard MJ, McNeil K, Atkinson C, Clark JC, White JF, Chilvers ER (2004) Use of 18FDG-pet to discriminate between infection and rejection in lung transplant recipients. Transplantation 77:1462–1464
42. Fischer BM, Lassen U, Hojgaard L (2011) PET-CT in preoperative staging of lung cancer. N Engl J Med 364:980–981
43. Bellani G, Amigoni M, Pesenti A (2011) Positron emission tomography in ARDS: a new look at an old syndrome. Minerva Anestesiol 77:439–447
44. Musch G (2011) Positron emission tomography: a tool for better understanding of ventilator-induced and acute lung injury. Curr Opin Crit Care 17:7–12

45. Jones HA, Schofield JB, Krausz T, Boobis AR, Haslett C (1998) Pulmonary fibrosis correlates with duration of tissue neutrophil activation. Am J Respir Crit Care Med 158:620–628

46. Jones HA, Clark RJ, Rhodes CG, Schofield JB, Krausz T, Haslett C (1994) In vivo measurement of neutrophil activity in experimental lung inflammation. Am J Respir Crit Care Med 149:1635–1639

47. de Prost N, Tucci MR, Melo MF (2010) Assessment of lung inflammation with 18F-FDG PET during acute lung injury. AJR Am J Roentgenol 195:292–300

48. Bellani G, Messa C, Guerra L, Spagnolli E, Foti G, Patroniti N, Fumagalli R, Musch G, Fazio F, Pesenti A (2009) Lungs of patients with acute respiratory distress syndrome show diffuse inflammation in normally aerated regions: a [18F]-fluoro-2-deoxy-D-glucose PET/CT study. Crit Care Med 37:2216–2222

49. Rodrigues RS, Miller PR, Bozza FA, Marchiori E, Zimmerman GA, Hoffman JM, Morton KA (2008) FDG-PET in patients at risk for acute respiratory distress syndrome: a preliminary report. Intensive Care Med 34:2273–2278

50. Schuster DP, Stark T, Stephenson J, Royal H (2002) Detecting lung injury in patients with pulmonary edema. Intensive Care Med 28:1246–1253

51. Rhodes CG, Hughes JM (1995) Pulmonary studies using positron emission tomography. Eur Respir J 8:1001–1017

52. Chen DL, Bedient TJ, Kozlowski J, Rosenbluth DB, Isakow W, Ferkol TW, Thomas B, Mintun MA, Schuster DP, Walter MJ (2009) [18F] fluorodeoxyglucose positron emission tomography for lung antiinflammatory response evaluation. Am J Respir Crit Care Med 180:533–539

53. Bayford RH (2006) Bioimpedance tomography (electrical impedance tomography). Annu Rev Biomed Eng 8:63–91

54. Bodenstein M, David M, Markstaller K (2009) Principles of electrical impedance tomography and its clinical application. Crit Care Med 37:713–724

55. Brown BH (2003) Electrical impedance tomography (EIT): a review. J Med Eng Technol 27:97–108

56. Costa EL, Chaves CN, Gomes S, Beraldo MA, Volpe MS, Tucci MR, Schettino IA, Bohm SH, Carvalho CR, Tanaka H, Lima RG, Amato MB (2008) Real-time detection of pneumothorax using electrical impedance tomography. Crit Care Med 36:1230–1238

57. Constantin J (2012) Lung imaging in patients with acute respiratory distress syndrome: from an understanding of pathophysiology to bedside monitoring. Minerva Anest. 79(2):176–184

58. Costa EL, Lima RG, Amato MB (2009) Electrical impedance tomography. Curr Opin Crit Care 15:18–24

59. Leonhardt S, Lachmann B (2012) Electrical impedance tomography: the holy grail of ventilation and perfusion monitoring? Intensive Care Med 38:1917–1929

60. Luecke T, Corradi F, Pelosi P (2012) Lung imaging for titration of mechanical ventilation. Curr Opin Anaesthesiol 25:131–140

61. Lundin S, Stenqvist O (2012) Electrical impedance tomography: potentials and pitfalls. Curr Opin Crit Care 18:35–41

62. Moerer O, Hahn G, Quintel M (2011) Lung impedance measurements to monitor alveolar ventilation. Curr Opin Crit Care 17:260–267

63. Muders T, Luepschen H, Putensen C (2010) Impedance tomography as a new monitoring technique. Curr Opin Crit Care 16:269–275

64. Gattinoni L, Carlesso E, Caironi P (2012) Stress and strain within the lung. Curr Opin Crit Care 18:42–47

65. Mead J, Takishima T, Leith D (1970) Stress distribution in lungs: a model of pulmonary elasticity. J Appl Physiol 28:596–608

66. Grychtol B, Wolf GK, Adler A, Arnold JH (2010) Towards lung EIT image segmentation: automatic classification of lung tissue state from analysis of EIT monitored recruitment manoeuvres. Physiol Meas 31:S31–S43

67. Hinz J, Hahn G, Neumann P, Sydow M, Mohrenweiser P, Hellige G, Burchardi H (2003) End-expiratory lung impedance change enables bedside monitoring of end-expiratory lung volume change. Intensive Care Med 29:37–43
68. van der Beek FB, Boermans PP, Verbist BM, Briaire JJ, Frijns JH (2005) Clinical evaluation of the Clarion CII HiFocus 1 with and without positioner. Ear Hear 26:577–592
69. Pulletz S, Adler A, Kott M, Elke G, Gawelczyk B, Schadler D, Zick G, Weiler N, Frerichs I (2012) Regional lung opening and closing pressures in patients with acute lung injury. J Crit Care 27:323–328
70. Costa EL, Borges JB, Melo A, Suarez-Sipmann F, Toufen C Jr (2009) Bohm SH, Amato MB: Bedside estimation of recruitable alveolar collapse and hyperdistension by electrical impedance tomography. Intensive Care Med 35:1132–1137
71. Gomez-Laberge C, Arnold JH, Wolf GK (2012) A unified approach for EIT imaging of regional overdistension and atelectasis in acute lung injury. IEEE Trans Med Imaging 31:834–842
72. Lowhagen K, Lundin S, Stenqvist O (2010) Regional intratidal gas distribution in acute lung injury and acute respiratory distress syndrome–assessed by electric impedance tomography. Minerva Anestesiol 76:1024–1035
73. Lowhagen K, Lindgren S, Odenstedt H, Stenqvist O, Lundin S (2011) A new non-radiological method to assess potential lung recruitability: a pilot study in ALI patients. Acta Anaesthesiol Scand 55:165–174
74. Zhao Z, Moller K, Steinmann D, Frerichs I, Guttmann J (2009) Evaluation of an electrical impedance tomography-based global inhomogeneity index for pulmonary ventilation distribution. Intensive Care Med 35:1900–1906
75. Zhao Z, Steinmann D, Frerichs I, Guttmann J, Moller K (2010) PEEP titration guided by ventilation homogeneity: a feasibility study using electrical impedance tomography. Crit Care 14:R8
76. Muders T, Luepschen H, Zinserling J, Greschus S, Fimmers R, Guenther U, Buchwald M, Grigutsch D, Leonhardt S, Putensen C, Wrigge H (2012) Tidal recruitment assessed by electrical impedance tomography and computed tomography in a porcine model of lung injury*. Crit Care Med 40:903–911
77. Wrigge H, Zinserling J, Muders T, Varelmann D, Gunther U, von der GC, Magnusson A, Hedenstierna G, Putensen C (2008) Electrical impedance tomography compared with thoracic computed tomography during a slow inflation maneuver in experimental models of lung injury. Crit Care Med 36:903–909
78. Borges JB, Suarez-Sipmann F, Bohm SH, Tusman G, Melo A, Maripuu E, Sandstrom M, Park M, Costa EL, Hedenstierna G, Amato M (2012) Regional lung perfusion estimated by electrical impedance tomography in a piglet model of lung collapse. J Appl Physiol 112:225–236
79. Adler A, Amyot R, Guardo R, Bates JH, Berthiaume Y (1997) Monitoring changes in lung air and liquid volumes with electrical impedance tomography. J Appl Physiol 83:1762–1767
80. Marquis F, Coulombe N, Costa R, Gagnon H, Guardo R, Skrobik Y (2006) Electrical impedance tomography's correlation to lung volume is not influenced by anthropometric parameters. J Clin Monit Comput 20:201–207
81. Bikker IG, Preis C, Egal M, Bakker J, Gommers D (2011) Electrical impedance tomography measured at two thoracic levels can visualize the ventilation distribution changes at the bedside during a decremental positive end-expiratory lung pressure trial. Crit Care 15:R193
82. Cereda M, Emami K, Kadlecek S, Xin Y, Mongkolwisetwara P, Profka H, Barulic A, Pickup S, Mansson S, Wollmer P, Ishii M, Deutschman CS, Rizi RR (2011) Quantitative imaging of alveolar recruitment with hyperpolarized gas MRI during mechanical ventilation. J Appl Physiol 110:499–511
83. Kauczor HU (2009) MRI of the lung. Springer, Berlin

84. Emami K, Stephen M, Kadlecek S, Cadman RV, Ishii M, Rizi RR (2009) Quantitative assessment of lung using hyperpolarized magnetic resonance imaging. Proc Am Thorac Soc 6:431–438
85. Hopkins SR (2004) Functional magnetic resonance imaging of the lung: a physiological perspective. J Thorac Imaging 19:228–234
86. Matsuoka S, Hunsaker AR, Gill RR, Jacobson FL, Ohno Y, Patz S, Hatabu H (2008) Functional MR imaging of the lung. Magn Reson Imaging Clin N Am 16:275–289
87. Fain SB, Korosec FR, Holmes JH, O'Halloran R, Sorkness RL, Grist TM (2007) Functional lung imaging using hyperpolarized gas MRI. J Magn Reson Imaging 25:910–923
88. Pinilla I, de Gracia MM, Quintana-Diaz M, Figueira JC (2011) Radiological prognostic factors in patients with pandemic H1N1 (pH1N1) infection requiring hospital admission. Emerg Radiol 18:313–319
89. Endo S, Shibata S, Sato N, Hashiba E, Tajimi K, Saito K, Kawamae K, Nakane M, Murakawa M (2010) A prospective cohort study of ALI/ARDS in the Tohoku district of Japan (second report). J Anesth 24:351–358
90. Wang S, Ruan Z, Zhang J, Jin W (2011) The value of pulmonary contusion volume measurement with three-dimensional computed tomography in predicting acute respiratory distress syndrome development. Ann Thorac Surg 92:1977–1983
91. Strumwasser A, Chu E, Yeung L, Miraflor E, Sadjadi J, Victorino GP (2011) A novel CT volume index score correlates with outcomes in polytrauma patients with pulmonary contusion. J Surg Res 170:280–285
92. Cianchi G, Bonizzoli M, Pasquini A, Bonacchi M, Zagli G, Ciapetti M, Sani G, Batacchi S, Biondi S, Bernardo P, Lazzeri C, Giovannini V, Azzi A, Abbate R, Gensini G, Peris A (2011) Ventilatory and ECMO treatment of H1N1-induced severe respiratory failure: results of an Italian referral ECMO center. BMC Pulm Med 11:2
93. Masclans JR, Roca O, Munoz X, Pallisa E, Torres F, Rello J, Morell F (2011) Quality of life, pulmonary function, and tomographic scan abnormalities after ARDS. Chest 139:1340–1346
94. Grieser C, Goldmann A, Steffen IG, Kastrup M, Fernandez CM, Engert U, Deja M, Lojewski C, Denecke T (2012) Computed tomography findings from patients with ARDS due to Influenza A (H1N1) virus-associated pneumonia. Eur J Radiol 81:389–394
95. Yoshida T, Rinka H, Kaji A, Yoshimoto A, Arimoto H, Miyaichi T, Kan M (2009) The impact of spontaneous ventilation on distribution of lung aeration in patients with acute respiratory distress syndrome: airway pressure release ventilation versus pressure support ventilation. Anesth Analg 109:1892–1900
96. Lu Q, Zhang M, Girardi C, Bouhemad B, Kesecioglu J, Rouby JJ (2010) Computed tomography assessment of exogenous surfactant-induced lung reaeration in patients with acute lung injury. Crit Care 14:135
97. Caironi P, Cressoni M, Chiumello D, Ranieri M, Quintel M, Russo SG, Cornejo R, Bugedo G, Carlesso E, Russo R, Caspani L, Gattinoni L (2010) Lung opening and closing during ventilation of acute respiratory distress syndrome. Am J Respir Crit Care Med 181:578–586
98. Mentzelopoulos SD, Theodoridou M, Malachias S, Sourlas S, Exafchos DN, Chondros D, Roussos C, Zakynthinos SG (2011) Scanographic comparison of high frequency oscillation with versus without tracheal gas insufflation in acute respiratory distress syndrome. Intensive Care Med 37(6):990–999
99. Beuhn A, Baugedo D, Riquelme F, Varas J, Retamal J, Besa C, Carbera C, Bugedo G (2011) Tidal volume is a major determinant of cyclic recruitment-derecruitment in acute respiratory distress syndrome. Minerva Anestesiol 77(4):418–426
100. Dakin J, Jones AT, Hansell DM, Hoffman EA, Evans TW (2011) Changes in lung composition and regional perfusion and tissue distribution in patients with ARDS. Respirology 16:1265–1272

Chest X-Ray in ICU: An Examination in Which There is Too Much Confidence. Possible Alternatives

Marco Vittorio Resta and Dario Niro

The resort to golden standard treatment is not always feasible in a critical patient, due to logistic organizing issues or the weakness of patient himself. In according to technological improvement, a progressive increase of bedside service quality has been observed.

In addition to hemodynamic monitoring this technological advance involved imaging too, meant as the opportunity to achieve excellent quality images in a short time.

Awaiting for the portable CT scan to come true (it is now limited to head and neck, therefore it is reserved to specific cases as the neurological ones), and awaiting for MRI units, increasingly accessible and most of all indispensable for their very high resolution, to become a safe place to monitor critical patients as you freely use to do with CT, awaiting for these epochal changes, we are attending to the advance of a readily applicable bedside method: ultrasonography.

Along this technological escalation, less-refined methods take up smaller and smaller room, being replaced or sustained by other approaches. Chest Radiology (CR) is among them.

Up to about 10 years ago, CR was the cornerstone of critical cardiopulmonary patient assessment, and in the last few years it had to give way in once exclusive fields to other more simple methods, sometimes cheaper and even better from a qualitative viewpoint.

M. V. Resta (✉) · D. Niro
Rianimazione e Terapia Intensiva, Piazza Malan 2,
20097, San Donato Milanese, MI, Italy
e-mail: Resta.marcomd@me.com

D. Niro
e-mail: darioniro@libero.it

B. Allaria (ed.), *Practical Issues in Anesthesia and Intensive Care 2013*,
DOI: 10.1007/978-88-470-5529-2_7, © Springer-Verlag Italia 2014

The aim of this CR application overview in critical units wishes areas overlapping other methodologies to be identified, highlighting added values and limits, and finding out a possible unique role of this imaging technique that will make it still necessary in critical units.

7.1 History

It was 1816 when René-Théophile-Hyacinthe Laennec invented the stethoscope, drawing his inspiration from a rolled notebook laid on the thorax of a patient, as an amplifier to perceive heartbeats (Fig. 7.1).

Since then, chest objective examination has achieved a main role in patient approach.

Simplicity and cheapness of examination made it fundamental to study patient who had to be submitted to lung and heart evaluation.

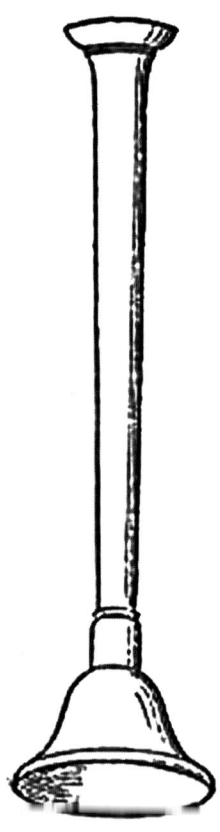

Fig. 7.1 Stethoscope representation

The critical patient did not escape this practice either, and auscultation became the first step in a likely acute condition setting, involving above all ventilatory and cardiac aspects.

However, in some particular occurrences even the more skillful medical ear began to be in difficulties to identify cardiopulmonary pathological patterns, also with the aid of respiratory-suppliers introduction that arouse pulmonary sounds not provided by traditional semeiotics. During this diagnostic improvement process, application of a further fundamental stage of medicine history came to important aid.

On November 8th 1895, Wilhelm Conrad Röntgen (Remscheid, March 27th 1845—Munich, February 10th 1923), a German physicist, discovered the electromagnetic radiation better known as X-rays.

Since then, the more and more advanced technology combined with the possibility of digitizing images has been enabling to put at disposal portable chest radiology equipments (CRX) for ages, with a image quality that is absolutely comparable to traditional instruments usually founded in radio-diagnostic services of most hospitals.

So we attended the bedside resort to cardio-pulmonary semeiotics and chest radiography for decades, to identify possible cardiothoracic issues in critical subjects taken into intensive care units. Only as the result of CT spread an imaging completion of these patients has been observed: they maintain such a level of unsteadiness that their transfer is often limited to very hard diagnostic challenge cases.

We had, therefore, to wait nearly till the end of the 1990s for ultrasound use in chest and above all lung (so far considered impenetrable due to the high air content) examination to start making its way in intensive care units.

The introduction of ultrasonograhy (US) for medical purposes dates back about to the 1970s. Then, radiologists started its employment in the diagnostic field. Only later, US became a shared wealth among radiologists, cardiologists, surgeons and finally anesthesiologists, thus opening new settings for the critical patient assessment.

Chest ultrasonography led to some changes in the approach to the patient, mainly affected by cardiopulmonary pathology, first in an emerging context and then in the even selected intensive care daily practice.

In the new setting, chest ultrasonography is surrounded by abdominal ultrasonography (most of all in vascular, traumatic or infective acute diseases) and the important role of both trans-thoracic and trans-esophageal echocardiography.

In the present context, we cannot propose to see how the fundamental supply provided by echocardiography to intensive care units stands, both as regards to the understanding of more and more complex hemodynamic patterns, and to the management of more and more critical ill patients with multiple co-pathologies.

It would be worth dealing separately with abdominal ultrasonography too, due to the complexity of clinical cases and the overlapping to other surgical spheres.

Therefore, chest ultrasonography outlook assessment continues to be interesting, particularly in the light of comparisons with CRX, that just arose an attractive debate and critical reviews in lots of the available literature.

7.2   CRX and Chest US Comparison in Critical Cases

7.2.1   CRX Thoracic Imaging

CXR use to assess patients in critical environment has acquired a key value along years. This primary role has been so highly emphasized that chest radiology represents the first step of intensive care therapy imaging in the anesthesiologist's common opinion, so it is considered a daily routine monitoring in some specialist intensive care units.

The great amount of guiding lines published along years about the correct execution and reading of radiograms (particularly the bedside ones performed by portable equipment) shows their importance and wide utilization.

For instance, the European guiding lines for radiographic imaging quality date to 1996 and show the main points that have to be searched for to perform a correct chest radiographic image and hence to read it adequately (Table 7.1) [1].

Suitable criteria about radiological practice by the American College of Radiology still date to the middle 1990s (last upgrade in 2011), taking into consideration the correctness of chest radiology resort depending on different pathologies.

The routinary resort to portable CRX or its employment to follow up clinical condition is very discouraged. On the contrary, bedside chest radiology on precise clinical query is encouraged (Table 7.2) [2].

Actually a committee of experts, on the basis of the last 20 years, literature review about CRX in cardiopulmonary patients, came to the conclusion that the resort to bedside CRX showed indeed a pathological or unexpected findings rate varying from about 40 to 60 %. However, limiting the analysis to routinary CRX, only percentages from 13 to 6 % showed unexpected findings (4.5 % in cardiothoracic surgery) and these reports brought about a change in the therapeutic approach only in about 2 % of patients.

Table 7.1 Image features modified from "European guidelines on correct quality of radiographic images" [1]

Performed at full inspiration and with suspended respiration
Number of ribs checked in respect to diaphragm: 6 before and 10 behind
Chest symmetry assessed by central position of spinous processes in respect to medial ends of the clavicles
Medial border of the scapulae outside the lung fields
Cage rib fully represented above the diaphragm
Vascular pattern visualization in the whole lung, particularly the peripheral vessels
Visualization of tracheal, cardiac, aortic, diaphragmatic, and fontal-costal sinus borders
Visualization of the retrocardiac lung and the mediastinum
Visualization of spinal processes behind the heart shadow

Table 7.2 Modified from "ACR appropriateness criteria" [2]

Disease and clinical condition	Suitable	Unsuitable
ICU routinely monitoring Unstable patient	Admittance specific query	Daily routine
Respiratory failure patient under mechanical ventilation	Specific query	Daily routine Only some subgroups could benefit by it
Intubated patient	At the time of tube positioning Specific query	Daily routine Monitoring
CVC positioning	At the time of tube positioning Specific query	Daily routine Monitoring
Cardiopulmonary disease Swan-Ganz positioning	At the time of tube positioning Specific query	Daily routine Monitoring
NGT positioning for enteral nutrition (EN)	At the time of tube positioning if the clinical examination is uncertain Specific query	Daily routine Monitoring
NGT positioning without EN	At the time of positioning Specific query	Daily routine Monitoring
Thoracic drainage	At the time of positioning Specific query	Daily routine Monitoring

Comparing CRX required on the basis of diagnostic suspicion or focused clinical problems results in quite different rates.

In this population of patients, such a finding to change the therapeutic approach is noticed in about 25 % of subjects.

No study showed care quality reduction or recovery times prolongation when a conservative behavior was kept in comparison to CRX execution.

The final advice is therefore not to consider CRX a routinary practice in acute cardiopulmonary patients.

CRX should always have to be required on the basis of clinical suspect in these subjects.

7.2.2 Chest Imaging in Pleural-Pulmonary Ultrasonography

Ultrasonography fits in with most features you look for in an ideal methodology: reliable, cheap (after the starting investment), safe and repeatable.

The more and more advanced technology enables now to rely at fair costs on equipment often light and easy to carry, resistant and supplied with integrated camera, very useful to provide the examination with related images (moreover a fundamental document in forensic medicine point of view).

Leaving out the explanation about physics of ultrasounds to a more specific context and aiming to simplify this technique in order to cause an adequate level of interest, here we wish just to give an overview about required equipment, pointing out its relative and sometimes apparent user-friendly character and describing some key principles about ultrasound examination that are more useful to arouse curiosity about the methodology's benefits than to provide the reader with information to teach it.

To sight the objective of ultrasonography learning satisfactorily, above all at a pleural-pulmonary level, the authors refer to many specific and high value courses now widely available and to main congresses by anesthesiology and reanimation scientific societies or to monothematic courses devoted to critical case ultrasonography.

7.2.3 Materials

First of all, you need an ultrasound system and one to three different probes to perform chest ultrasonography. Selecting the equipment, initially you can look for one left by another specialist (cardiologic units usually upgrade their more obsolete devices frequently), as long as provided with at least one cardiologic sectorial probe, even better a convex type one (see description below). If you may ask for new equipment, on the same quality image, portability is certainly an important added value since it facilitates bedside examination and maybe it can enable the equipment's move to critical patients in wards or emergency units. With regard to probes, their main features have to be high definition and low penetration for pleural studies (more superficial tissue), while high penetration to the detriment of lower definition for deeper structures. These features usually match high frequency line-probe (e.g. 8 MHz linear) for pleura and medium (e.g., 5 MHz convex) or low (e.g., 3.5 MHZ sectorial) frequency for other tissues (Fig. 7.2). Generally, a 5–7 MHz range is hoped for pleural-pulmonary US probes.

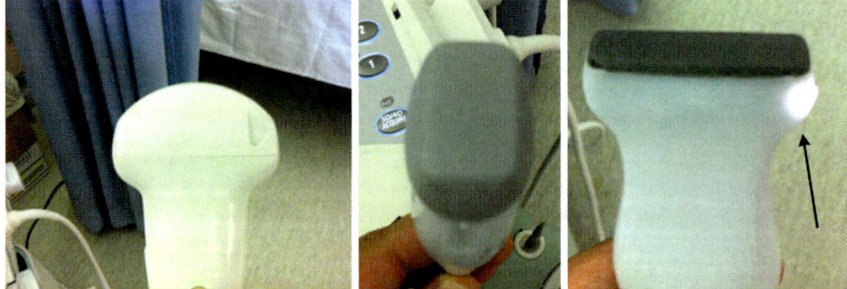

Fig. 7.2 US probes. Different kind of ultrasound probes. *Left to right*: Convex—Sectorial or cardio type—Linear or vessel probe. On the right side of the vessel probe, a light can be seen (*arrow*), representing the marker that is essential for probe orientation (toward patient's head if longitudinally aligned and toward the back if sagittally aligned)

Chest ultrasonography is able to study both static and dynamic conditions such as effusions, consolidation (pneumonia or atelectasis), pneumothorax, interstitial-alveolar syndrome, and diaphragmatic pathologies by making the most of probes with different features.

If all three probes are at one's disposal, echography becomes a key factor even to abdomen and heart examination, completing the valuable contribution of this technique in intensive and critical care units.

Another ultrasounds added value is their assistance in central and peripheral vein access positioning, in critical case or post-intubation airways control, intra-procedural on percutaneous tracheotomy, effective control on extemporary evacuation or draining tube positioning in the course of pleural effusion or finally in bioptic practice.

All these applications require a line-probe to pleural and vessel visualization and a convex probe to different proceedings.

7.2.4 Application

However, in such a limited context it is not possible to go into details about ultrasonographic approach.

Maybe a sort of ultrasound objective examination could be created, to let us understand how and where pleural-pulmonary images have to be looked for, still as an attempt of great simplification.

The examination is usually carried out on patient's back, even if the positioning on one's side lets the dorsal regions, otherwise not very visible, more easily to be explored.

There are many equivalent approaches, depending on different sources of teaching.

As a rule, it is important to define an examination pattern and keep it for all the patients.

The lung is conventionally divided into three main areas each subdivided in turn into a dorsal and a ventral region (Figs. 7.3, 7.4 and 7.5), in order to standardize approach and sense of direction during examination and to compare it with other pulmonary imaging techniques.

The first one explores in front the lung (Fig. 7.3).

This is the best area to look for possible pneumothorax in a supine patient, as the air arranges on high.

The second one (Fig. 7.4) shows the least ultrasonographic restrictions, as it is lacking in rough bone structures that reflect ultrasounds completely. The patient can be positioned with his arm behind the head, amplifying intercostal spaces, to optimize the intercostal window (like all the bones ribs reflect ultrasounds fully, producing a conical-shaped shadow at the back).

In this region, thickenings hidden by the cardiac shadow can be easily identified on CRX, mainly on the left side.

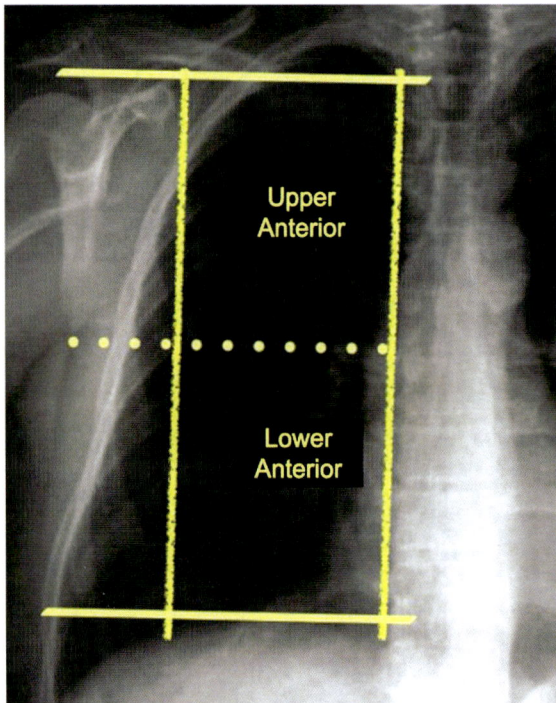

Fig. 7.3 Anterior chest. The anterior region of the rib cage has to be defined at ultrasound chest examination. This area is divided into an upper and a lower part by a halving line. It is delimited medially by the parasternal line, laterally by the anterior armpit line and below by the diaphragm (it has to be identified by ultrasonography and "curtain-sign" appearance). Liver and spleen are located positioning the marker toward the patient's head, longitudinally aligned (parenchymatous pattern) and then you can try to identify the lung, entering from the left corner of the screen and covering the liver image. Diaphragm looks like a hyperechoic line. The field is delimited above by the clavicle

The third area (Fig. 7.5) is the most interesting to be explored, since the least visible on CRX. The greatest trouble is in case of a non-collaborative patient, since free and raised trunk positioning is complicated and a sitting posture is not readily achieved and maintained.

Once areas to be explored have been defined, the examination must start looking for diaphragm and lung images along the caudal region (the probe is pointed perpendicularly to ribs—longitudinal axis—and probe marker toward patient's head, corresponding to the screen left corner). "The curtain sign" is the dynamic sign that identifies this area. It is referred to liver (or spleen) vanishing during inspiration and reappearance during expiration, due to the expanded lung that lies over in front of the probe. On UltraSound imaging, the liver and spleen look like gray, granular (iso-echoic), and compact areas with brighter shoots—the vessels.

Fig. 7.4 Lateral chest. The lateral pulmonary region is defined above by the anterior armpit line and behind by the posterior one. The diaphragm is below and the armpit hollow is above. The region is halved into an upper and a lower part

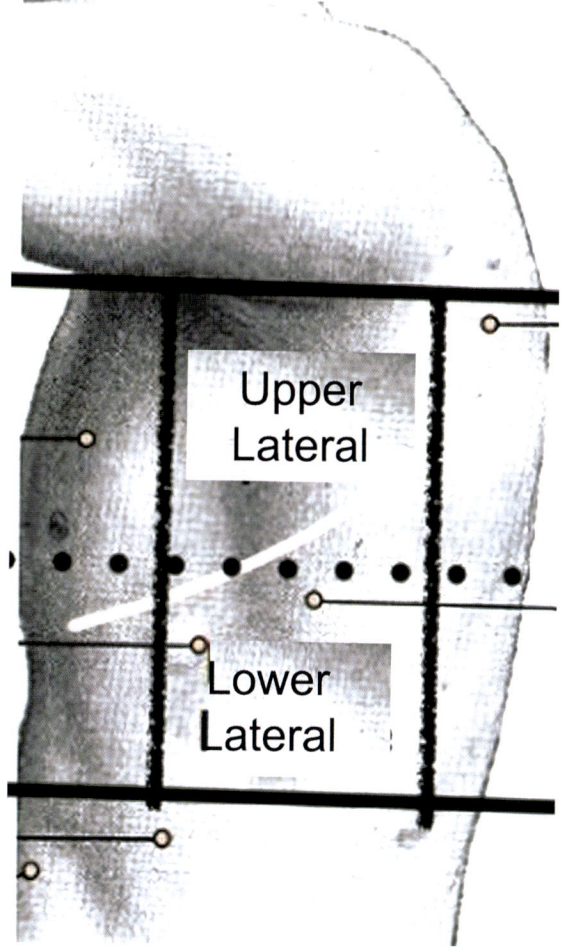

If the probe is correctly positioned, the movement covers the view from left to right.

Starting here it is easy to identify effusions or consolidation areas, more typically laid in the most caudal regions of the lung.

Whereas another approach provides for starting examination from apical regions, recognizing the pleural line that seems like a thin hyperechoic (bright white) line, still well defined by positioning the probe in a longitudinal section with its marker toward patient's head and identifying two conical-shaped shadows from two ribs. The hyperechoic area between the two conical-shaped shadows is the pleural line (Fig. 7.6 and Table 7.3).

This image is called "Bat sign". The pleural line is nothing but the interface between pleural and visceral sheets of the lung sliding one above the other. In case of underlying airy tissue (potentially unharmed lung), hyperechoic lines follow one

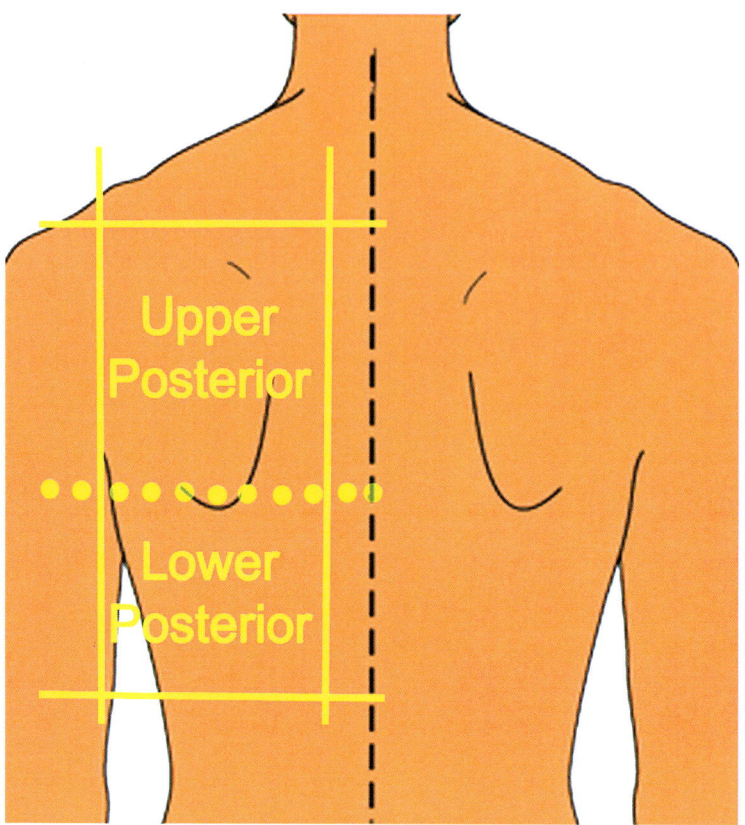

Fig. 7.5 Posterior chest. Posterior region. The scapula sets an important limit to ultrasound examination representing an anechoic area since the bone fully reflects the ultrasound beam producing a complete conical-shaped shadow. All the structures behind cannot be explored. It is defined laterally by the posterior armpit line, medially by the paravertebral line and below by the diaphragm. The splitting line is the one joining the armpit and the paravertebral lines midpoints.

another at regular intervals under the pleural line (A-Lines): they represent mirror-like artifacts, expression of a normal pattern. Pleural line examination enables the so-called "Gliding" or "Sliding sign" assessment, describing the pleural and visceral sheets flowing, an important clue to identify a breathing lung on the wall. Really, this area can be studied by monodimensional mode too (M-mode, a time-dependent dynamical ultrasonography function: it enables to measure movements in all the regions under an exact point of the ultrasound beam in a given moment), looking for an important sign, the so-called "seashore sign" (Fig. 7.7a).

This finding is formed by two overlapping areas that represent, respectively, the movement of structures upon the pleural line (upper zone) and the airy lung (lower zone) that looks like a homogeneous granular image.

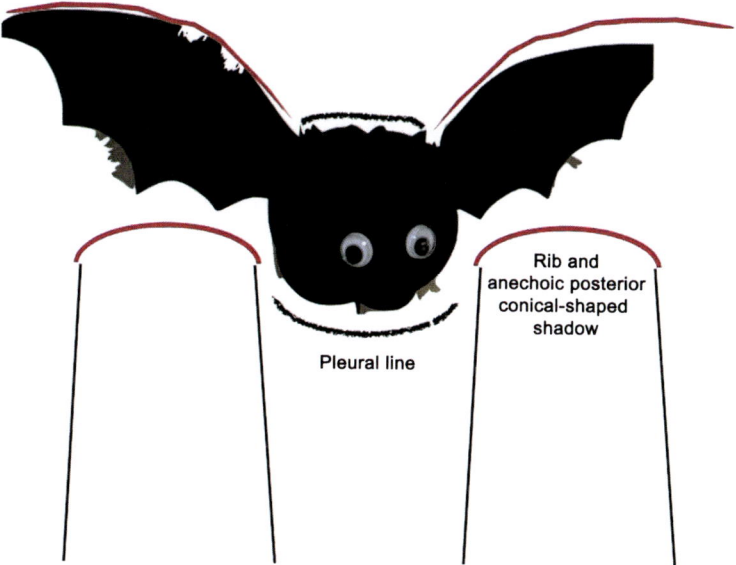

Fig. 7.6 Bat sign. The Bat sign image has to be searched for to identify the pleural line. Bat wings ideally depict the two ribs subtended to the longitudinally positioned probe. The conical-shaped shadow behind confirms this finding. Bat body corresponds to a hyperechoic line representing the pleural line. Hyperechogenicity describes the very light airy film interposed between the pleural sheet and the visceral one

In some pathological conditions the sign disappears, particularly pneumothorax where seashore sign disappearance and stratosphere sign appearance (Fig. 7.7b) are observed, i.e., the lung ultrasound image down below pleural line vanishes. The M-mode image looks like a line set, a sort of barcode (hence the term "barcode sign"). Moreover, the point the lung moves away from chest wall (lung point identification) can be found by a skilled surgeon: it looks like a sliding sign reappearance area or a stratosphere to seashore sign crossing on M-mode. So in this approach examination goes on toward diaphragm, a hyperechoic line beneath which liver and spleen may clearly be seen (Fig. 7.8).

Passing by different zones, pleural effusion may be observed. It looks like an anechoic dark area due to the complete absorption of ultrasound beam or like an area indicative for thickenings (atelectasis or focus of pneumonia), resembling isoechoic parenchymal tissue ("tissue-like" structures) with hyperechoic strengthening mainly in the presence of entrapped air that takes the typical hyperechoic appearance (Fig. 7.8). Correspondence with CT imaging is often high (Fig. 7.9).

In pathological conditions, the same pleural line is enriched by linear "comet tail" images, also called B-Lines (normally 2 to 4 in pleural line), that are important to define interstitial-alveolar syndrome, characterized by interstitial or intraalveolar edema.

Table 7.3 Chest US basic terminology

Name	Probe positioning	Main use
Longitudinal	Probe perpendicular to ribs	Linear Probe Pleural line recognition Sliding—PNX study Costosternal fracture study Convex-sectorial probe parenchyma study effusion visualization and measurement
Transverse	Probe parallel to ribs (intercostal space)	It enables a CT-like sharp image. It is useful to complete images achieved by the other scanning level
Bat sign and A-LINE	Image taken by a longitudinally positioned probe over the ribs (marker toward the patient's head). It is consisting of two ribs image laterally on the right and on the left, and of relating conical-shaped shadow. They look like two concavities downwards. A hyperechoic image may be easily seen between the two ribs. Pleural line "mirror-reoccurring" in the deepest lung region is a refraction artifact that produces A-LINES	It enables a CT-like on sharp image. It is useful to complete images achieved by the other scanning level. A-lines absence is a probable lung tissue lack expression
Gliding or Sliding sign	Image taken as for Bat sign. It is the hyperechoic line corresponding to the "bat" body. The sliding, representing the facing pleural layers movement, may be easily seen in a normal condition	Absence is an important sign of a breathless lung. If absent, it can indicate PNX
Lung point	Image taken by a high frequency probe (the region that has to be explored is superficial). It can be identified by pleural line study both in bidimensional and M-mode. It describes a shift from the sliding sign absence state to its appearance or from M-mode stratosphere sign to the shore one	PNX diagnosis (pathognomonic)
Seashore sign	It is taken by M-mode longitudinal probe. It is represented by horizontal lines, i.e., layers from skin toward the pleural lines and then a granular-like image up to the end of the screen, typical of lung parenchyma. It vanishes in case of PNX	PNX assessment

(continued)

Table 7.3 (continued)

Name	Probe positioning	Main use
Stratosphere sign	It is taken by M-mode longitudinal probe. It is represented by horizontal lines that occupy the whole screen, indicative for lung parenchyma absence. It appears in case of PNX	PNX assessment
B-lines	Hypoechoic "comet-tail" lines, originating from the pleural line and deepening to the deepest regions of the lung. From 2 to 4, they are physiological	Alveolar-interstitial syndrome. Their absence is suggestive of PNX because they are bound to non-airy lung tissue

7.3   Main Clinical Patterns That may be Investigated by CRX and Pleural-Pulmonary US

7.3.1   Thickenings (Atelectasis and Pneumonia)

7.3.1.1 CRX

Most of the lung opacity images on RX in critical care units relapse in this pathological pattern.

Anyone submitted to general anesthesia, especially as old, smoker or obese, is very likely to develop an atelectasic area, mainly at the left lower lung lobe.

Differential diagnosis with a pulmonary infective process is the most important diagnostic issue. The lower lobes, above all on the left, are the more affected by inflammatory process, at least during the opening phases.

Left opacity and diaphragmatic outline disappearance must arouse radiological suspicion of atelectasis.

Air bronchogram investigation may be diriment in this way (Fig. 7.10).

Lack of air on the inside of the atelectasis make you think of obstruction deserving a bronchoscopic washing.

"Cavitation sign" may also be helpful in differential diagnosis between infective thickening and a different kind of atelectasis.

Only integration with clinical examination and inflammatory indexes will be able to confirm the diagnostic suspicion.

The main problem is that air bronchogram reading, as many other pathological images, is strongly challenged by RX quality particularly in the supine patient. Table 7.4 summarizes the main factors (more or less corrigible) that differentiate a standard RX from a bedside one.

Although conditions predisposing to a good RX have been optimized, a third of CRX appears not to be reliable when compared to corresponding CT images [3, 4].

Different studies report a 38 % CRX sensibility in finding out thickened areas, with a 49 % diagnostic accuracy [5].

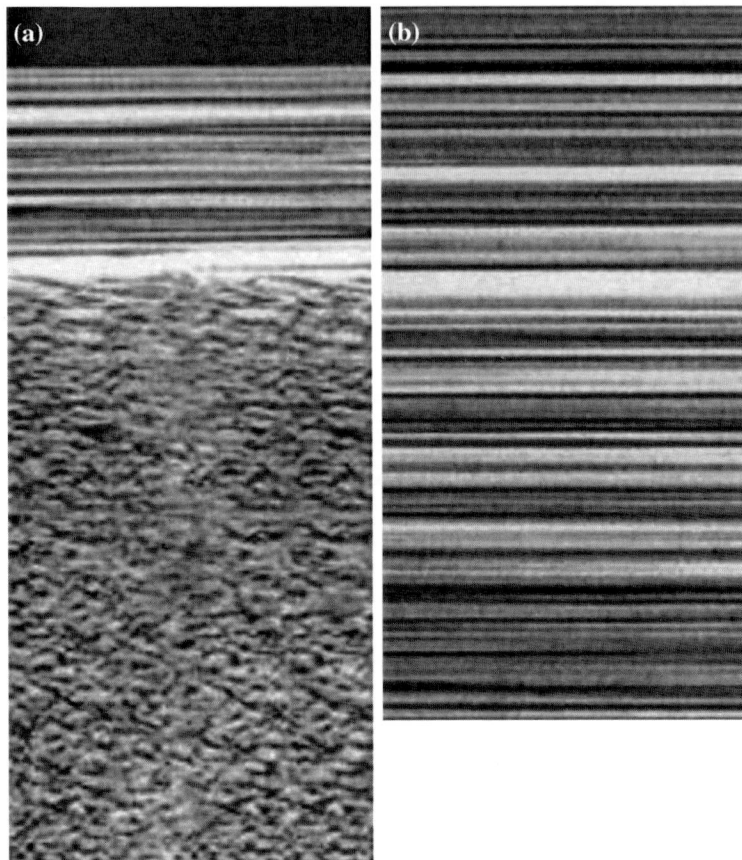

Fig. 7.7 a Seashore sign. Seashore sign image on M-mode. From *top to bottom*: skin, subcutaneous tissue, muscle, and pleural line can be seen in correspondence to horizontal lines. Immediately below, a granular-like image representing the lung parenchyma can be observed. **b** Stratosphere sign. Stratosphere sign image on M-mode. As in Fig. 7.7a, layers from skin to pleural line can be identified back to back. Loss of underlying lung tissue and air interposition—reflecting ultrasounds entirely by definition—produce an artifact as if the first image was repeated endlessly. Therefore, a barcode-like image is created, hence the name "Bar-code sign" too

Actually, CRX represents a good monitoring system of a suspected infective disease development under pharmacological treatment, rather than the ideal examination to diagnose pneumonia [6].

7.3.1.2 US

In critical patients US sensibility in detecting thickenings is near 100 %, with a diagnostic accuracy referred to the ability to find out pathological areas in 94 % of cases [5–7].

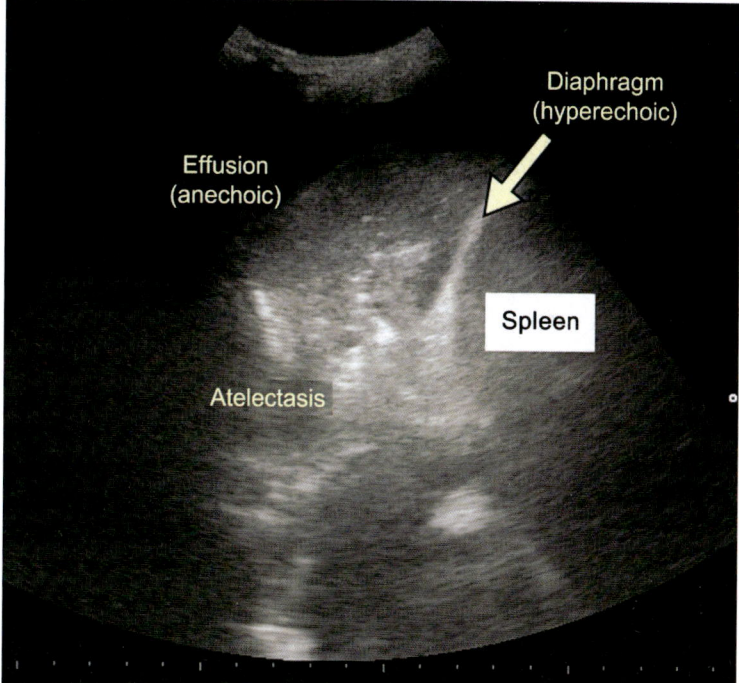

Fig. 7.8 Effusion atelectasis. Longitudinally aligned left pleural basis US scan. A more solid zone with hyperechoic points on the inside can be highlighted over the diaphragm (hyperechoic line down on the right in the figure). This region stands for atelectasis of the lung pressed by a quite clear great effusion, i.e., the black area (anechoic) all around the hyperechoic one. Fig. 7.8 is the CT reference image

Atelectasis can be divided in central and peripheral by pleural-pulmonary ultrasonography. The first has to be attributed to airways obstruction, the second is produced by lung parenchyma compressed by effusions, pneumothorax, injuries, or a mass. The thickened tissue depicts a homogeneous-type image with ultrasonographic characteristics or anechogenicity compared to hepatic parenchyma.

In the hands of a skilled operator, ultrasonography allows to distinguish two different conditions inside the atelectasic area, that may be helpful in the differential diagnosis between airways secretory hindrance atelectasis or extrinsic compression and the probably infective-kind thickening. Actually, the sight of echoic-walled tubular structures filled with liquid is expression of pulmonary vessels or bronchi full of mucous material, indicative of obstructive or compressive atelectasis patterns. If that is the case, it is referred to as "ultrasonographic liquid bronchogram." The contrary, "ultrasonographic airy bronchogram" by analogy with CRX or CT bronchogram represents an inflammatory sign. The image looks like a hypo- or anechoic area, or a mixed hypo/hyperechoic one with

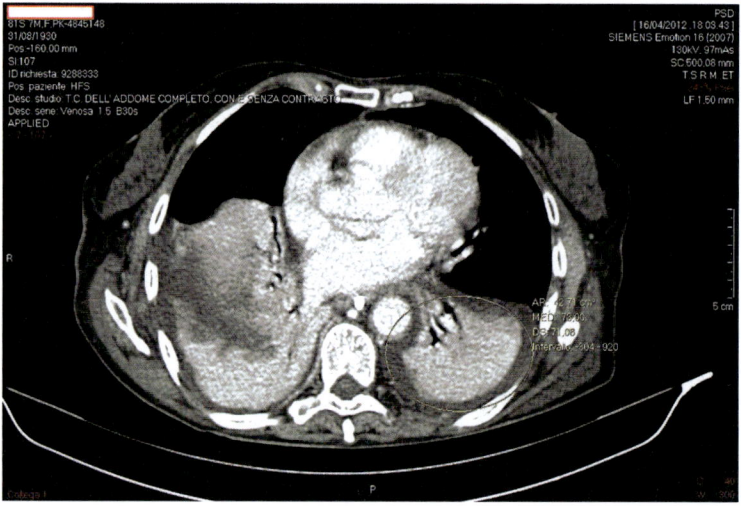

Fig. 7.9 CT atelectasis. CT image of the same area examined by chest US and shown in Fig. 7.6. A tight linkage between the two images can be noted

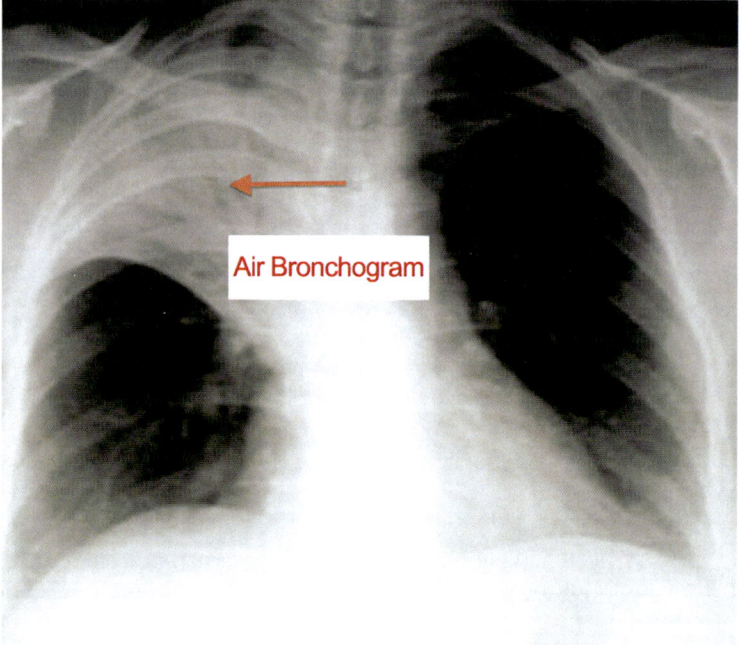

Fig. 7.10 Air bronchogram. Air bronchogram of right medial-apical pneumonia on CRX

Table 7.4 Bedside CRX main issues

Issue	Correctable	Not very correctable
Chest wall movement Movement artifacts RX during inspiration	Sedated and/or curarized patient: respiratory curve reading training for radiologist technicians in order to identify the inspiratory phase	Previously sedated, non–intubated and troubled patient at the risk of respiratory depression if sedated
A-P correct view or need for L–L views	Patient positioning before RX	Obliged positions. Supination Lateral decubitus
Film and beam position Reduced recommended distance between beam source and radiograph seat. No tangential rays in respect to the lung	Radiodiagnositic performance	Obliged front beam at a reduced distance due to the equipment features. Obliged posterior film. Aid may come from beds compatible with RX equipment with a cassette placed beneath the chest region. In this case, a correct patient positioning enables a higher quality image

softened margins. In the inside hyperechoic lines can be recognized, expression of bronchi still filled with air.

The so-called "shred sign" is another clue of pneumonia. Really, pathological areas of the lung look like hyperechoic shreds or strips in the sound pulmonary parenchyma.

The great ease in the application of this technique knocks down the diagnosis period, dodging the interval between technician call and reporting.

7.3.2 Effusions

7.3.2.1 CRX

CRX accuracy in recognizing effusion is poor (69–67 %) [8, 9], and sensitivity is not above 65 % [5].

Small effusions often escape RX examination.

As the effusion's extent increases RX pattern changes, first putting on a sprinkling appearance and then a diaphragmatic image attenuation, costal-phrenic sinus vanishing and pulmonary vessels visibility reduction (Fig. 7.11).

Air bronchogram persistence can help maintain a differential diagnosis between thickening and effusion, but lung collapse due to extrinsic effusion constraint may produce confusing images, simulating patterns consistent with an atelectasic process too. You could almost state that is actually the consensual atelectasis to make effusion nearly always quite evident. The volume assessment is often difficult too, over- o underestimated. CT itself is frequently inclined to overestimate effusion, involving an obliged supine decubitus.

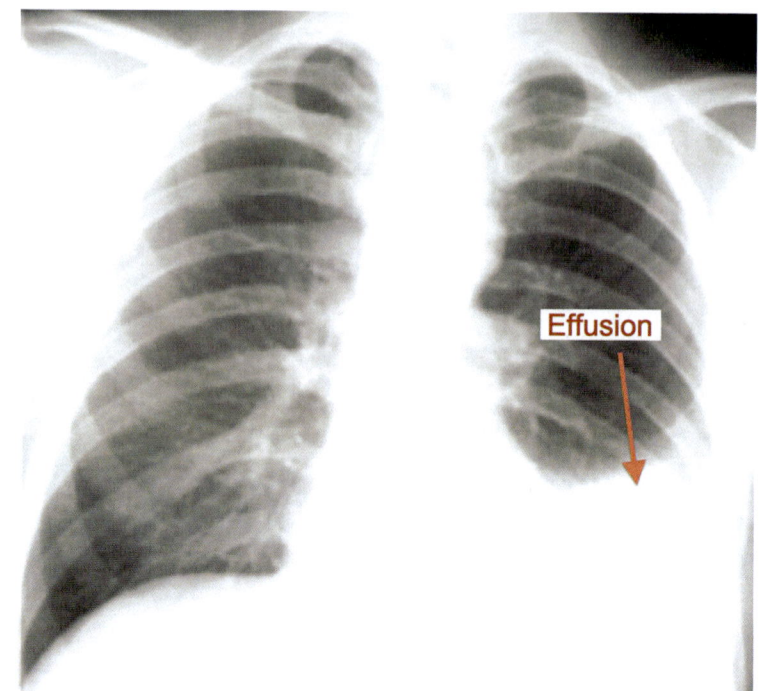

Fig. 7.11 Left basal effusion on CRX

7.3.2.2 US

In pleural effusion diagnosis chest US shows very high sensitivity and specificity rates of 90–100 %, recognized by most of the literature [5–10].

Chest US is able to identify the slightest effusion too (about 10 ml).

Effusion looks like a hypoechoic layer often combined with consensual hyperechoic images typical of lung atelectasis.

As well as the high accuracy of effusion identification, pleural ultrasonography allows the possible drainage treatment too, still in the same diagnostic context. Therefore, during the same clinical act you can find an introductory diagnostic phase, a dimensional assessment with check for possible drainage criteria by effusion volume evaluation, the effects on pulmonary parenchyma (compression and consensual atelectasis), and eventually the therapeutic management (echo-guided drainage). In a supine patient, a measured distance between the lung (it is often floating within the effusion) and the caudal thoracic wall ≥50 mm is usually correlated to a more than 500 mL extent effusion. You do not need to assess the inspiratory or expiratory phase. Effusion quantification seems to be less accurate for a volume lower than 500 mL and greater than 1 L (but this is so evident that it does not raise any difficulties about a possible drainage indication). Another measuring approach is the calculus of an area as deep as the greatest effusion extent (cm) assessed in a supine position on the paravertebral line, and showing as surface the section evaluated by the US area calculation software program, measured at the medium point of the previous distance.

Therefore the calculus is: effusion length by surface measured on the medium point of the length [11]. Once volume and area have been identified, echography can be employed for ultrasound-guided centesis, if any.

During a non ultrasound-guided thoracocentesis practice, a variable percentage from 7 to 15 % of patients expose to pneumothorax. Introducing pleural-pulmonary ultrasonography as an intraprocedural guide, this rate falls to 0.5 % [7].

7.3.3 Pneumothorax

7.3.3.1 CRX

Nearly all the patients admitted to ICU show conditions potentially favoring PNX onset. PNX is not uncommon as main iatrogenic complication in about 25 % of ventilated patients (high PEEP with or without peak pressure >40 mmHg, high current volumes), particularly with attendant clinical diseases such as pneumonia, ARDS, emphysema, or in patients who need central venous catheter placement [6].

In such a situation, PNX can be found most frequently in an anteromedial and sub-pulmonary position, at the edge of diaphragm, more seldom in an apical, lateral, or posteromedial position.

Despite clinical findings or indirect signs such as subcutaneous emphysema, PNX cannot often be confirmed by CRX examination. Even to assess how and where PNX has to be drained, it is therefore necessary to perform RX from a different view (i.e., latero-lateral) or, especially and most often, a resort to CT involving all the transfer correlated issues of these deeply unstable patients [6].

According to different studies, CRX sensitivity and specificity in PNX diagnosis are 26 and 100 %, respectively [4].

7.3.3.2 US

PNX finding at ultrasound examination looks like the result of physiological signs suppression of lung tissue presence.

"Sliding" and B-lines disappearance due to the lack of transmitting parenchyma can be seen.

M-mode use should make the "seashore sign" absence and the "stratosphere sign" appearance evident. Carrying out examination from the most apical regions (whatever the patient positioning as the air localizes upwards) and going toward the more sloping ones, scanning all the way down the lung, it could allow to find out the "lung point" both at the pleural line level and on the M-mode. "Lung point" represents where lung goes back against the wall and it is pathognomonic for PNX. It can be seen on the pleural line as the point sliding comes back.

It is the crossing point from stratosphere to shore sign on M-mode (Fig. 7.12). Whereas its presence is pathognomonic for PNX, its lack is not an absence clue because it could not be found in case of complete lung collapse. Subcutaneous

Fig. 7.12 M-mode lung point. Lung point sign on M-mode. Seashore sign representing a sound lung can be easily observed on the left. Stratosphere sign representing the sub-pleural area with no lung parenchyma can be seen on the right of the dividing line (the very lung point)

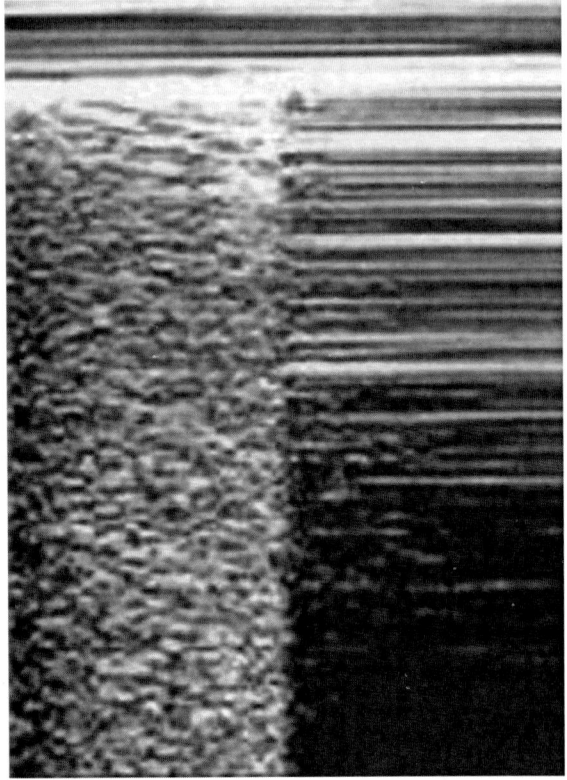

emphysema consensual to serious PNX can challenge examination due to massive air interposition between probe and tissue.

Whereas the pulmonary US learning curve is usually rather quick, PNX diagnosis requires experience.

According to different studies, US sensitivity and specificity in PNX diagnosis are 80–85 and 97–100 %, respectively [4, 5].

7.3.4 Alveolar-Interstitial Syndrome

7.3.4.1 CRX

In serious inflammatory or infective processes such as pneumonia, ARDS, pulmonary edema, up to septic shock status, you can frequently find out water-overloaded conditions, due to the basic disease that alters alveolar permeability and damages the alveolar-capillary barrier or as a result of the reanimation phase that often needs generous water volumes to warrant an adequate flow. It is still referred to as water-overloaded for diseases such as heart failure or fluidic overloading.

These overloading conditions, inevitably giving rise to a generalized lung tissue edema picture, can be primarily divided in hydrostatic edema pattern (pump failure or overload) and altered permeability edema pattern (ARDS, sepsis/serious sepsis, septic shock, inhalation syndrome, gas—embolism etc.).

The venous vessels diameter increase is the initial radiographic sign for hydrostatic impairment, and it has to be interpreted as an indirect clue of the left ventricle end diastolic pressure (LVEDP) increase. However, supine position in which most CRX examinations are carried out can alter these findings. Bronchial wall thickening, A–B–C Kerley striae appearance, frosted glass image and eventually effusion clouding development particularly in the sloping lung regions are further facts of this phase. However, the differentiation between interstitial edema and infective process is not always obvious on CRX examination. Only daily monitoring and a quick change under treatment suggest edema instead of consolidation. Edema due to LVEDP increase looks like an alveolar, bilateral, and often symmetric opacification on CRX examination. However, minimal position changes, recruitment operations, and concurrent cardiac patterns can make images asymmetric and so the differential diagnosis more complex.

It seems difficult to set alveolar edema too, being easily mistaken for infective consolidation or hemorrhagic alveolar imbibition.

7.3.4.2 US

In state of lung damage with an increase of parenchyma level to the detriment of airy zones, the standard lung parenchyma image undergoes well identifiable changes on US examination. From pleural line, B-lines (2–4 normal vertical lines) significantly increase. The number of new B-lines is proportional to airy tissue loss. In interstitial edema condition, B-lines are less close (about 7 mm away one another—B line 7 mm pattern) whereas in alveolar edema pattern they are more close (about 3 mm "comet tail" medium distance—B line 3 mm pattern). The finding of the former B line type corresponds to a thickened interlobular septa image by comparison with CT (pulmonary fibrosis). Thicker B-lines correspond on the other hand to so-called frosted glass CT images, frequently observed in pulmonary edema, overloading and ARDS.

An interesting comparison study about lung auscultation, CRX and US diagnostic effectiveness to find out pathological events in alveolar-interstitial syndrome has shown very high pulmonary US sensitivity and specificity compared to auscultation and CRX, and a 95 % diagnostic accuracy (Table 7.5) [10].

7.3.5 RX and US Conclusions

In critical patients you can easily run up against clinical diseases such as PNX, consolidation, alveolar-interstitial syndrome (ARDS, pulmonary edema, fibrosis). Routinely, ultrasonography by US bedside objective examination can be a valid alternative to daily CRX, being added or even proving to be better for diagnosis.

Table 7.5 Comparison study about lung auscultation, CRX and US diagnostic effectiveness. Modified from [10]

Disease	Parameters	Auscultation	CRX	US
Effusion	Sensitivity	42	39	**92**
–	Specificity	90	85	**93**
–	Diagnostic accuracy	61	47	**93**
Consolidation areas	Sensitivity	8	68	**93**
–	Specificity	**100**	95	**100**
–	Diagnostic accuracy	36	75	**97**
Alveolar-interstitial syndrome	Sensitivity	34	60	**98**
–	Specificity	90	**100**	88
–	Diagnostic accuracy	55	72	**95**

Best values are bold. US benefits are evident in all the diseases
Comparison among
Sensitivity (likelihood of an anomaly positive confirmation)
Specificity (likelihood of an anomaly negative confirmation)
Diagnostic accuracy (ratio between the positive predictive value PV [likelihood of a real positive positivity] and the negative predictive value NV [likelihood of a real negative negativity] as regards to false positives FP and false negatives FN
(NV + PV)/(PV + NV + FP + FN)

Non-invasivity, money-saving (after initial purchase), high specificity and sensitivity, quite short training, and the possibility of performing even probable therapeutic handling associated to the confirmed disease without waste of time, all make US something which cannot be almost renounced in modern ICU.

The possibility of completing by an ultrasound study the hemodynamic unstable critical patient setting too, adds great value to the methodology.

Thinking about echography in daily routine becomes therefore interesting, taking a reality such as Lichtenstein as a starting point (the country is one of the more active promoter for US employment in critical environment), by algorithm application like the one suggested in dyspnoeic patient and shown in Fig. 7.13 (modified from Lichtenstein et al. [12]).

7.3.6   Notes About US

US shows some important restrictions, although its specifications make it close to the ideal methodology.

First of all it is operator dependent.

The learning curves are quite short, above all for effusion identification, consolidation (although experience is needed to discriminate between pneumonia area with an air bronchogram and atelectasis region), alveolar-interstitial syndrome.

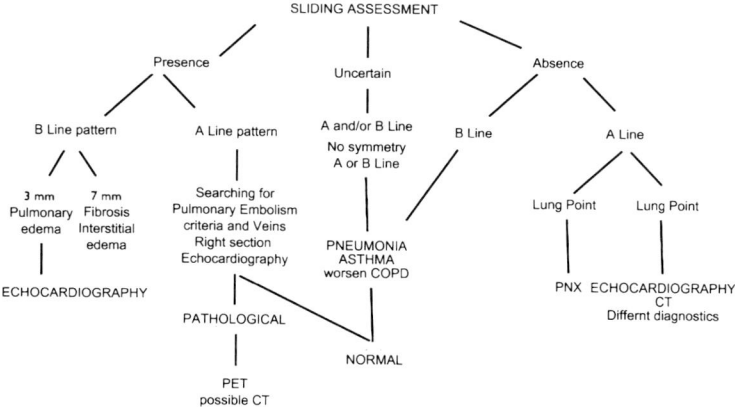

Fig. 7.13 Chest US objective examination proposal in the dyspnoic patient, modified from [12]

Only PNX remains a clinical condition that takes more time and learning curves up to 2–3 months (about twice as much as the other clinical diseases) [13].

The necessity to have at one's disposal a daily and prolonged access to ultrasound scanner not to extend the learning period too much is a further consequence.

Second, diseases such as obesity with interposition of large fat tissue areas or subcutaneous emphysema can make image interpretation very hard but even nonassessable.

Starting ultrasound examination by describing the acoustic window quality is a good practice. If quality is poor, the exam could be heavily challenged.

At the end, ultrasound probe may become source of infections like all the devices touching the skin, particularly in patients that are often treated by multiple complicated antibiotic therapies.

It is advisable to avoid gel packet use for several patients, to minimize this potentially serious problem in an already critical environment due to infective aspects, particularly if there is no care in escaping the probe surface to get in touch with the gel container. If you want to perform routine ultrasound objective examination in all the patients, providing every bed with a gel bottle is a good practice.

Ultrasound system keyboard contact reduced to a sorry state and possibly limited to clean hands is another important care, since it is one of the greater sources of transmission. By the way, there are devices provided with washable keyboards or keyboard covers. Since probes are the main source of infection, it is a good practice not to put them away in the case or on the ultrasound system after examination so that they will not be contaminated. Probes would have to be cleaned just after the examination as appointed by manufacturer not to damage surfaces, and they only would be put away once dry.

Table 7.6 Central venous catheter (CVC) positioning. Modified from [14]

Access	Formula
Right subclavian vein	(Patient height cm/10)—2 cm
Left subclavian vein	(Patient height cm/10) + 2 cm
Internal right jugular vein	(Patient height cm/10)
Internal left jugular vein	(Patient height cm/10) + 4 cm

A CVC positioning reference table is reported. The table shows access sites and relating formulas to calculate catheter skin-side length according to the patient height

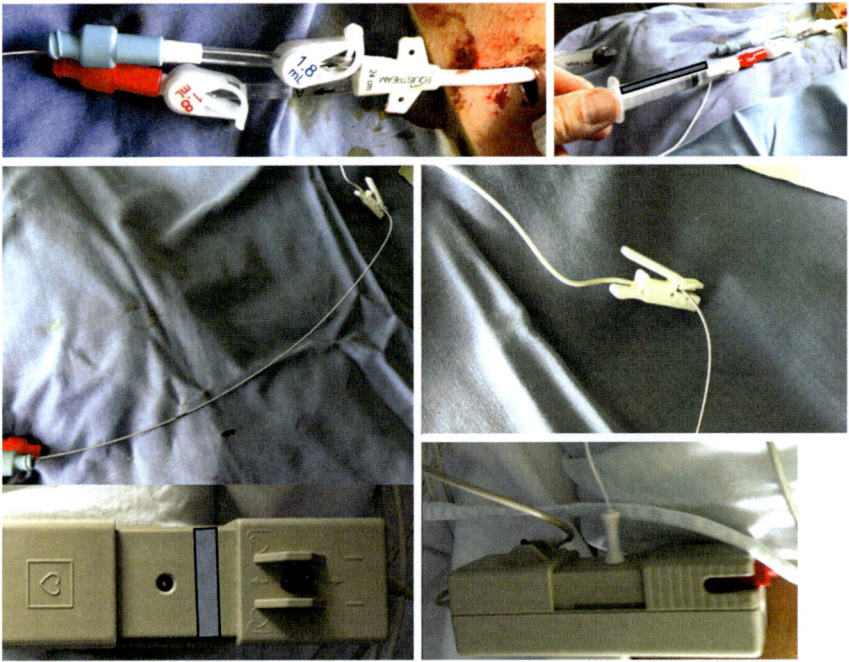

Fig. 7.14 ECG-guided CVC positioning practice. *Top* to *bottom* and *left* to *right*: Spindle inside the CVC Alternative liquid spindle kit. Spindle connected to a clip for multi-parametric screen ECG reading. Clip detail. Switch: this equipment enables to keep patient ECG on a reading state (black switch on the right, right position) and to read endocavitary ECG if necessary (switch moved on the left). Different kits allow one or the other reading, unplugging the electrode from the patient and connecting it to the cable. Patient (*red clip*) and CVC (*white cable*) connected to the switch

7.3.7 CRX and Central Venous Catheterism

CRX execution still plays an important role to check positioning of some devices, i.e., central venous access, thoracic drainage, and endotracheal tube, particularly to control positioning and to exclude more serious complications such as post-procedural iatrogenic PNX or to leave one of the pulmonary hemi-systems out during a selective bronchial intubation. However, with regard to CVC (central venous catheter) positioning, ultrasound technique combination associated to significant side effects decrease and the endocavitary CVC ECG rediscovery to find out the central venous catheter's tip, have limited CRX role in this field too.

Certainly, CVC positioning by ECG guide is not proved to be more effective than CVC length assessment by indirect measurement or formulas (tables or RX evaluation) (Table 7.6) [13, 14]. However, being sure of the puncture (by an echo-guided approach) and two parameters like endocavitary ECG and CVC distance reference tables according to puncture point and patient's height, enable to get a good certainty level and to postpone a RX check-up later, if any. This allows the catheter to be immediately used and RX to be performed later, maybe combining CVC control and a previously organized CRX to check lung parenchyma or another device control such as a thoracic drainage or a nasogastric tube. The technique is very easy and it provides for reading through a proper kit the endo-cavitary ECG signal by connecting the spindle inside the catheter during posi-tioning and the multi-parametric monitor on ECG second lead. Kits that allow to read endocavitary ECG even by a liquid spindle (physiologic saline in already positioned CVC) carrying electrical signal to the monitor have been recently introduced. Figure 7.14.

Curves reading is immediate and it allows CVC to proceed toward the correct position (just before the atriocaval junction) avoiding it to be too low (right atrium—AD) or too high (superior vena cava—SVC). Figures 7.15 and 7.16.

7.3.8 CRX and NGT

NGT (nasogastric tube) assessment is still a field where CRX keeps the supremacy above any other technique.

However, even in this practice—anything but not very noble, in the light of recent attention drawn by literature to the importance of enteral nutrition (ERAS protocol)—you need to proceed with caution in relying on CRX, due to false positive risks. Actually, the risk of placing nasogastric probe (NGP) into the trachea makes a post-positioning radiological check compulsory, especially if the aim is to start enteral nutrition or drug administration.

Really, an assessment by sounds auscultation during air insufflation is abso-lutely insufficient because of the great false positive risk due to sounds trans-mission to epigastrium through the lungs too (very high aspiration risk).

Gastric material sample shows a very high safety level but only NGP visuali-zation in the stomach or beyond can make sure about a correct positioning.

So CRX is always necessary to confirm NGP correct positioning definitively. Running means of contrast into NGP is often advisable, due to the critical patient condition and the likely presence of air and intestinal loops overlapping gastric image on CRX examination.

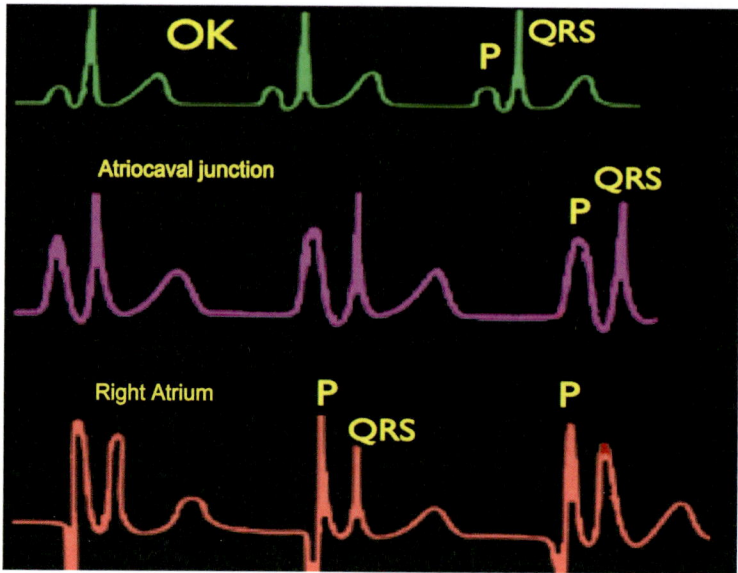

Fig. 7.15 Endocavitary ECG tracing read on the second lead of a normal multiparametric monitor ECG trace. From top to bottom:Normal tracing, correct positioning. Sharp and high *P*-wave. Atriocaval junction. The catheter has to be withdrawn by 1–2 cm up to tracing 1 reappearance. Biphasic *P*-wave. CVC distal end is into the right atrium. The catheter has to be decisively withdrawn up to tracing 1 reappearance

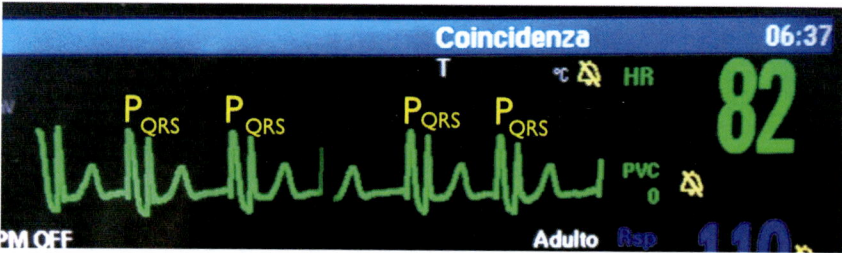

Fig. 7.16 Real CVC tip tracing into the atriocaval junction. In this particular case, the catheter was a permanent and tunneled dialysis CVC. Distal end of these catheters is advised to be into the atriocaval junction, as close as possible to the right atrium. This one was optimally positioned, as subsequently confirmed by scopy too

7.4 Conclusions

Although CRX has been holding on a key role in critical patient cardiopulmonary assessment for decades and skilled radiologists are still able to supply important information from CRX, many interfering factors are leading the technique on the fringe of ICU routine practice. Image quality, delay between execution and image or report availability, interpretative doubtful points and inaccessible areas are conditions that could be readily avoided by wider and wider ultrasound system use. Even though it is an easy method, chest ultrasonography still needs basic ultrasound knowledge acquisition about both the way of getting images and their interpretation. In addition, a long training is necessary and this could be achieved only by having at one's disposal an ultrasound system and at least a convex probe.

In the presence of many highly qualified courses, this context has absolutely no pretensions to supply knowledge that could even only introduce to chest ultrasonography, but it just wishes to point out the simple method and its wide ICU application.

The attempt is to make the specialist so curious that he could take into account the possibility to attend one of these courses devoted to ultrasound neophytes and at the same time to awaken his own administration offices about the even medicolegal benefits of having at ICU's disposal an ultrasound equipment.

Ultrasound facility in supporting CVC management (e.g., in operating rooms) is not of minor importance also in hospitals without an ICU, taking into account that ultrasonography resets complications nearly to zero during a jugular vein access, reducing the infection risk too.

Finally, on account of CRX benefits, even taking into consideration the most severe survey, the existing quite ready CT accessibility is the last tile for the more and more often CRX abandonment.

However, it still remains a useful aid usually in combination with clinical practice and other techniques (endocavitary ECG or auscultation), particularly if an ICU devoted ultrasound system is not immediately available and in small institutes where CT access is still difficult especially during summer time or at night.

References

1. ftp://ftp.cordis.lu/pub/fp.5-euratom/docs/eur16260.pdf
2. www.acr.org
3. Wiener MD et al (1991) Imaging of the intensive care unit patient. Clin Chest Med 12:169–198
4. Rouby JJ et al (2000) CT scan ARDS study group: regional distribution of gas and tissue in acute respiratory distress syndrome: II physiological correlations and definition of an ARDS severity score. Intensive Care Med 26:1046–1056
5. Xirouchaki N et al (2011) Lung ultrasound in critically ill patients: comparison with bedside chest radiography. Intensive Care Med 37:1488–1493
6. Maffessanti M et al (2010) Radiologia toracica in terapia intensiva. Radiol Med 115 (supp):S34–S44
7. Sperandeo M et al (2008) Role of thoracic ultrasound in the assessment of pleural and pulmonary diseases. J Ultrasound 11:39–46
8. Fishman JE et al (2005) Thoracic imaging in the intensive care unit. Appl Radiol 34:8–17
9. Henschke CI et al (1996) Accuracy and efficacy of chest radiography in the intensive care unit. Radiol Clin North Am 34:21–31

10. Lichtenstein D et al (2004) Comparative diagnostic performances of auscultation, chest radiography and lung ultrasonography in acute respiratory distress syndrome. Anesthesiology 100:9–15

11. Remerand F et al (2010) Multiplane ultrasound approach to quantify pleural effusion at the bedside. Intensive Care Med 36:654–655

12. Lichtenstein D et al (2008) Relevance of lung ultrasound in the diagnosis of acute respiratory failure—The BLUE protocol. Chest 134:117–125

13. Lee JH et al (2009) Comparison of bedside central venous catheter placement techniques: landmark vs electrocardiogram guidance. Br J Anesth 102:662–666

14. Czepizak CA (1995) Evaluation of formulas for optimal positioning of central venous catheters. Chest 107:1662–1664

Continuous Renal Replacement Therapy (CRRT) in Intensive Care

8

Filippo Mariano

Since preliminary experiences of Kramer with arteriovenous hemofiltration at low blood flow in 1977 [1], technological improvements led to develop a dedicated hardware (monitors, filters) for Continuous Renal Replacement Therapy (CRRT).

After some technical aspects of CRRT, this brief review will focus on two crucial points of high clinical impact on CRRT practice such as dose of dialysis and anticoagulation of extracorporeal circuit.

8.1 CRRT: An Overview of the Different Techniques

Dialysis circuit consists of : (1) the blood circuit; (2) the dialysate circuit. The core of dialysis process is the filter, where a semipermeable membrane separates the blood and dialysate compartments. Dialysis membrane rules the exchanges of water and solutes between blood and dialysate compartments driven by diffusive and convective fluxes (Fig. 8.1).

The different dialytic methodologies differ in a different assembly of the components, that is in a increasing degrees of technical complexity. They ranges from SCUF, in which there is a loss of water and solutes by exclusive convective motion without replacement liquid infusion, to continuous hemodiafiltration (CVVHDF) in which there are an exchange of solutes with both convective and diffusive motions, and a replacement liquid infusion.

F. Mariano (✉)
Department of Medicine, Nephrology and Dialysis, Citta' della Salute e della Scienza di Torino, CTO Hospital, Via G. Zuretti 29, 10126 Turin, Italy
e-mail: filippo.mariano@hotmail.it

B. Allaria (ed.), *Practical Issues in Anesthesia and Intensive Care 2013*,
DOI: 10.1007/978-88-470-5529-2_8, © Springer-Verlag Italia 2014

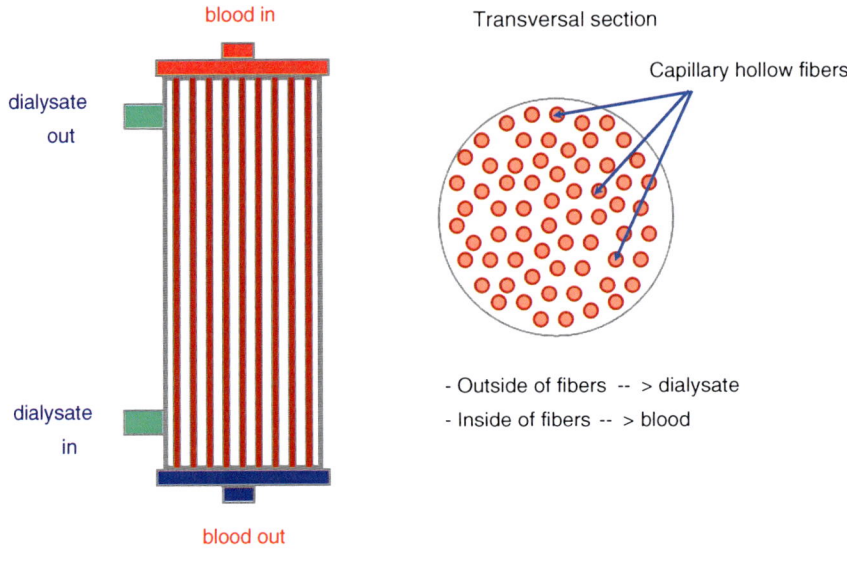

Fig. 8.1 The filter of dialysis

8.1.1 Filters for CRRT

Filters for CRRT are hollow fiber filters with synthetic membrane, in polysulfone, polyethersulfon, polyamide, or polymethylmetacrilate.

Filters for CRRT are characterized by a membrane exchange area of 0.8–2 mq, and by an inlet blood flow of 100–300 ml/min. The membrane is highly permeable, with a *cut-off* for diffusible solutes of 20–40,000 Da. By these filters, convective motion of solutes throughout membranes allows a sustained clearance of middle and middle–high-molecular weight substances (1,000–30,000 Da). In addition, by these filters convective exchange can be coupled with a dialysate flow, allowing also a diffusive exchange of solutes.

The ability of a molecule to pass through a semipermeable membrane is expressed as sieving coefficient value (SC, see formula in Fig. 8.2).

Fig. 8.2 Formula of sieving coefficient

$$SC = \frac{(Cuf\_i + Cuf\_o)/2}{(Cpl\_i + Cpl\_o)/2}$$

Legenda:
SC   = sieving coefficient
Cuf_i   = concentration of solute in inlet dialysate
Cuf_o   = concentration of solute in oulet effluent
Cpl_i   = concentration of solute in inlet plasma
Cpl_o   = concentration of solute in outlet plasma

Several hydraulic factors such as blood flow, transmembrane pressure, and filtration fraction (FF) affect SC during dialysis. In particular, SC varies inversely proportional to the FF. In order to avoid a marked reduction of SC due to an excessive concentration of blood and plasma proteins along fibers, FF is optimal for values of 15–20 % of blood flow. At these FF values, phenomena of fouling of membrane are limited, and the membrane can maintain a constant SC for whole treatment duration. As a matter of fact, membranes such as polymethylmethacrylate also have an adsorption capacity. Therefore, with polymethylmethacrylate molecules trapped in the membrane are not found in ultrafiltrate.

8.1.2 SCUF-Slow Continuous Ultrafiltration

- SCUF needs a pump in blood circuit and a pump in ultrafiltrate circuit (optional)(two- or one-pump circuit).
- SCUF do not use infusion replacement fluid or dialysate.
- Ultrafiltrate rate is modulated by patient's hemodynamic tolerance.
- Indicative flow rates: blood pump flow rate: 80–150 ml/min; ultrafiltrate flow rate 10–30 ml/min.
- Indications:. Los of excess fluid in overloaded patients not responsive to diuretic therapy (edemigene syndromes and congestive heart failure).
- Comments: Depurative capacity is very poor, and it is proportional to amount of ultrafiltrate.

8.1.3 CVVHF-Continuous Veno-Venous Hemofiltration

- CVVH needs a pump on blood circuit, a pump for ultrafiltration, and a pump for replacement fluid in dialysate circuit (three-pumps circuits). The method is exclusively convective, and it optimally works with a FF of 15–20 % of blood flow.
- In CVVHF replacement fluid can take place after dialysis filter (post dilution CVVHF), before the dialysis filter (pre dilution CVVHF), or before and after the filter (pre/postdilution CVVHF).
- In post dilution CVVHF an important hemoconcentration of blood along dialysis fibers occurs. Circuit clotting risks are greater, and in general post dilution CVVHF needs higher amount of anticoagulant than predilution CVVHF.
- In predilution CVVHF solute dilution occurs before filter exchanges. However, solute clearance is lower than that predicted by theory, probably for the diffusion of solutes across the membrane of erythrocytes in circuit line after predilution site. For example, in the case of urea with Qb of 150 mL/min and a sample predilution of 75 ml/min, measured clearance reduction is equal to

30 %, compared with a theoretical reduction of 40 % (an increase about 10 % of urea clearance has been demonstrated).

- Indicative flow rates:
  Postdilution CVVHF: blood pump 150–200 ml/min; ultrafiltrate 20–40 ml/min.
  Predilution CVVHF: blood pump 100–150 ml/min; ultrafiltrate 30–60 ml/min.

8.1.4   CVVHD: Continuous Veno-Venous Hemodialysis

- Method is exclusively diffusive, and requires a pump for blood circuit, a pump for inlet dialysate and a pump for outlet dialysate (three-pumps circuits).
- Dialysate is usually set at low flow rate, not exceeding 30 % of blood flow value. As a result, saturation of small- to medium-sized molecules in the effluent is equal to 100 %.

8.1.5   CVVHDF: Continuous Veno-Venous Hemodiafiltration

- CVVHDF is mixed method combining diffusion and convection. In addition to dialysate, CVVHDF uses an infusion fluid solution in pre and/or postfilter. Predilution CVVHDF (infusion fluid in prefilter) provides same hemorheology benefits described for predilution CVVHF.
- CVVHDF is the best compromise to getting high clearance of both small and medium-sized molecules. In fact, CVVHDF by adding a diffusive component is more efficient than CVVHF (pure convection) in removing low-molecular weight substances. On the other side, in comparison to CVVHD CVVHDF shows a good clearance for substances with a molecular weight close to membrane cut-off, i.e., between 5,000–30,000 Da,
- CVVHDF is the currently most used method in CRRT.

8.1.6   HV-HF: High Volume Hemofiltration

- HV-HF uses high exchange volumes, generally reaching 50–70 L/day.
- To ensure these volumes of ultrafiltrate, in HV-HF blood flow rate are usually 200–250 mL/min and are coupled with high permeability and high surface filters (>2 sqm).
- Infusion is usually done simultaneously in both pre and postdilution to get an excellent convective clearance of high-molecular weight substances, and to take advantage of the predilution effects on filter duration.

8.2   Dose of Dialysis

The dose of dialysis, like every other therapy, is intended as a dosage of a drug, which in turn depends on specific indications, on therapeutic efficacy and on side effects presence. In this context, first the dose of dialysis in ICUs is conditioned by catabolic state and patient's muscle mass, by presence of sepsis, of comorbidities, of electrolytic disorders and hydration state.

RRT lasting 4 h and 3 times a week at high dialytic efficiency usually allows survival in chronic uremic patients. However, when these patterns of short dialysis protocol were applied in ICUs patients they suffered from poor dialysis tolerance and insufficient dialysis dose. In these patients, mortality was significantly increased in comparison to patients treated with intermittent daily long treatments [2]. In fact, short treatments were abandoned for prolonged and continuous intermittent treatments [3].

8.2.1   Prescribed and Delivered Dialysis Dose

Delivered dialysis dose is different from prescribed dose, because the latter always overestimates the dose actually delivered. As recently confirmed by the International Collaborative Multicentre DOse REsponse Initiative (DoReMi) [4], the difference is the "down-time" from therapy that is dialysis time window in which CRRT machine does not work [4]. The down-time during dialysis can be due to bag and/or circuit exchanges (for early coagulation, interruption for diagnostic/ therapeutic procedures and other), during periods of inactivity or low efficiency dialysis for vascular access problems (real dialysis flow rate lower than prescribed), or even in the dialysis prescription errors. In quantitative terms, the difference between the prescribed and delivered dose is usually significant, reaching the 30–40 % of the total daily prescribed dose [4, 5].

8.2.2   Calculation of Dialysis Dose

The exact calculation of delivered dialysis dose needs the direct measurement of solutes in effluent, in order to calculate solutes mass transfer and clearance. Since these measurements are not feasible in clinical practice, taking into account SC of urea is equal to 1 the urea effluent concentration is considered equal to blood concentration. Therefore, volume of effluent is clearance of urea, the low-molecular weight nitrogen catabolite. However, the concept of a direct relationship between effluent volume and urea clearance has some important limitations: (1) there is no proof that toxicity in acute uremic patients is due to urea, or that urea is a good marker of uremic toxicity; (2) where urea was a good marker, measurement of dialysis dose should be done in patients with a stable urea generation and predictable urea distribution volume, conditions not appropriate for critically ill ICU patients; (3) if it is correct that effluent volume is equal to clearance in postdilution CVVHF, this is not the case in predilution CVVHF, or in HV-HF (at high flow rate exchanges); (4) clearance of metabolites in medium–high-molecular weight range (1,000–10,000 Da) is meaningful only in hemofiltration/hemodialfiltration, and concerned only with low protein binding solutes.

Keeping in mind all these limitations, in clinical large trials effluent dose is the usual way to calculate the dialysis dose. Dialysis dose is usually expressed as L/h or ml/Kg/hour, or better with ml/Kg/day (in the latter case, also PIRRT could be compared with continuous treatments) [6].

8.2.3 Dialysis Dose and Survival

A relationship between dialysis dose and survival was first reported in 1996 by Paganini et al. [7]. By stratifying clinical severity of disease and dialysis dose in 842 patients treated with intermittent hemodialysis or CRRT, Paganini et al. demonstrated that survival of the extreme less serious cases and more serious ones were not affected by the dialysis dose, and that in these patients mortality was related to severity of illness score regardless of the dose of dialysis. In contrast, in patients with intermediate illness score, survival improved proportionally to the increased dialysis dose [7]. In 2000 a randomized monocentric trial involving 425 patients Ronco et al. confirmed a significant increase in survival with increasing dialysis dose, and established a dialysis dose of 35 ml/Kg/h as optimal survival target [8].

However, more recently two large polycentric randomized studies involving more than 2,000 patients in United States and Australia/New Zealand (ATN Study and RENAL Study) [9, 10] compared a dialysis dose "normal" (20–25 ml/Kg/day) to a "more intensive" dialysis dose (35–40 ml/Kg/day). Both 2 trials failed to demonstrat any advantage with increasing dialysis dose [9, 10]. In details:

– ATN study: comparison in CVVHDF between a prescribed "normal" dose of 20 ml/Kg/hour (hemodynamic unstable patients) or intermittent 3 times a week HDF (hemodynamically stable patients) versus an "intensive" dose of 35 ml/Kg/h in CVVHDF (hemodynamically unstable patients) or daily intermittent HDF (hemodynamically stable patients) [9]. Intensive dose did not demonstrate any added benefit to normal dose (cumulative mortality rate in intensive and normal dose groups: 53.5 vs. 51.5 %, p 0.10), including analysis done in subgroups of septic patients and of those treated with vasopressor amines [9].

– RENAL Study: comparison in CVVHDF between a prescribed "normal" dose of 25 ml/Kg/h versus an "intensive" dose of 40 ml/Kg/h [10]. Mortality at 90 days was 44.7 % in "normal" dose versus 44.7 % in "intensive" dose (p 0.99).

Keeping in mind that in patients with AKI in ICU uremia per se is an independent risk factor of mortality [11]; nowadays, suggested prescription of dialysis dose for patients in ICU with AKI (in CRRT or in PIRRT) is 20–25 ml/kg/h, or better expressed as 480–600 ml/Kg/day [5, 12].

8.3   Anticoagulation of Extracorporeal Circuit

In critically ill patients, the main limit of application of CRRT remains the need of an efficient anticoagulation of the extracorporeal circuit to prevent its premature clotting. Even if in most cases systemic anticoagulation is an invasive procedure, there are many good reasons to obtain a clinical effective anticoagulation of extracorporeal circuit (Table 8.1).

However, bleeding is really of clinical significance as its incidence is high (varies from 4 to 23 %). A bleeding from cruel or surgical wounds, or from tracheostomy tube, gastrointestinal tract or upper respiratory tract mucosa during suction maneuvers are serious complications. When bleeding occurs it will always affect heparin anticoagulation protocol in a restrictive diagram [13].

During the development of extracorporeal circulation hirudin extracted from leeches was the first applied anticoagulant. Then, at the end of 1920s heparin extracted from pig intestinal mucosa was available in pure enough quantity.

After more than 90 years from its appearance unfractionated heparin (UFH) and low-molecular weight heparin (LMWH) are still the most systemic anticoagulant used in the world in maintaining patency of extracorporeal circuit. However, alternative anticoagulation methods designed to avoid bleeding as heparin main side adverse effect has been proposed and applied with mixed success. These alternative methods include systemic anticoagulation methods (heparinoids, thrombin inhibitors, nafamostat, prostacyclin) and regional methods (saline flushes, protamine-heparin, citrate) (Table 8.2).

Undoubtedly regional anticoagulation methods are the most interesting, because in this case anticoagulation is virtually restricted to extracorporeal circuit. Among these methods, citrate is now emerging as an effective, safe, and feasible technique. In recent KDIGO guidelines citrate is suggested as choice anticoagulant during RRT in ICUs [14].

8.3.1   Unfractionated Heparin and Low-Molecular Weight Heparin

UFH is a mixture of branched glycosaminoglycans ranging from 3,000 to 30,000 Da with a mean molecular weight of 15,000 Da (about 45 monosaccharide

Table 8.1 Consequences of a premature loss of extracorporeal circuit

The premature loss of coagulation reduces the actual dialysis time and increases down-time
A high rate of circuit clotting means anemia and needs more frequent blood transfusions
A high coagulation rate of circuit leads on the long term:
to an increased workload of the nursing staff
to an increased stress during work
to an increased general cost of RRT

Table 8.2 Types of extracorporeal circuit anticoagulation

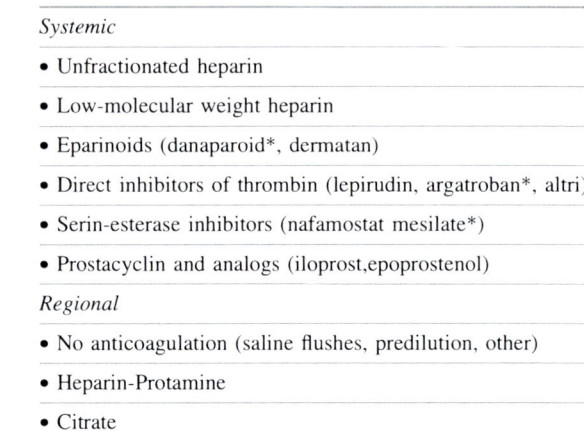

Systemic
• Unfractionated heparin
• Low-molecular weight heparin
• Eparinoids (danaparoid*, dermatan)
• Direct inhibitors of thrombin (lepirudin, argatroban*, altri)
• Serin-esterase inhibitors (nafamostat mesilate*)
• Prostacyclin and analogs (iloprost,epoprostenol)
Regional
• No anticoagulation (saline flushes, predilution, other)
• Heparin-Protamine
• Citrate

unit). On the contrary, LMWH is a more homogeneous glycosaminoglycans composition with a mean molecular weight of 5,000–6,000 Da (less than 18 monosaccharide units) (Fig. 8.3).

Anticoagulant activity of UFH is mainly due to its interaction with antithrombin III (ATIII) and subsequent formation of heparin–antithrombin complex (Heparin-AT) with ATIII consumption. Heparin-AT complex changes ATIII inhibitory activity on thrombin, physiologically slow and progressive, in a rapid and

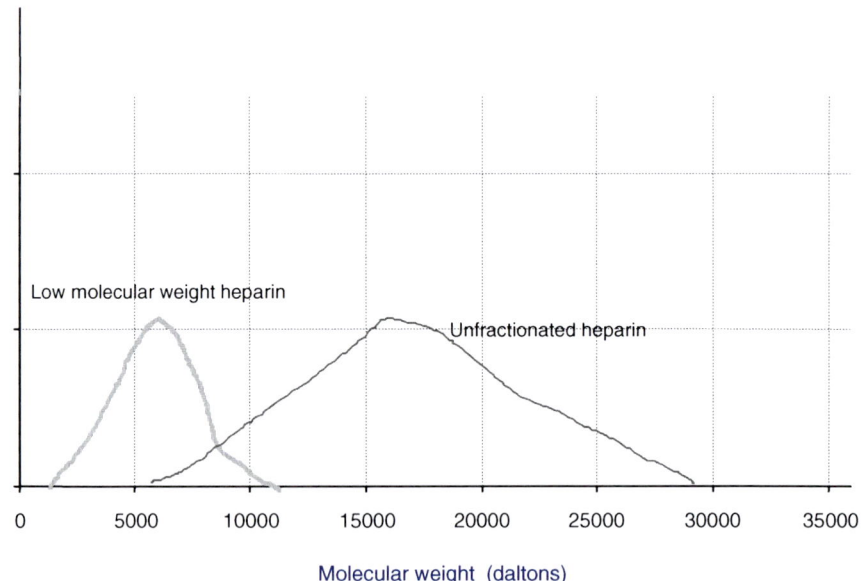

Fig. 8.3 Unfractionated heparin and low-molecular weight heparin

irreversible inhibition on thrombin. Heparin binds ATIII by a well defined pentasaccharide sequence, which has been recently synthesized and constitutes the new heparinoid anticoagulant fondaparinux.

As to differentiate between UHF and LMWH, it should be highlighted that: (1) inhibitory activity to thrombin needs the formation of a trimolecular complex given by heparin-ATIII complex (via the pentasaccharide sequence specific binding) and thrombin (via non-specific charge binding between heparin and thrombin); (2) thrombin is about 10 times more sensitive to inhibition of heparin-ATIII complex compared to factor Xa, thus thrombin is the main target of anti-coagulation activity of UHF; (3) inhibitory activity to factor Xa requires only the specific binding between the heparin-ATIII complex by pentasaccharide sequence; (4) by administering a bolus dose of UFH, only one-third of the dose can bind to ATIII to form the complex heparin-ATIII.

Therefore, LMWH (less than 18 monosaccharide molecules) loses the ability to inhibit thrombin (LMWH is not able to tie together thrombin and heparin), but keeps the ability to inhibit factor Xa by pentasaccharide sequence.

As to elimination of UFH, heparin high-molecular weight molecules have two mechanisms of clearance: (1) a cellular clearance, due to the binding of heparin to endothelium and macrophage receptors, which in turn promote the removal of heparin from bloodstream by a fast and saturable mechanism; (2) a renal clearance, characterized by a slow elimination kinetics and not saturable mechanism. Based on this elimination kinetics, LMWH (and the fraction of UFH of lower molecular weight) has only the renal clearance. In addition during CRRT LMWH clearance by filter is negligible even with highly permeable membranes [15].

Acute Phase Reactants proteins can affect in vivo UFH anticoagulant activity. As a matter of fact, UFH is a polyanion able to bind in an aspecific way many plasma proteins. This aspecific binding reduces UFH anticoagulant activity, and unpredictably contributes to so-called phenomenon of "UFH resistance".

Apparent biological half-life of UFH is dose-dependent, and varies from 30 min after a bolus dose of 25 U/Kg up to 60 and 150 min observed after a bolus dose of 100 and 400 U/Kg, respectively. LMWH has a more predictable and much longer half-life, tending to accumulate over time. Curiously, after administration of UFH the part of low-molecular weight heparins present in UFH mixture tends to accumulate more and more. As a result, using UFH continuously over days anti-coagulant activity of heparin will change with a decrease of antifactor-IIa/anti-Xa activity ratio.

From these physiological basis it comes out that in patients with AKI in CRRT without residual diuresis the use of UFH leads to anticoagulant effects not easily predictable.

In last 10 years in western countries LMWH is becoming the standard anti-coagulant in chronic hemodialysis patients [15]. Conversely, LMWH in ICUs in patients treated with CRRT has failed to demonstrate any advantage (drug safety and filter life) in comparison to UFH [16–18]. In addition, daily costs of LMWH anticoagulant, including assays, are higher by about 10 % than of UHF anticoagulant [19].

Recommended dose of UFH in patients on CRRT is 1,000–2,500 IU as initial bolus, followed by 5–10 IU/Kg/h with a PTT target of 1–1.4 times.

Recommended dose of LMWH (nadroparin, enoxaparin, and dalteparin) in patients at bleeding risk should reach a anti-Xa activity target of 0.25–0.35 IU/ml.

8.3.2 Regional Citrate Anticoagulation

Citrate has been used in hemodialysis for the first time in 1960 by Morita et al. [20]. Thirty years later citrate, revised by Mehta et al. has been successfully applied as RCA in critically ill patients on CRRT [21]. Nowadays, 20 years after first experience in ICU impact of RCA on renal and intensivist practice is real and increasing. RCA is supposed to spread more and more because of increasing experience of staff, of availability of dedicated monitors and materials and of operational protocols simple and adaptable to the patient needs.

RCA is mainly popular in North America and Northern Europe. Since 1999 in Calgary (Canada) a standard system of anticoagulation with heparin alternative to RCA has been implemented for all CRRT [22]. Based on pediatric registry of CRRT in North America, 56 % of CRRT sessions are now done with RCA [23]. In the same way, in Italy RCA is in rapid development, although the available data are few. In a survey of dialysis practice of the year 2007 in Northwest Italy (4.5 million inhabitants with global data concerning all ICUs) anticoagulant heparin was by far the most widespread (5,296 on 7,842 days of dialysis, 67.5 % of cases) [24]. However, in patients at high risk of bleeding RCA was performed in 18 % of cases [24] in 2007, but it reached 25 % of all treatments in 2009 (unpublished data).

Based on these data an increase of RCA indications has been suggested by recent guidelines recommending RCA as standard anticoagulant for extracorporeal circuit in ICUs [14].

8.3.2.1 Extracorporeal Circuit During Regional Citrate Anticoagulation

Citrate is infused at the beginning of extracorporeal circuit. Citrate binds ionized calcium (iCa ++) and magnesium. In extracorporeal circuit citrate usually reaches a concentration of 3–5 mmol/L, whereas iCa ++ concentration decreases at 0.4–0.2 mmol/L. Since enzymes of coagulation cascade are iCa ++-dependent, blood clotting capacity inversely decreases. It should be noted that filter membranes are freely permeable to citrate (molecular weight 192 Da). Therefore, of whole citrate entering in filter a part (at about half as Ca ++-citrate complex) is lost in effluent (or dialysate), and the remaining part enters to patient by circuit venous line. During RCA inlet dialysate is Ca ++-free, and Ca ++ (iCa ++ or complexes Ca ++-citrate) is lost in effluent. Infusion of Ca ++ at the end of circuit line is only meant to replace the amount of Ca ++ lost in effluent, which is directly proportional to effluent volume (Fig. 8.4) [25].

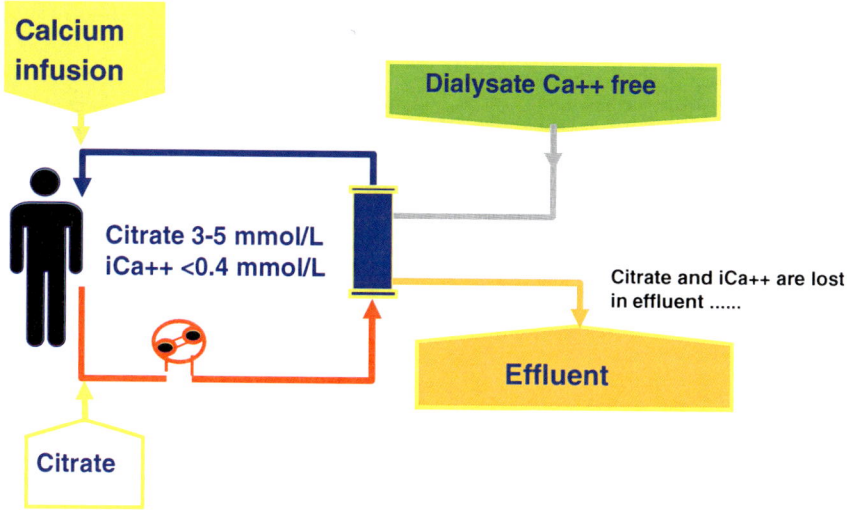

Fig. 8.4 Regional citrate anticoagulation during CVVHDF (or HF/HD)

The amount of citrate (as Ca ++-citrate complexes) entering patient through circuit venous line is rapidly metabolized to bicarbonates in liver, muscle, and kidney.

8.3.2.2 Efficacy and Safety of Citrate

In comparison to heparin citrate is capable of maintaining the circuit patency for equal time, if not longer [12, 22, 26, 27]. A comparison among different studies is not easy, because they are monocentric and evaluated different populations. Circuit life can be affected both by factors inherent to studied patient such as procoagulant patient capacity, platelet counts, levels of ATIII, sepsis, or by factors inherent to dialysis such as membrane type, convective flux, filtration fraction, predilution, vascular access efficiency, blood flow rate, and type of monitoring and alarm circuit intervention.

In addition, during RCA circuit survival is strongly affected by citratemia reached in extracorporeal circuit varying from 2 to 5 mmol/l (mean citratemia 4 mmol/L) [21–23, 25–27]. As a matter of fact, for increasing values of citratemia (from 2 to 6 mmol/L) values of iCa ++ inversely decrease (from 0.5 to 0.1 mmol/L). At level of 6 mmol/L of citratemia iCa ++ concentration is 0.1 mmol/L, and blood coagulation is inhibited.

8.3.2.3 Metabolism and Kinetics of Citrate

After infusion plasma citrate is rapidly uptaken by liver, kidney, and muscle. Citrate enters citric acid cycle, generates bicarbonate and consumes H^+. In quantitative terms, liver is the most important metabolic site of citrate.

Table 8.3 Metabolic alteration clinical data

• Increased citratemia	–	Increased citratemia
(= failure of citrate metabolization)	–	Increased anion gap
	–	Total Ca/iCa ++ > 2.5
	–	Hypocalcemia/
	–	Hypomagnesiemia
• Excess of buffer	–	Metabolic alkalosis
(= from metabolized citrate)		
• Excess di sodium-citrate	–	Hypernatremia
• Inappropriate calcium infusion	–	Hypo/hypercalcemia

During RCA some metabolic alterations can arise including: (1) an excessive citrate metabolism with systemic alkalosis; (2) accumulation of citrate for impaired metabolism, with hypocalcemia/hypomagnesemia, or total Ca ++/iCa ++ ratio >2.5 (or better demonstrated by citratemia dosage) [25]. When citrate accumulates iCa ++ concentration decreases whereas total Ca ++ concentration is constant. Therefore, total Ca ++/iCa ++ ratio increase is more accurate marker of citrate accumulation than iCa ++ decrease; (3) hypernatremia, most often seen in the past with old protocols of RCA (Table 8.3).

In general, in all studies assessing metabolic alterations during RCA (cumulative total of 770 patients) metabolic tolerance was good, with no significant

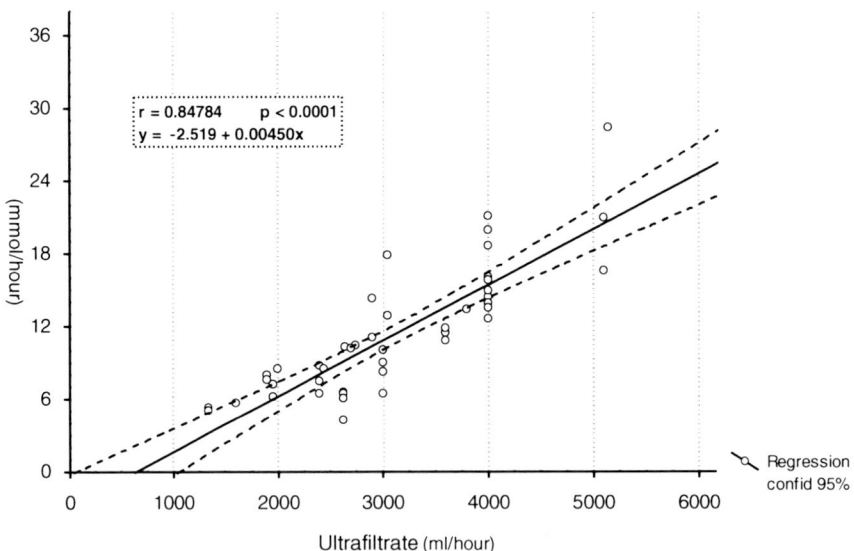

Fig. 8.5 Absolute citrate loss is directly related to effluent volume

electrolyte and acid-base alterations [25–27]. Risk of hypernatremia is usually prevented by using dialysate solutions containing lower sodium concentration, such as 120–132 mEq/L, and by providing a dialysate flow rate as high as able to enhance diffusive clearance of Na^+ [12, 25–27].

In addition, in populations at risk of citrate accumulation the optimization of diffusive clearance in order to increase citrate loss in effluent allowed an excellent acid-base control [12, 25]. Citrate losses in effluent can be usefully exploited to reduce its metabolic load to patient. As shown in Fig. 8.5, in CVVHDF at blood flow ranging from 100 to 150 ml/min and at effluent flow ranging from 1,200 to 5,000 ml/hour, losses of citrate in effluent were directly related to effluent volume, and can reach up to 70 % of citrate amount passing the filter [25].

References

1. Kramer P, Wigger W, Rieger J, Matthaei D, Scheler F (1977) Arteriovenous haemofiltration: a new and simple method for treatment of over-hydrated patients resistant to diuretics. Klin Wochenschr 55:1121–1122
2. Schiffl H, Lang SM, Fischer R (2002) Daily hemodialysis and the outcome of acute renal failure. N Engl J Med 346:305–310
3. Vinsonneau C, Camus C, Combes A et al (2006) Continuous venovenous haemodiafiltration versus intermittent haemodialysis for acute renal failure in patients with multiple-organ dysfunction syndrome: a multicentre randomised trial. Lancet 368:379–385
4. Vesconi S, Cruz DN, Fumagalli R et al (2009) Dose Response Multicentre International collaborative Initiative (DO-RE-MI Study Group). Delivered dose of renal replacement therapy and mortality in critically ill patients with acute kidney injury. Crit Care 13(2):R57
5. Kellum JA, Ronco C (2010) Dialysis: results of renal: what is the optimal CRRT target dose? Nat Rev Nephrol 6:191–192
6. Granado RC, Macedo E, Chertow GM et al (2011) Effluent volume in continuous renal replacement therapy overestimates the delivered dose of dialysis. Clin J Am Soc Nephrol 6:467–475
7. Paganini EP, Tapolyai M, Goormastic M (1996) Establishing a dialysis therapy/patient outcome link in intensive care unit acute dialysis for patients with acute renal failure. Am J Kidney Dis 28(3):S81–S89
8. Ronco C, Bellomo R, Homel P et al (2000) Effects of different doses in continuous veno-venous haemofiltration on outcomes of acute renal failure: a prospective randomised trial. Lancet 356:26–30
9. VA/NIH Acute Renal Failure Trial Network (2008) Intensity of renal support in critically ill patients with acute kidney injury. N Engl J Med 359:7–20
10. RENAL Replacement Therapy Study Investigators (2009) Intensity of continuous renal-replacement therapy in critically ill patients. N Engl J Med 361:1627–1638
11. Metnitz PG, Krenn CG, Steltzer H et al (2002) Effect of acute renal failure requiring renal replacement therapy on outcome in critically ill patients. Crit Care Med 30:2051–2058
12. Mariano F, Tedeschi L, Morselli M, Stella M, Triolo G (2010) Normal citratemia and metabolic tolerance of citrate anticoagulation for hemodiafiltration in severe septic shock burn patients. Intensive Care Med 36:1735–1743
13. van de Wetering J, Westendorp RG, van der Hoeven JG et al (1996) Heparin use in continuous renal replacement procedures: the struggle between filter coagulation and patient hemorrhage. J Am Soc Nephrol 7:145–150

14. Khwaja A (2012) KDIGO clinical practice guidelines for acute kidney injury. Nephron Clin Pract 120:179–184

15. Davenport A (2009) Review article: Low-molecular-weight heparin as an alternative anticoagulant to unfractionated heparin for routine outpatient haemodialysis treatments. Nephrology 14:455–461

16. Reeves JH, Cumming AR, Gallagher L, O'Brien JL, Santamaria JD (1999) A controlled trial of low-molecular-weight heparin (dalteparin) versus unfractionated heparin as anticoagulant during continuous venovenous hemodialysis with filtration. Crit Care Med 27:2224–2228

17. Jeffrey RF, Khan AA, Douglas JT, Will EJ, Davison AM (1993) Anticoagulation with low molecular weight heparin (Fragmin) during continuous hemodialysis in the intensive care unit. Artif Organs 17:717–720

18. de Pont AC, Oudemans-van Straaten HM, Roozendaal KJ, Zandstra DF (2000). Nadroparin versus dalteparin anticoagulation in high-volume, continuous venovenous hemofiltration: a double-blind, randomized, crossover study. Crit Care Med 28:421–425

19. Mariano F (2012) Il citrato: un diverso approccio mentale all'anticoagulazione del circuito extracorporeo. G Ital Nefrol 19:27–32

20. Morita Y, Johnson RW, Dorn RE, Hall DS (1961) Regional anticoagulation during hemodialysis using citrate. Am J Med Sci 242:32–43

21. Mehta RL, McDonald BR, Aguilar MM, Ward DM (1990) Regional citrate anticoagulation for continuous arteriovenous hemodialysis in critically ill patients. Kidney Int 38:976–981

22. Bagshaw SM, Laupland KB, Boiteau PJ, Godinez-Luna T (2005) Is regional citrate superior to systemic heparin anticoagulation for continuous renal replacement therapy? A prospective observational study in an adult regional critical care system. J Crit Care 20:155–161

23. Symons JM, Chua AN, Somers MJ et al (2007) Demographic characteristics of pediatric continuous renal replacement therapy: a report of the Prospective Pediatric Continuous Renal Replacement Therapy Registry. Clin J Am Soc Nephrol 2:732–738

24. Mariano F, Pozzato M, Canepari G et al (2011) Renal replacement therapy in intensive care units: a survey of nephrological practice in northwest Italy. J Nephrol 24:165–176

25. Mariano F, Morselli M, Bergamo D et al (2011) Blood and ultrafiltrate dosage of citrate as a useful and routine tool during continuous venovenous haemodiafiltration in septic shock patients. Nephrol Dial Transplant 26:3882–3888

26. Morgera S, Schneider M, Slowinski T et al (2009) A safe citrate anticoagulation protocol with variable treatment efficacy and excellent control of the acid-base status. Crit Care Med 37:2018–2024

27. Oudemans-van Straaten HM, Bosman RJ, Koopmans M et al (2009) Citrate anticoagulation for continuous venovenous hemofiltration. Crit Care Med 37:545–552

Loss of Self-Regulation in Interstitial Fluid Dynamics of Septic Patients, and Oedema Development Patterns

9

Emanuela Biagioni and Massimo Girardis

Imagine if in the drawer of the night table next to our patients there was a recent picture of them: we would often look at it, in order to see what is changing in them and how. When we first let our patients' relatives in ICU one of our major concerns is to prepare them to see their loved ones subject to a series of medical treatments that may be difficult to understand and accept. However, rarely has anyone been impressed by an orotracheal tube or by a central catheter, the most frequent question being instead "Why is he so swollen... look at his face, his hands... I could barely recognize him... will he return like he was before?" This question often catches us unprepared. We are accustomed to see our patients get some kilos in a few hours, without even noticing it, so we usually answer: "It's normal, do not worry, we had to give him a lot of liquids. Oedema is the less concerning of his current issues. You will see: he will regain his former shape when he will recover". But the question remains: is this always true? In the next paragraphs, we will describe the patterns behind the formation of oedema in patients with severe sepsis, the pivotal role of endothelial cells, the aftermaths of oedemas in organ functions and some possible present and future therapeutic treatments.

E. Biagioni · M. Girardis (✉)
Intensive Care Unit, University Hospital of Modena, L.go del Pozzo 71,
41125 Modena, Italy
e-mail: Girardis.massimo@unimo.it

E. Biagioni
e-mail: emanuela545@katamail.com

B. Allaria (ed.), *Practical Issues in Anesthesia and Intensive Care 2013*,
DOI: 10.1007/978-88-470-5529-2_9, © Springer-Verlag Italia 2014

9.1   Endotelium: A "Variable" and Very "Busy" Tissue

Visible changes occurring in our patients can be compared to structural and functional—though less visible—alterations of single cells and tissues—such as red blood cells, neutrophil granulocytes and, in particular, the endothelial system. In critical patients in general, and in septic ones in particular, the response of the host against a pathogen cause involves a multitude of cells and systems. Its final effect is that of modifying vascular homeostasis through the endothelium [1].

The endothelium is composed of around 1 trillion cells; it covers the internal surface of the whole vascular tree (4–7,000 m^2, almost a soccer pitch) and must be considered an organ in itself (it weighs 1 Kg). It has very diverse features and functions that are very likely to change over time. Positioned between plasma and tissues, the main features of the endothelium are to help blood coagulation, to fight inflammations, to preserve vascular tone and, moreover, to allow for the exchange of fluids and solutes through vascular permeability regulation [1, 2].

9.1.1   Endothelium and Coagulation

A healthy endothelium inhibits the aggregation of platelets through inducible or constituent production of nitrogen oxide (NO) and prostacyclin (PGI$_2$). Furthermore, the endothelial reception for vitamin C (EPCR) facilitates the activation of plasmatic protein C; this transforms the enzymatic property of thrombin to activate its habitual substrates (fibrinogen and platelet receptors) in an activity of indirect inhibition [3]. Endothelial cells also play a pivotal role in controlling fibrinolysis, because they are the main tissue activators of plasminogen (t-PA) and other fibrinolysis' activators, such as urokinase (u-PA) [3, 4]. In physiopathology of sepsis, the endothelium plays a pivotal role, in particular as far as the loss of balance of the haemostatic system is concerned. When the endothelium is stimulated—e.g. by the inflammatory response to an infection, but also by a trauma—it gives start to coagulation cascade and releases the plasminogen activator inhibitor (PAl-1). Similarly, the activation of specific cytokines (IL-1, IL-6 and TNFα) reduces the endothelial expression of glycosaminoglycan by acting as a pro-coagulant, inhibiting the activation of anti-thrombin [5]. The main consequence of that is an endothelial unbalance of the haemostasis, with an evident pro-coagulant trend, in patients suffering from infection and systemic inflammatory response. This trend determines the formation of micro-thrombi at the microcirculatory level and, therefore, an inadequate tissue perfusion and oxygenation leading ultimately to cell dysoxia. This explains the potential protective activity of anti-thrombotic drugs (e.g. antithrombin, heparins, recombinant activated protein C) in patients suffering from severe sepsis. As we already know, though, none of these anticoagulation drugs has proven efficient in reducing sepsis mortality rates, at least according to the rules of current medicine, based on evidence.

9.1.2   Endothelium and Vascular Tone

At a parietal level, the endothelium is responsible for the modulation of vascular tone through NO production. NO is a powerful systemic vasodilator. NO production is carried out both directly and indirectly, through the activation of an inducible enzyme (nitroxide synthase). NO causes vasodilation by activating sensitive potassium calcium channels; these channels hurdle endogen and hexogen vasoconstrictor agents. Other vasodilation factors produced by the endothelium are the hyperpolarising factor (EDHF) and (PGI$_2$). Endothelial cells also produce vasoconstrictive substances such as prostaglandins (PGH2), endotheline-1 (ET-1) and thromboxane A2 (TXA2) [6]. It is widely known that endothelial NO production regulation in patients suffering from infections and sepsis is strongly compromised, the phenomenon is jeopardised in various tissue districts and this leads to irregular organ perfusion. In general, during the early stages of sepsis we can observe an increase in local NO production due to inducible upregulation of NO-synthetase, determined by systemic inflammatory response. However, this situation changes over time, depending on the microorganism and on the host's response; and this generates a new situation with low-perfusion and high-perfusion tissues. Attempts to control the mechanisms behind district NO overproduction in sepsis with monoclonal antibodies have failed.

9.1.3   Endothelium and Oedema

Endovascular endothelium behaves like a semipermeable membrane, which regulates the passage of small and medium size molecules through arteries, capillaries and venules. The passage of these solutes is carried out on a trans-cellular basis (e.g. vesicular transportation of albumin) or on a paracellular one (by exploiting the junctions between endothelial cells). Junctions are made of transmembrane proteins that leave a rather wide space for the passage of solutes (i.e. adherens junctions (AJ)) or a tighter one (i.e. tight junction (TJ)). The forces that regulate capillary filtration (that is to say, the direction and flow of movement of water and solute from the endovascular space to the interstitium and vice versa) are the hydrostatic pressure and the colloidal osmotic pressure.

Hydrostatic pressure depends on arterial pressure and on pre- and post-capillary resistances, and represents the force the blood exerts on blood vessel walls. Vascular endothelium can respond to certain stimuli through an increase in intracellular levels of Ca^{++} and protein kinase C. The liberation of these substances at cytoplasmic level modulates intracellular transmission, and this leads to the contraction of smooth muscle cells. As a result, hydrostatic pressure and permeability increase, leading to an improvement in filtration levels.

The key factor preventing the passage of fluids from the endoluminal space to the interstitial one is the colloidal osmotic pressure of the endovascular fluids [7–9] which is, in the systemic district, simply colloidal pressure (also known as oncotic

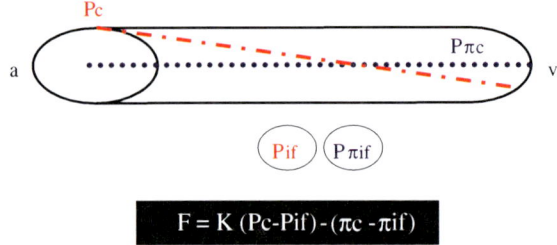

Fig. 9.1 Capillary filtration and osmotic-hydrostatic balance

$$F = K\,(Pc\text{-}Pif)\text{-}(\pi c\,\text{-}\pi if)$$

pressure) because the endothelial membrane is permeable to the main osmotically active solutes: their movements follow those of fluids thanks to diffusive mechanisms, which are regulated by the presence of a concentration gradient. When the oncotic pressure overcomes the hydrostatic one in the endovascular space, fluids can start moving in the opposite direction (reabsorption). In physiological conditions, the filtration of liquids and solutes exceeds reabsorption in the venous capillary system (5–7 l in 24 h). This excess of fluids enters systemic circulation through lymphatic capillaries, covered by a subtle layer of endothelial cells, whose characteristics—similar to those of venules—facilitate reabsorption [9] (see Fig. 9.1).

9.2 Endothelium and Sepsis: Why Does My Patient Swell?

Essential prerequisite for fluid homeostasis is the structural and functional integrity of the endothelium. Any phenomenon producing an alteration of endothelial mechanisms can cause imbalances in the process of capillary filtration leading to the development of tissue oedema. Microorganisms and bacterial endotoxins can determine, in addition, direct endothelial damage with structural alterations that increase permeability, allowing for the passage of circulating elements from one side to the other. Moreover, infectious processes and the inflammatory response increase the concentration of circulating cytokines, such as IL6, IL8 and TNFα, determining endothelial alterations that, ultimately, lead to a complete dysregulation of cellular functions. In the case of infections, in addition, one of the pathophysiological functions of the endothelium is to activate neutrophils through the release of chemotactic substances. Neutrophils bind to the endothelial cell through adhesion molecules expressed on the surface of the cell itself (ICAM-1, ELAM-1 and selectins). The intracellular response of the endothelial cell to the binding of neutrophils is an increased permeability leading to the passage of blood cells and other macromolecules [6, 10]. It follows an increase in the presence of liquid with a high protein content in the interstitium, causing oedemas. Thanks to the use of direct immunofluorescence, some studies have identified the presence of damaged endothelial cells in circulation during a septic shock, and their concentration is closely related to the severity of the condition and the survival probability of the patient [11]. The study of sepsis and other typical conditions of patients with critical endothelial damage justifies the recent interest in the possibility of measuring the degree of endothelial dysfunction. This term is generally defined as the imbalance between vasoconstriction and vasodilation in the circulatory apparatus in the area affected by endothelial damage and oedema. At the present time, no currently existing marker of endothelial damage has proved sufficiently accessible and reliable to be recommended in clinical use [12].

The appearance of interstitial oedema, according to the mechanisms described above, assumes great importance in the pathophysiology of sepsis-induced organ dysfunction. The development of oedema leads to an increase in the distance between cells and capillaries making it difficult to maintain adequate oxygenation of more distant cells from the capillary axis. This phenomenon is associated, during sepsis, with other alterations (see above) that reduce tissue perfusion, thus exposing some organs at high risk of cell dysoxia followed by cellular apoptosis and finally organ dysfunction [13, 14]. Reperfusion injury associated with ischaemia due to deficient perfusion further stimulates the production by endothelial cells of oxygen radicals leading to inflammatory cascade and increased permeability.

9.3   Endothelium, Oedema and Sepsis: What Can I Do?

The development of tissue oedema, typical of patients with sepsis determines, among other things, a state of relative hypovolemia with altered haemodynamic conditions characterised by reduced cardiac output and average perfusion pressure. In order to ensure adequate oxygen supply to the tissues and to improve the macro-haemodynamic condition, the therapeutic strategy suggested by the guidelines of the Surviving Sepsis Campaign provide for a volume expansion by means of colloid or crystalloid solutions and produced by the central venous pressure [15]. Bear in mind that despite the demonstrated effectiveness of fluid resuscitation in patients suffering from septic shock in emergency departments, doubts remain as to its efficacy in patients with severe sepsis as well as in the case of septic shock in surgical patients. In addition, a positive fluid balance is associated with an increased risk of death in patients hospitalised in intensive care with septic shock. With reference to the open question on whether it is preferable to use crystalloids or colloids, a randomised controlled study of nearly 800 patients with severe sepsis showed that resuscitation with synthetic colloids, as compared to Ringer's acetate, is associated with an increased risk of death in the first 90 days, as well as with an increase in the need to resort to renal extracorporeal purification techniques [16].

The evidence that the endothelium plays an important pathophysiological role has also suggested the possibility of considering this "organ" a therapeutic target for improving the survival of critically ill patients, and there are a number of targeted therapies aimed at restoring microvascular and endothelial homeostasis [17–20]. Intravenously administered methylene blue is able to act by means of the guanosine monophosphate system in the inhibition of nitric oxide synthase, thus reducing the production of NO.

Some studies suggest that the infusion of methylene blue in patients with refractory septic shock can improve the values relating to mean arterial pressure and cardiac output determining a better endothelial response to endogenous and exogenous vasoconstrictors. There are serious concerns about the effects produced by the inhibition of NO production at the level of the splanchnic area, where excessive vasoconstriction can cause poor organ perfusion. Also, the effects on the pulmonary circulation may be negative, especially at high doses as they may limit hypoxic vasoconstriction. At present, there is no evidence on what the right dose of methylene blue may be, and treatments with methylene blue should be considered a rescue therapy in refractory septic shock [21].

According to recent theories, the overproduction of NO during a septic shock would be a "positive" adaptive response to the pathogenic agent to improve organ perfusion and to prevent micro-capillary thrombosis. During oxidative stress, such as the activation/endothelial damage in patients with sepsis, neutrophil activation produces superoxide, a cytotoxic agent that contributes to the consumption of NO by reacting with its radical form and forming a highly reactive molecule, i.e. peroxynitrite [1, 19]. A number of studies have evaluated the efficacy of drugs providing NO groups (e.g. nitro-glycerine), but despite the interesting pathophysiological hypothesis, results are not yet conclusive to recommend their use in clinical practice.

Another molecule capable of acting with a protective anti-inflammatory and antioxidant effect at endothelial level seems to be selenium. Some researchers have shown low levels of selenium in patients with oxidative stress and a recent meta-analytic study, which included 10 randomized controlled trials, showed that exogenous administration of selenium in critically ill patients is associated with a reduced risk of death [21]. However, a randomized controlled trial published in 2007 showed no advantage in the use of selenium in patients with septic shock [22]. Selenium has been included in the guidelines for the treatment of patients with severe sepsis and septic shock by the German Sepsis Network with indication of level C [23] but, in the light of recent clinical trials, its effects in patients with septic shock must be defined more precisely [24].

Regarding the problem of endothelial injury and oedema development, it has recently been demonstrated in animal models that the use of a specific recombinant protein called Slit, which belongs to the control system of the endothelial permeability, together with the receptor called Robo, allows a reduction of endothelial lesions and in particular endothelial permeability determined by endotoxins and cytokines [25]. This approach appears promising and surely, if these effects will be demonstrated also on humans, the use of specific therapies to reduce the development of interstitial oedema will have wider applications in the treatment of critically ill—septic and non-septic—patients in the future [26].

9.4 Conclusion

Attempts to effectively intervene on sepsis mechanisms by correcting the dysfunction and the pathological activation of microcirculation—and, therefore, of the endothelium—represent the most fascinating challenge for physicians and researchers dealing with these patients. However, to date there is no evidence that specific therapeutic strategies aimed at controlling micro-vascular endothelium may, in patients suffering septic shock, provide clinical benefits and increased survival probability. As for oedema and sepsis, the news is even worse: we know that the formation of oedema is a constant in patients with sepsis, we know that the development of oedema can cause the deterioration of organ functioning due to deficient perfusion and cellular oxygenation and we know that, unfortunately, today there is no effective drug nor winning strategy. In the light of all this, the concern expressed by the wife of my patient was well grounded and maybe I should worry a little more too.

References

1. Parodi O, De Chiara B, Campolo J, Sedda V, Roubina E (2006) Endothelial dysfunction and oxidative stress in sepsis. G Ital Nefrol 36:69–73
2. Dejana E, Mantovani A (1993) Anatomia funzionale. In: Dejana E, Mantovani A (eds) Fisiopatologia dell'endotelio vascolare. Piccin, Padova, pp 7–21
3. Bazzoni G, Dejana E, Mantovani A (2007) Funzioni specifiche delle cellule endoteliali. In: Bazzoni G, Dejana E, Mantovani A L (eds) 'Endotelio, fisiopatologia, basi molecolari, implicazioni terapeutiche. Piccin, Padova, pp 15–23
4. Dejana E, Mantovani A (1993) Regolazione della coagulazione e della fibrinolisi. In: Dejana E, Mantovani A (eds) Fisiopatologia dell'endotelio vascolare. Piccin, Padova, pp 32–40
5. Levi M, Van Der Poll T, Schultz M (2012) New insights into pathways that determine the link between infection and thrombosis. Neth J Med 70:114–120
6. Calò L, Semplicini A (1998) Funzione dell'endotelio normale. In: Calò L, Semplicini A L (eds)'Endotelio vascolare aspetti morfofunzionali fisiopatologici e terapeutici. Piccin, Padova, pp 19–39
7. Bazzoni G, Dejana E, Mantovani A (2007) Anatomia funzionale caratteristiche generali. In: Bazzoni G, Dejana E, Mantovani A L (eds)'Endotelio, fisiopatologia, basi molecolari, implicazioni terapeutiche. Piccin, Padova, pp 1–13
8. Berne RM, Levy MN (1995) La microcircolazione e i linfatici. In: Berne RM, Levy MN (eds) Fisiologia. Casa editrice Ambrosiana, Milano, pp 498–10
9. Huxley VH, Scallan J (2011) Lymphatic fluid: exchange mechanism and regulation. J Physiol 589:2935–2943
10. Schnoor M, Lai FPL, Zarbock A, Klaver R, Polaschegg C, Schulte D, Weich A, Oelkers JM, Rottner K, Vestweber D (2011) Cortactin deficiency is associated with reduced neutrophil recruitment but increased vascular permeability in vivo. J Exp Med 208:1721–1735
11. Mutunga M, Fulton B, Bullock R (2001) Circulating endothelial cells in patients with septic shock. Am J Respir Crit Care Med 163:195–200
12. Paulus P, Jennewein C, Zacharowski K (2011) Biomarkers of endothelial dysfunction: can they help us deciphering systemic inflammation and sepsis? Biomarkers 16(51):511–521
13. Henrich M, Gruss M, Weigand MA (2010) Sepsis-induced degradation of endothelial glycolcalix. Sci World J 18(10):917–923

14. De Backer D, Donatello K, Taccone FS, Ospina-Tascon G, Salgano D, Vincent JL (2011) Microcirculatory alterations: potential mechanism and implications for therapy. Ann Intensive Care 19(1):27

15. Dellinger RP, Levy MM, Carlet JM, Bion J, Parker MM, Jaeschke R, Reinhart K, Angus DC, Brun-Buisson C, Beale R, Calandra T, Dhainaut JF, Gerlach H, Harvey M, Marini JJ, Marshall J, Ranieri M, Ramsay G, Sevransky J, Thompson BT, Townsend S, Vender JS, Zimmerman JL, Vincent JL (2008) Surviving sepsis campaign: international guidelines for management of severe sepsis and septic shock: 2008. Intensive Care Med 34:17–60

16. Perner A, Haase N, Guttormsen AB, Tenhunen J, Klemenzson G, Aneman A, Madsen KR, Moller MH, Helkjaer JM, Poulsen LM, Bendtsen A, Winding R, Steensen M, Berezowicz P, Soe-Jensen P, Bestle M, Strand K, Wiis J, White JO, Thornberg KJ, Quist L, Nielsen J, Andersen LH, Holst LB, Thormar K, Kjaeldgaard AL, Fabritius ML, Mondrup F, Pott FC, Moller TP, Winkel P, Wetterslev J (2012) Hydroxyethyl starch 130/0.42 versus ringer's acetate in severe sepsis. N Engl J Med 367(2):124–134

17. Ruiz C, Hernandez G, Ince C (2010) Diagnosis and treatment of the septic microcirculation. In: Vincent JL (ed) Yearbook of intensive care and emergency medicine. Springer, Berlin, pp 16–26

18. Boyd JH (2010) Targeted treatment of microvascular dysfunction. In: Vincent JL (ed) Yearbook of intensive care and emergency medicine. Springer, Berlin, pp 16–26

19. Trzeciak S, Cinel I, Dellinger RP, Shapiro RI, Arnold RC, Parrillo JE, Hollenberg SM (2008) Resuscitating the microcirculation in sepsis: the central role of nitric oxide, emerging concepts for novel therapies, and challenges for clinical trials. Acad Emerg Med 15(5):399–413

20. Aird WC (2004) Endothelium as an organ system. Crit Care Med 32(5):271–279

21. Juffermans NP, Vervloet MG, Daemen-Gubbels C, Binnekade MdJ, Groeneveld ABJ (2010) A dose-finding study of methylene blue to inhibit nitric oxide actions in the haemodynamic of human septic shock. Nitric Oxide 15(4):275–280

22. Heyland DK (2007) Selenium supplementation in critically ill patients: can too much of a good thing be a bad thing? Crit Care 11:153

23. Reinhart K, Brunkhorst FM, Bone H-G, Bardutzky J, Dempfle C-E, Forst H, et al (2010) Prevention, diagnosis, therapy and follow-up care of sepsis: 1st revision of S-2 k guidelines of the German sepsis society (Deutsche Sepsis-Gesellschaft e.V. (DSG)) and the German Interdisciplinary association of intensive care and emergency medicine (Deutsche Interdisziplinäre Vereinigung für Intensiv- und Notfallmedizin (DIVI)). Ger Med Sci 8: Doc14

24. Forceville X, Laviolle B, Annane D, Vitoux D, Bleichner G, Korach J-M, Cantais E, Georges, H, Soubirou J-L, Combes A, Bellissant E (2007) Effects of high doses of selenium, as sodium selenite, in septic shock: a placebo-controlled, randomized, double-blind, phase II study. Crit. Care 11:R73

25. London NR, Zhu W, Bozza FA, et al (2010) Targeting Robo4-dependentslit signalling to survive the cytokine storm in sepsis and influenza. Sci Transl Med 2:23ra19

26. Lee WL, Slutsky AS (2010) Sepsis and endothelial permeability. N Engl J Med 363(7):689–691

How to Prevent and Effectively Treat Postoperative Shivering

10

Marco Dei Poli

The continuous progress of the anesthetic and surgical techniques and the increase of sophisticated monitoring systems of physiological functions have expanded by far the surgical indications, for both elective and urgent, in patients with compromised or even critical conditions.

Scientific surveys show that 5–30 % of perioperative adverse events occur in the hours that immediately follow the dismission from the operating room, and mostly involve the respiratory and cardiovascular system.

In these conditions a careful monitoring is mandatory: admission to specially equipped structures as environment of critical care units could be recommended.

The monitoring of these patients consist in periodic postoperative evaluation of consciousness, of the respiratory, cardiovascular, neuromuscular function, of temperature, pain, diuresis, surgical drainage conditions: treatment of complications could ensue, for instance nausea, vomiting, bleeding, arrhythmias, and shivering.

Shivering is defined as *muscular involuntary oscillatory activity, involving one or more muscle groups, which increases the metabolic production of heat.*

Typically presents in the immediate postoperative period, with an incidence ranging between 63 % and 66 % [1]. Male gender, young adult age, duration of general anesthesia and kind of surgery seem to be determinant factors [2]. A moderate perioperative hypothermia not always heralds the appearance of the Postoperative Shiver (PS), but obviously favors it in direct proportion with the appearance of hypothermia itself. The incidence is ultimately dependent on the type of drug used in the course of anesthesia: the halogenated gases, the pentothal, and small amounts of opiates (perioperatively administered) facilitate its beginning, the opposite occurring

M. Dei Poli (✉)
IRCCS Policlinico San Donato, Piazza Malan 1, 20097, San Donato Milanese, Italy
e-mail: deipolimd@gmail.com

B. Allaria (ed.), *Practical Issues in Anesthesia and Intensive Care 2013*,
DOI: 10.1007/978-88-470-5529-2_10, © Springer-Verlag Italia 2014

with the use of propofol [3]. A vigorous shiver can increase the production of heat up to 600 % compared to the basal level. However, a doubling of production of heat is the energetic work that can be sustained for prolonged periods. Shivering often doubles or even triple the VO_2 and determines production of CO_2 (even if in a lower amount compared to the VO_2 increase). The increase of metabolic requests may predispose to complications these patients with heart failure, coronary artery disease, limited respiratory reserve, or chronic respiratory diseases, for increased cardiac work, decreased cardiac output (up to myocardial ischemia in coronaropathic patients), increased glycolytic metabolism resulting in lactic acidosis.

The PS creates considerable discomfort in patients, and some consider the feeling of coldness that accompanies it worse than surgical pain. It may also occasionally disturb monitoring (in particular ECG and pulse oximeter), compli-cate nursing procedures, increasing the risk of accidental trauma and/or damage of devices, determine increase of intraocular pressure and of the Intracranial Pressure (ICP), and is particularly troublesome for pregnant women during labor and delivery.

Postoperative shivering is less frequent in elderly patients because the advanced age itself renders the thermoregulatory homeostasis less efficient.

For the shivering intensity is reduced in elderly and fragile patients it is unlikely that shivering itself could worsen their outcome, in terms of mortality and morbidity.

The PS is rarely associated with clinically relevant hypoxemia, since the decrease PaO_2 has an inhibitor effect on this type of response. The cardiac mor-bidity associated with moderate perioperative hypothermia is mediated by a mechanism finer than PS, probably the marked increase in plasma catecholamines that could be registered in course of perioperative hypothermia.

In this brief discussion it will be firstly reviewed the physiological basis of thermoregulation and shiver, followed by a model of approach and evaluation of postoperative shivering.

10.1 Thermoregulation Physiology

Mammals and birds are homoeothermic species, as they need to keep the internal body temperature (Core or Central Temperature, CT) almost constant, within a range that consents the maintaining of the homeostasis of environment and internal functions. The thermoregulatory system operates so that the central temperature never rises >0.2 °C over the physiological value of 37 °C.

The brain uses both positive and negative feedback to minimize the effects of thermal changes, comparing them with default value; when these changes occur, effector mechanisms increase the production of heat from metabolism or increase the environmental heat loss.

The lateral spinothalamic tract was traditionally viewed as the exclusive afferent pathway to the hypothalamic centers of thermoregulation. Modern evidences suggest that most of these afferent fibers terminate in the reticular formation, and that the thermoregulatory neurons could be located in different brain regions, including the ventral medial hypothalamus, midbrain, bulb, and spinal cord [4]. The mammals thermoregulation system consists of three components that will be examined below.

10.1.1 Thermoreceptors and Afferent Pathways

This component is essentially composed by three structures:

Spinal cord: is concerned with the perception and modulation of thermal signals, and its temperature modulates all effector responses, as demonstrated by marked reduction of frequency and intensity of the shiver in the regions localized distally to a traumatic spinal section. The neurotransmitters involved in spinal cord activities are norepinephrine, serotonin, acetylcholine, and dynorphin.

Brain stem: contains temperature regulation sites that are not associated with a specific anatomical region, but scattered and distributed ventrally in the trunk and in the reticular formation: they connect to hypothalamus in a nonspecific polysynaptic (norepinephrine, serotonin, Ach, histamine, dopamine); animal experiments suggest that responses to heat increase are regulated by the tonic inhibitory activity of the midbrain (Ach, enkephalins) and pons (norepinephrine, serotonin, Ach).

Nucleus raphe magnus and locus subcoeruleus: the raphe magnus (bulbar) contains a relatively high proportion of thermo responsive serotonergic neurons, especially reactive for a rise of the temperature; the locus subcoeruleus (pontine) contains the largest brain aggregate of noradrenergic neurons, and both are responsible of the thermal signals transmission activity from skin receptors to the hypothalamus, and seem to be more involved in the modulation of the signals than in their generation.

10.1.2 Signal Integration Centers and Responses Elaboration

The preoptic area of the anterior hypothalamus is considered to be the area mainly involved in afferent thermoceptive signal integration and in autonomic and behavioral handling of the efferent response; many of the excitatory impulses come to this region from the hippocampus, so involving the limbic system to the thermoregulatory activities. The activity level of these neurons is also regulated by the waking state and the activity of the suprachiasmatic nucleus, so explaining the changes of core temperature in sleep and circadian rhythms in general. Preoptic neurons do not only recognize the local temperature but they compare it with signals coming through afferent sensitive ways (thermal and not!). Electrophysiological studies suggest that some hypothalamic nuclei in the anterior region present both sensor and integrative activities, and that there is a direct proportion between frequency of electric shock and thermosensitivity range.

10.1.3 Autonomic and Behavioral Effector Pathways

The effector mechanisms determine the range of ambient temperature values that the body can tolerate while maintaining a normal body temperature. Each effector has its own threshold and dedicated control, for which there is a progression in the activated responses and their entities according to the needings. When these mechanisms are inhibited, the tolerance range is reduced: the body temperature remains constant unless an intervention of other effectors with opposing effect.

The effector systems include the cutaneous vasomotor activity, the not-shivering thermogenesis, the shiver, and the sweating: these are activated by integrated central signals channeled toward a common efferent impulse. Usually, energy-saving mechanisms (vasoconstriction) are activated early and reach their maximum before energetically expensive processes are activated (shivering). The mechanism quantitatively more important is represented by behavioral adjustment (appropriate dressing, changes of the environmental temperature, adoption of positions that expose skin surfaces, involuntary movements).

The cutaneous vasoconstriction is the most commonly used vegetative effector mechanism; the loss of metabolic heat mainly takes place by convection and radiation from the skin surface, and vasoconstriction reduces such loss. The cutaneous blood flow is divided in two components, nutritional (particularly capillaries) and thermoregulatory mainly through arteriovenous shunt.

The latter are anatomically and functionally distinct from the capillaries, that provide nutritional contribution to the skin, so the vasoconstriction does not compromise the delivery of substrates and O_2 to peripheral tissues. The arterio-venous shunt have ≈ 100 μm diameter, therefore, given the same length, can convey a quantity of blood 10,000 times greater than a nutritional capillary (that has a diameter of 10 μm). The control of bloodstream through the shunt tends to be of "on/off" type: the α-adrenergic terminations of the sympathetic nervous system locally control the vasoconstriction, so that the perfusion amount is only minimally regulated by the concentration of circulating catecholamines.

Thermogenesis without shivering (not-shivering thermogenesis) increases the production of metabolic heat (measured as VO_2) without generating mechanical heat [5]. It is very active in children and infants (can double heat production), only minimally in adults. Its sources are the skeletal muscle and the brown adipose tissue; the latter owes its name to the macroscopically visible dark coloration, resulting from the enormous mitochondrial density therein. The activation of the process takes place thanks to $\beta 3$-adrenergic nerve endings, which locally activate a uncoupling protein [6].

Sweating is mediated by postganglionic cholinergic endings, thus being an active process that may be inhibited by anticholinergics (i.e., atropine) and determines dissipation of 0.58 kcal/gm of evaporated sweat. The loss of fluids that ensues in untrained individuals could be up to 1 l/h, doubling in athletes.

It is important to underline that sweating is the only mechanism that allows dissipation of heat in an environment where the temperature is greater than body temperature. The acute vasodilation is mediated by an unidentified factor released by sweat glands, which could be of proteinaceous type, and is not inhibited by any standard substance [7]; in conditions of extreme environmental heat, the bloodstream through the whole skin surface (for a thickness of 1 mm) may reach 7.5 l/min, equivalent to 1.5 times the cardiac output at rest. The activation threshold of the vasodilator mechanism is similar to perspiration threshold, but the control may be less prompt: the maximum cutaneous vasodilatation is delayed until the body temperature is well above that activating the greatest intensity of sweating.

10.2 Dependence of Thermoresponsivity on the Waking State

Although it is not possible to converge a heat stimulus on a single cellular element, at hypothalamic level, thermosensitive cell groups are present, and can be considered thermoresponsive.

These units can be activated by a direct thermal stimulus or by other interneurons that respond to skin thermal stimulation or to areas that are distant from the central nervous system. The thermoresponsivity of these areas is not constant, but significantly varies during time, and depends on the vigilance state and on cortical activity.

A recent work has demonstrated the potential of the waking state to combine with environmental temperature in determining the appearance of thermosensitivity or thermoresponsiveness of cells.

The cells of anterior preoptic region of the hypothalamus seem to be responsive to changes in skin temperature: every variation in the discharge frequency of these cells is associated with EEG pattern change. Responses from units in the ventro medial part of rostral medulla (which consists in the nucleus raphe magnus and adjacent regions of the brainstem) are not specific for temperature oscillations, but reflect changes in EEG-EMG activity, the latter determined by a variety of factors, including the thermal and nociceptive stimuli. Similar results (no thermal response observed within a given EEG pattern) were seen in response to stimulation of the subcoeruleus locus.

10.3 Physiology of Shiver

The shiver is elicited by a reduction in temperature at the level of the preoptic hypothalamic region, its signals descending along the efferent medial forebrain bundle. Historically, the origin of the central descending pattern of the shiver was situated in the posterior hypothalamus.

There is not enough experimental evidence that the anterior preoptic hypothalamus could suppress the shiver through inhibition of the posterior hypothalamus, as previously thought. Modifications in temperature are able to change the neuronal activity at the level of the reticular midbrain formation, of the dorso-lateral pons and of the medulla: influences on the descending spinal cord, which increase muscle tone, are secondary to this activity.

It is not demonstrated whether reticulospinal neurons receive their synaptic impulses directly from the anterior hypothalamic preoptic region or from posterior hypothalamus.

The α-spinal motoneurons and their axons are the common final pathway for coordinated motor activity and shiver. One hypothesis suggests that the excitability of motoneurons is inversely proportional to the cell size.

During continuous stimulation of the skin or of the spinal cord by a thermal low intensity signal, the motoneurons are progressively recruited depending on their size, starting from small γ-motoneurons, then the small α-tonic motoneurons, and finally, the biggest motoneurons. The latter are likely to play a synchronous electrical activity compared to the smaller ones. The motoneurons synchronization during the shiver is probably mediated by frequent inhibitory activity through the Renshaw interneurons. The reflex activation of α-motoneurons through the γ-motoneurons of muscle spindles (instability of the feedback system of the stretch reflex) is another potential, but controversial, mechanism that could determine rhythm and discharge frequency of α-motoneurons.

10.4 Temperature Control During General Anesthesia

Heat can be dispersed into the surrounding environment in four ways: radiation, convection, conduction, and evaporation. Radiation and convection account for the most part of the perioperative heat losses (radiation first): all surfaces with temperature values greater than absolute zero (−273 °C) radiate heat, and likewise all surfaces absorb radiant heat from surrounding surfaces, with a transfer rate directly proportional to the fourth power of the absolute temperature difference (Δt) between the surfaces. Conduction is instead directly linked to Δt between two adjacent surfaces and the strength of thermal insulation that separates them; generally it is a negligible mechanism during surgery, since the patient is in direct contact only with the foam pad (excellent thermal insulator) that usually covers the operating table. Heat lost by direct conduction toward the air molecules is limited by the formation of a still layer, adjacent to the skin, which acts as an insulator; when this layer is disturbed by air currents, its insulating properties are considerably reduced and therefore the heat loss increases. This mechanism is defined as "convection" and its entity is directly proportional to the square root of air velocity and is the basis of the common "blast of cold air" phenomenon. The speed of the air flow in the operating room is typically 20 cm/s and this only slightly increases heat loss, compared to what would happen if the air was completely still. However, the intensity of the convective motions greatly increases in the operating rooms equipped with laminar air flow: in this case heat loss is limited by the insulation provided by the surgical drapes.

Sweating is rare during anesthesia, and in its absence evaporation from the skin surface in adults is 10 % of metabolic heat production; small children, instead, lose a larger proportion of heat with this mechanism for the lesser thickness of the skin surface, up to 1/5 metabolic heat in premature infants; the amount of heat lost through the respiratory system (perspiration) is almost insignificant compared to evaporation through the surgical wound.

10.5   Thermoregulatory Changes in the Perioperating Period

The behavioral thermoregulation is impossible during general anesthesia, because patients are unconscious and in condition of muscle paralysis. All the currently used general anesthetics alter the neurovegetative body temperature control: the threshold for heat is slightly increased, the threshold for cold is markedly reduced: so the interthreshold range is broader, compared to its normal values (≈ 0.2 °C) up to 2–4 °C.

Drugs such as propofol, alfentanil and dexmedetomidine cause a slight linear increase of the sweating threshold, combined with a marked and linear lowering of thresholds for vasoconstriction and shivering. Even isoflurane and desflurane slightly increase perspiration threshold, but they reduce the threshold for cold in a nonlinear way; as a result, volatile anesthetics inhibit vasoconstriction and shivering to a lesser extent, compared to propofol at low concentrations.

The cooling rate is similar during general and local anesthesia, but after the latter rewarming is slower, as vasodilation and the residual myoresolution prevent the production and the maintenance of heat. Greater reductions of body temperature occur in case of cachexia, trauma, burns, hormonal changes, and infants (mass reduction/body surface area).

Average body temperature begins to decrease when the heat transferred to surrounding environment exceeds the production of heat itself (that, during anesthesia, is about 0.8 kcal/kg/h). As human body specific heat is ≈ 0.83 kcal/kg, there is a reduction of approximately 1 °C/h when the heat transferred to environment exceeds the metabolic production for a factor of 2.

At the end of surgery, patients are often hypothermic, despite adequate intraoperative body temperature control.

Hypothermia comes from a combination of altered thermoregulation due to anesthetics, cold operating room environment (in which heat is lost in several ways and moments), evaporation during the preparation of skin, humidification of dried inspired gas in respiratory circuitry, convection and radiation from the skin and wounds (see previous paragraph). Moreover the core temperature decreases, for infusion of fluids at room temperature.

The slight accidental hypothermia (core temperature reduction <36 °C) concerns ≈ 50 % of patients in the immediate postoperative period and, in relation to their size, it may take 2–5 h for the full restoration of normothermia [8]. Subjects with increased risk of developing postoperative hypothermia are children, elderly, individuals with BMI < 20, patients suffering from endocrine system diseases.

Hypothermia complicates the postoperative period through different patho-physiological mechanisms [9, 10]:

- Increased sympathetic tone and peripheral vascular resistance;
- Reduction in venous capacitance;
- Increased risk for cardiac ischemia and arrhythmias [11];
- Vasoconstriction mediated reduction of the reliability of pulse oximetry, of NIBP (noninvasive blood pressure) and IBP (invasive blood pressure) monitoring, of neuromuscular function monitoring;
- Tissue hypoperfusion causing tissue hypoxia and metabolic acidosis, and possibly compromising the perfusion of the grafts;
- ΔA-aO$_2$ and Hb affinity for O$_2$, and reduced transfer of oxygen to peripheral tissues;
- Platelet sequestration, reduction of the platelet functionality, and decreased activity of clotting factors bleeding risk;
- Hyperglycemia, reduced effectiveness of immune responses with increased incidence of postoperative infections;
- Every 1 °C causes a reduction in the MAC of the inhalational anesthetics of 5–7 %, so the level of anesthesia deepens;
- Lengthening of the half-life of muscle relaxants and sedatives, for reduced organ perfusion and subsequent reduction of their metabolism;
- In case of severe hypothermia there is alteration of genesis and propagation of action potentials in the heart, followed by lengthening of the PR, QRS, and QT, with occurrence of the so-called Osborn J wave. At ≤28 °C a ventricular fibrillation may spontaneously generate.

10.6 Thermoregulatory and Non-Thermoregulatory Shiver

The main cause of the onset of PS is represented by the thermoregulatory response [12] to post operatory hypothermia [13]. As previously pointed out, body temperature is normally maintained within a swing of maximum 0.2 °C, compared to a target set at central level, thanks to efferent mechanisms such as sweating, vasoconstriction, and shivering.

In the intraoperative period several factors, in particular anesthetic drugs, reduce of 2–4 °C the threshold of vasoconstriction and shivering activation. Consequently, the patients frequently become hypothermic. After surgery, if the Tc reaches values lower than the threshold of response to cold, vasoconstriction, and shivering are stimulated: the level of Tc that activates the first mechanism, is approximately 1 °C higher than the one that activates the so-called thermoregulatory shiver.

Typically even normothermic patients, in absence of vasoconstriction, could present the so-called shivering like tremor, where fever is one of the possible pathogenetic mechanisms, through the action of endogenous pyrogens, in only partially known ways [14].

Damaged tissues release the majority of these cytokines; fever is characterized by a synchronous increase in the thermoregulatory thresholds response (up regulation of the "set-point"); shivering associated with fever is often preceded by vasoconstriction of arteriovenous shunts already during anesthesia.

An alternative explanation to the spontaneous muscle activity, in normothermic post-surgical patients, is represented by the non-thermoregulatory shiver [15], which is attributed to various causes, such as reduction of the sympathetic noradrenergic activity [16], poor pain control, administration of anesthetic drugs, loss of descending control reflexes, suppression of adrenal activity, any respiratory alkalosis, and, as mentioned above, release of endogenous pyrogens after a tissue damage [17], vasoplegia during spinal or epidural anesthesia [18].

In particular, it has been demonstrated that an insufficient pain control [19] in the postoperative period facilitates the beginning of shivering, being an important stimulus for the spontaneous muscle activity. Adequate analgesia largely prevents grade 1 and 2 (see Table 10.1) non-thermoregulatory tremor, increasing patient comfort, and concomitantly reducing the negative psychological impact of pain perception itself.

Many drugs are active in the prevention and treatment of postoperative shiver; which ones of these act specifically against the non-thermoregulatory shiver is yet to know, but it is clear, however, that the analgesic drugs may have a indirect effect at least in this sense, probably dose-dependent, regardless of the action on the inhibitory thermoregulatory shivering.

10.7 Patterns of Abnormal Postoperative Tremor

Postoperative shivering is very common in hypothermic patients during recovery from general anesthesia.

According to the conventional interpretation of PS, the drug-induced thermoregulation inhibition suddenly disappears, allowing the shivering threshold to increase toward normal level. The discrepancy between the persistent low body

Table 10.1 Postoperative shivering classification

Grade 0	No shivering
Grade 1	Piloerection and/or peripheral vasoconstriction without visible muscular activity
Grade 2	Visible muscular activation in a single muscular group
Grade 3	Visible muscular activation without generalized shivering
Grade 4	Whole body surface, generalized shivering

temperature and current "almost normal" threshold activates the common thermoregulatory shiver.

However, a more recent study suggested that specific surgery-related factors (such as stress or pain) may contribute to the genesis of postoperative tremor, because it was impossible to identify any Shiver-Like Tremor activity (SLT) in normothermic volunteers. Pain may facilitate SLT, both in postoperative patients and in women in spontaneous labor at term. Any increase in the thermoregulatory set point (fever) in the early postoperative phase can determine the normal thermoregulatory shivering in normothermic patients, or even in hyperthermic once.

The surgical stress may increase the thermoregulatory set point during the postoperative period: even in absence of signs of clinical infection, the 25 % of postoperated patients can reach core temperatures of 38 °C, and 50 % of them 38.4 °C [4]. Of course, there are many other reasons for these patients to develop fever, such as infections, pulmonary atelectasia, release of pyrogenic toxins from inflamed/damaged tissues.

Three patterns of muscle activity were observed in hypothermic volunteers during emergency anesthesia conducted with isoflurane: the first one was a tonic stiffening, appearing as a direct effect of anesthesia with isoflurane, not dependent on temperature.

At end-tidal concentration of isoflurane ≈ 0.3 % a second pattern occurred: synchronous, tonic increasing–decreasing activity.

The latter is by far the more frequent pattern, very similar to the cold-induced shiver in anesthetized volunteers, known as "genuine" thermoregulatory shivering.

The third observed pattern was a spontaneous electromyographic clonus, which occurred with hypothermia, associated to an end-tidal isoflurane concentration between 0.4 and 0.2 %.

During epidural anesthesia synchronous increasing–decreasing pattern occurred; however, abnormal electromyographic (e.g., cloni) pattern were not identified.

Despite possible alternative etiology in specific patients, "normal" response to central (core) and peripheral (skin) hypothermia remains by far the most common cause of postoperative shiver.

10.8 Management

10.8.1 Which Monitoring Systems for Temperature Should We Use?

The infrared tympanic thermometer presents the advantage of low invasiveness, speed of measurement, low cost, and good sensitivity. Tc should be continuously monitored during the application of MTH.

The gold standard for Tc evaluation, to be reserved for conditions that need a continuous temperature monitoring, is the central venous temperature measurement; alternatives to such method, in order of decreasing effectiveness, are:

- Esophageal temperature measurement;
- Bladder temperature measurement (may be not reliable if urine output <0.5 ml/kg/h);
- Use of rectal probe (rectal temperature can not quickly follow core temperature changes, with up to a ≤1.5 °C difference).

10.8.2 Targets

Selecting patients on age (oldest and youngest first), physical constitution, type of intervention and duration, bleeding, fluidic los,s and comorbidities (endocrinopathies in particular), the measurement of body temperature should be carried out entering and at discharge from the recovery room (level A recommendation of SIAARTI (Italian Society of Anesthesiologists) 2010 guidelines); normothermia during postanesthetic period must be reached and maintained with passive and if necessary with active mechanisms (level A recommendation). Its maintenance is the key intervention for prevention and treatment of postoperative shiver.

In case on unresolving shiver, a pharmacological approach is indicated, despite patient's normothermia (level A recommendation).

If the patient is normothermic, positioning a passive heating system (that reduce heat dispersion) will be sufficient [20]; insulating blankets (e.g., cotton) reduce heat dispersion only of 30 %, obviously insufficient to prevent hypothermia and consequent PS in patients undergoing general anesthesia; in awake patients, wool blankets are preferable, since they trap a thicker layer of air and allow more heat retention.

In case of hypothermia, we must use drugs and active heating methods such as forced air systems [21], heated water devices [22], and electric covers [23]. Methods that minimize convective heat losses are the most effective in prevention of intraoperative hypothermia. The different methods are compared in Table 10.2.

10.9 Pharmacological Modulation of the Shiver

Several classes of pharmacologically active substances, including catecholamines, cholinergic drugs, endogenous peptides, as well as NMDA (n-methyl-D-aspartate) receptor antagonists, are likely able in handling the central thermoregulatory control mechanisms.

The desirable properties for a drug, active in prevention of PS, include ready availability and minimal side effects.

We will discuss in this section the changes induced by these molecules in thermosensitivity, as well as the mechanism of action of drugs used in postoperative shivering control.

Table 10.2 Comparison between active-warming devices

Method	Advantages	Disadvantages
Forced air systems	Rapid warming, no burning risk, high-capacity system	Environment warming; expensive system
Circulating-water garments	Good warming capacity, low burning risk, no environmental warming	Potential water loss, infective risk; cumbersome
Water mattress	No environmental warming, no surgical wound contact	Low capacity, pressure-ulcer risk
Electrical mattress	Silent, no environmental warming, no surgical wound contact	Slow warming, high burning risk in case of system damage, low capacity
Radiating warming	Rapid warming, good capacity (related to the distance from the patient)	Cumbersome, not usable in the operating room, environmental warming, high burning risk
Warmed infusions	Direct effect on core temperature; first choice if charging >1 l/h	Insufficient warming capacity in case of small infusion amounts

In particular, randomized, double-blind, placebo-control studies have demonstrated the effectiveness of meperidine [24, 25], clonidine [26–28], tramadol, nefopam [29, 30], and ketamine.

10.9.1 Clonidine

It is an agonist of the α2-adrenergic receptors at brainstem level, whose stimulation induces the activation of inhibitory interneurons, that reduce the sympathetic nervous system discharge (reduction of peripheral resistances, of Heart Rate (HR), of MAP, reduction of vascular renal resistances) and thus, the shiver genesis; when epidurally administered, clonidine reduces the level of transmission of the pain signal, acting at the spinal presynaptic α2-and post-junctional receptors level: the resulting analgesic action eliminates one of the causes of the shiver itself, and therefore reduces its incidence. Pain relief is obtained only in body regions innervated by the spinal segments, in which analgesic concentrations of the drug are reached. Thus, clonidine is able to reduce the threshold of vasoconstriction and shiver of 0.5 °C, by acting at central level (the center of shiver is under the inhibitor control of the preoptic hypothalamic region).

Labeled uses of the drug are: oral administration in the management of arterial hypertension (either alone or in combination), and in the treatment of Attention Deficit Syndrome/Hyperactivity Disorder (ADHD); continuous epidural infusion as adjunctive therapy in severe pain control in oncologic patients non-responsive to opioids (or those who have developed tolerance); transdermal route administration in the management of arterial hypertension.

Off-label uses could be the withdrawal from nicotine or heroin, severe pain, dysmenorrhea, vasomotor symptoms associated with menopause, ethanol addiction, prophylaxis of migraine, glaucoma, clozapine-induced salivation, insomnia associated with ADHD in children, pediatric La Tourette syndrome, aggressive behavior disorders; postoperative shiver control; clonidine is finally used as an adjuvant in diagnosis of GH deficiency.

Clonidine can be administered subcutaneously, im or slow iv (1 vial diluted in 10 ml of saline), placing the patient in supine position to prevent the occurrence of orthostatic hypotension; each vial contains 150 µg of active ingredient, the maximum dosage is 600 µg/daily; when administered in continuous infusion (c.i.), the speed must be maintained between 0.2 and 0.5 γ/kg/min. In postoperative shivering control we use iv boluses of 75 µg, at the intervention end we can administer 1.5–3 mg/kg in continuous infusion. and up to 200–300 µg in cardiac surgery.

10.9.2 Remifentanil

Powerful short-acting μ opioid, approved for clinical use since 1996, contains an ester link that allows its metabolization by nonspecific esterases located in blood and muscles: consequently, it has an extremely brief plasma half-life, with sudden action cessation. The half-life is estimated at ≈ 1.3 min, thus avoiding the accumulation of medication; a deficit of pseudo-cholinesterase do not seem to alter the pharmacokinetics of remifentanil, not being a good substrate for these enzymes. From a pharmacodynamic point of view acts as a μ receptor agonist for opioids and its action is antagonized by naloxone.

The cardiovascular effects, consisting in reduction of MAP and HR, are mediated by stimulation of the vagal nerve, and inhibition of sympathetic activity (not histamine effect); side effects are common to other opioids, mainly represented by respiratory depression, nausea, vomiting, constipation, itching, and, sometimes, dose depending muscle stiffness.

Continuous intravenous infusion of remifentanil is useful for analgesia in annoying and painful procedures conducted in spontaneous breathing, and deep analgesia can be obtained with minimal effects on cognitive functions; remifentanil also provides sedation and adequate analgesia during the execution of blocks in locoregional anesthesia, and in association with the use of a topical anesthetic, may allow the inhibition of reflex responses and facilitate "awake" intubation. The use of remifentanil in general anesthesia improves intraoperative hemodynamic stability, and reduces the incidence and duration of breathing depression in the postoperative period.

The drug appear not so effective as meperidine in reducing the incidence of postoperative shivering, although its epidural administration can be effective in obstetrical locoregional anesthesia.

A recent review [31] of RCT compared the use of remifentanil in general anesthesia with other opioids (fentanyl, sufentanil, alfentanil): remifentanil was associated with deeper intraoperative anesthesia and analgesia; high doses administered in a short period of time can cause muscle stiffness (trunk and chest mostly) and/or closure of the vocal cords making mask ventilation difficult; it does not appear to be associated with an increased incidence of awareness.

The use of remifentanil determines rapid recovery and low incidence of respiratory depression in the postoperative period; however, its use has been associated with greater incidence of PS and no advantage in the prevention of Postoperative Nausea and Vomiting (PONV). So it could be most favorably used for procedures that implicate a rapid recovery time and not causing severe pain. Patients treated with remifentanil often require additional analgesic therapies, and this may depend on several reasons: rapid development of tolerance, hyperalgesia, and shorter duration of analgesic effect for the rapid metabolism.

These mechanisms may, alone or in combination, at least partially explain the increased incidence of PS associated with the use of remifentanil compared with other opioids: the opioids inhibit thermoregulatory responses, including the shiver; for a given level of postoperative hypothermia, the shiver may occur earlier in order of the particular pharmacokinetics of remifentanil. Another explanation could be the not thermoregulatory significance of shiver associated with pain, which is less effectively controlled by remifentanil, compared to other opioids.

The appearance of acute tolerance, often early after administration of narcotics with shorter action duration, must be taken in mind.

We must therefore pay particular attention to postoperative analgesia and effective and appropriate intraoperative heating when using remifentanil for the execution of general anesthesia.

10.9.3 Nefopam

It is a non-opioid analgesic with potent antishivering properties which inhibits the reuptake of 5-HT, norepinephrine and dopamine; it slightly reduces the body temperature.

Its analgesic action is of central nature, as demonstrated by experiments on mice (acid acetic test, hot plate test, the phenyl benzoquinone test), and is expressed in the spinal and supraspinal cord. Its antishivering action occurs instead, at least partially, at pontine level [32, 33].

Nefopam does not cause respiratory depression in the postoperative period, and differently from other drugs reduces the activation threshold of PS without changing the vasoconstriction and sweating threshold [34].

The daily dosage of nefopam varies between 30 and 90 mg PO (each tablet contains 30 mg of nefopam hydrochloride), or 20 mg iv/im diluted in saline or dextrose, every 6–8 h (the injection should be performed with the patient lying down, allowing rest for 15–20′). The dosage used in the prevention of PS is 0.15 mg/kg or 20 mg iv in the immediate postoperative period [35], possibly in association with alfentanil (20 µg/kg or 1.2–1.3 µg iv), association that increases the threshold reduction level of PS itself [36].

10.9.4 Tramadol

It is a non-opioid antishivering analgesic medication which acts with a mechanism similar to nefopam: it inhibits the reuptake of 5-HT (serotonin), norepinephrine, dopamine, and facilitates the release of 5-HT.

Probably, the α2-adrenergic receptors in brain play a role in the action of tramadol on postoperative shivering: the α2-adrenergic agonists determine neuronal hyperpolarization, probably increasing the conductance to K^+ through Gi-coupled proteins. This suppresses the neuronal discharge, which is related to the range of thermosensitivity; moreover, the activation of α2-adrenoceptors suppresses the entry of Ca^{2+} inside the cell, and this reduces the release of neurotransmitters.

The accumulation of Ca^{2+} on the cell surface stabilizes the neuronal membrane and reduces the frequency of discharge of the rear hypothalamus units committed to heat production.

Tramadol may be orally administered (rigid capsule of 50 mg or oral drops solution of 10 g/100 ml), rectally (suppositories 100 mg), slow intravenous, intramuscular or subcutaneous (ampoules 50 mg/1 ml or 100 mg/2 ml), without exceeding the maximum dose of 400 mg in any way of administration (although in refractory cancer pain you can reach 600 mg/die dosages or more).

The administration of 1 mg/kg i.v. is effective in PS control, reducing the threshold of 0.8 °C [37].

10.9.5 Dexmedetomidine

It is an α2-adrenergic receptors agonist, with anesthetic and sedative action, probably due to activation of G-proteins of brainstem receptors, resulting in inhibition of norepinephrine release; activation of peripheral α2b-receptors occurs by exposure to high doses or rapid iv infusion, determining vasoconstriction.

Labeled uses of dexmedetomidine are the sedation in intubated and mechanically ventilated patients in the first days of ICU stay, and sedation before and/or during surgical procedures or other invasive procedures in non-intubated patients.

The off-label indications are the premedication in case of general anesthesia induced with barbiturates; anesthetic adjuvant in ophthalmic surgery; treatment of PS [38]; prevention of cardiovascular adverse effects and delirium associated with the use of ketamine.

Dosage should be calibrated on desired clinical effect; randomized clinical trials have demonstrated efficacy and safety comparable to benzodiazepines in continuous infusion, lasting no longer than 5 days; for sedation in the ICU, for sedation during procedures or for analgesia during fiberoptic awake intubation a loading dose of 1 γ/kg/min in 10' is recommended, followed by a maintenance dose of 0.2–0.7 γ/kg/min. Doses >1.5 γ/kg/min do not improve efficacy, but exacerbate the risk of hemodynamic compromission. Effective dose in preventing PS is 1 mcg/kg iv during the intraoperative period [39, 40].

Patients receiving dexmedetomidine show a greater hemodynamic stability at extubation and during recovery of general anesthesia; MAP and HR are well controlled, the impact of nausea and vomiting is reduced, the depth and duration of sedation is increased [41].

10.9.6 Ketamine

Ketamine is a general anesthetic. It is a non-competitive antagonist of the NMDA glutamate receptor; it is used for the induction and maintenance of general anesthesia; the off-label use includes analgesia, sedation, PS treatment [42, 43].

At sub-anesthetic doses it causes analgesia and modulation of the central sensitization phenomena, hyperalgesia and opioid tolerance; reduces the spinal polysynaptic reflex activity.

Dosage should be adjusted to the desired effect and routes of administration are im or iv: for the induction of general anesthesia the off-label dosages are 4–10 mg/kg im or 0.5–2 mg/kg iv; for the anesthesia maintenance additional doses are given, about 50 % of the induction dose, or a continuous iv infusion of 0.1–0.5 mg/min. For sedation/analgesia im doses of 2–4 mg/kg, or iv of 0.2–0.75 mg/kg, followed by continuous infusion of 2–7 γ/kg/min are recommended.

Pediatric dosages: when sedation is required for invasive/annoying procedures oral doses of 5–8 mg/kg, in a single administration (diluted in 0.2–0.3 ml/kg of a chosen beverage) 30′ before the procedure; to reach a level of sedation/analgesia the im dose is of 2.5 mg/kg, or 0.5–1 mg/kg iv followed by infusion of 5–20 γ/kg/min.

For the control of PS: iv dose of 0.25–0.5 mg/kg [44] that may be increased up to 0.75 mg/kg.

The drug is associated with the higher incidence of adverse effects in the group of drugs used in PS control: increase of MAP and HR, postoperative agitation, hallucinations, vivid dreams, drooling are the most common; uncommon effects are laryngospasm, breathing depression, increased intraocular pressure, tonico-clonic seizures, skin rash, rarely associated with arterial hypotension, bradycardia, cardiac arrest, anaphylactic reactions, nausea and vomiting. Such effects are directly related to the speed of administration and to the dosage, and can be minimized using the im route.

10.9.7 Hydrocortisone

Hydrocortisone is used as anti-inflammatory agent since a very long time: it affects the fat, proteic, carbohydratic and purinic metabolism, interferes with the electrolyte balance and exerts a direct calorigenic effect, that may be useful in preventing and mitigating postoperative shivering.

A recent double-blind randomized controlled trial conducted on patients undergoing knee arthroscopy under general anesthesia (nitric oxide, isoflurane, and remifentanil) has tested and proven the effectiveness of a 1–2 mg/kg single dose of hydrocortisone, administered approximately $10'$ before the end of anesthesia, in preventing the onset of PS [45].

Shivering was observed in 82 % of the controls, while only in 32 % of patients who received 1 mg/kg of hydrocortisone (hydrocortisone group 1) and in 20 % of patients who were given 2 mg/kg of hydrocortisone (hydrocortisone group 2). The global incidence of PS was similar in patients in the hydrocortisone group 1 and 2.

The exact mechanism by which the drug acts preventing the PS is not known, some animal studies suggest an anabolic effect with increased hepatic levels of ATP; exposure to high temperatures for a long period of time (8 weeks) causes a depression of plasma levels of endogenous hydrocortisone, indicating a possible thermoregulatory role.

Its effect could even be mediated by changes in the metabolism of thyroid hormones or NO synthase activity.

A single dose of 100–200 mg of hydrocortisone do not determine adverse hemodynamic nor immunological alterations, does not alter the surgical wounds healing process, and is also able to reduce the incidence of infections in the postoperative period.

10.9.8 Pethidine or Meperidine

Meperidine is an analgesic opiate receptors agonist that mainly exerts its action at the level of the central nervous system; it produces analgesia, sedation, euphoria, dysphoria, sometimes respiratory depression and other central effects such as miosis, abolition of the corneal reflex, muscle involuntary contractions up to epileptiform access.

When administered iv during general anesthesia, the cardiovascular effects could be a reduction of cardiac output and an increase in Central Venous Pressure (CVP), without significant changes in HR. It shows atropine-like and spasmolytic properties on smooth muscle.

Compared to other opiates, particularly morphine, meperidine is associated with spasm of biliary tract, colecystokinetic activity, and minor constipation, having a comparable analgesic activity.

Meperidine is mainly used in treatment of moderate to severe postoperative pain, for neoplastic pain or during labor, as well as in eclampsia and pre-eclampsia syndromes, in anesthetic premedication for inducing state of basal narcosis.

As an analgesic, meperidine is administered im or subcutaneous, in 25–100 mg doses, or by slow intravenous infusion at 25–50 mg per dose; in children, it is administered im in 0.5–2 mg/kg doses. In obstetrical environment it is used 50–100 mg im or sc (repeatable after 1–3 h), as soon as contractions assume a regular interval.

For pre-anesthesia (in adults) 50–100 mg are administered 60' before surgery.

Meperidine shows potent antishivering properties [46], resulting, for an equi-analgesic action, more useful for that than the pure κ-receptors agonists: it is able to reduce the threshold for activation of PS and of vasoconstriction of at least two times [47]. The effect is, at least in part, due to the interaction with the κ-receptors agonists, and may also be due to the agonist action on the α2b-receptors, on which meperidine acts at relevant clinical concentrations [48]. The local anesthetic and central anticholinergic action are also well documented. Since thermoregulation requires the involvement of different systems, including serotoninergic, adrenergic and cholinergic (the "redundancy" of the system reflects the importance of this homeostatic mechanism), we can assume that it may act at multiple levels in determine the antishivering effect.

For the treatment of PS a 25–50 mg or 0.5 mg/kg iv bolus is recommended [49].

10.9.9 Magnesium Sulfate

It is mainly used for the prevention and treatment of seizures, during eclamptic or pre eclamptic state or for hypertensive encephalopathy; a labeled use is replenishment in deficiency states associated with tetany, in supraventricular hyperkinetic and ventricular arrhythmias (in particular ventricular fibrillation and torsades de pointes), in the digitalis intoxication and in the acute phase of myocardial infarction.

It is administered intravenously (usually using 40 ml of 10 % solution or 20 ml of 20 %), in a discontinuous infusion, modulating the dose according to age, weight, clinical condition, not exceeding 30–40 g in 24 h, monitoring the magnesemia, which must be close to ≈ 6 mg/dl.

Vasodilation, sweating, and reduction of MAP and HR, arrhythmias, syncope, respiratory depression, very rarely cardiac arrest, represent its side effects. Other effects can be hyporeflexia, flaccid paralysis, hypocalcaemia with signs of tetany, fever; at level of the injection site can occur infections, thrombophlebitis, extravasations, and hypervolemia.

Magnesium (Mg^{2+}) is an antagonist of Ca^{2+} channels, and a non-competitive antagonist of the receptors of N-methyl-D-aspartate (NMDA); it was associated with excellent cardio and neuroprotection in experimental ischemia models [50], and is effective in treatment of PS, after general anesthesia [51], since it reduces the shivering threshold.

Magnesium exerts not only a central action: it is also a muscle relaxant and this probably counteracts the increase in intensity of PS associated with progressive hypothermia. It also produces peripheral vasodilation, which improves blood flow to the skin, further reducing the incidence of PS.

The dose used in general anesthesia for the prevention of BP is a bolus of 30–80 mg/kg administered in about 30', followed by an infusion of 2 g/h until the end of the procedure.

During spinal anesthesia doses of 50 mg/kg, administered in 15′ and followed by a continuous infusion of 15 mg/kg/h are used until the end of the intervention [52, 53].

10.9.10 Ondansetron

It is an antiemetic and anti-nausea drug, highly selective antagonist of $5HT_3$ receptors, very powerful.

Its action is probably of both central and peripheral type. Normally, the release of serotonin at the level of the small intestine activates vagal afferents that determine $5HT_3$ receptor stimulation, and induce the reflex of vomiting; at central level this is induced by the stimulation, through serotonin, of area postrema, located on the floor of the fourth ventricle.

Ondansetron inhibits both these mechanisms. Moreover it shows antishivering properties, both in patients undergoing general anesthesia [54], or during spinal or epidural anesthesia [55].

In both cases, an iv bolus of 8 mg does not induce changes in hemodynamic profile of the patient.

The mechanism through which ondansetron prevents PS could be related with inhibition of serotonergic reuptake at the level of the anterior hypothalamic pre-optic region; $5HT_3$ receptors influence both the production and loss of heat: their stimulation produces vasodilation and hypotension.

The antishivering effect of ondansetron is independent from intraoperative core hypothermia (the redistribution of heat from core to periphery that occurs in the first 20–30′of a general anesthesia, resulting in the reduction of 1 °C of the BT), suggesting that its action is taking place at central level.

After regional anesthesia, however, inhibition of thermoregulation usually occurs, with reduction of vasoconstriction and shivering threshold, proportional to the number of blocked segments: every extension in height of the block determines a reduction of 0.15 °C in body temperature.

The correlation between PS and the level of block is modified using ondansetron.

References

1. Lienhardt A et al (1992) Postoperative shivering: analysis of main associated factors. Ann Fr Anesth Reanim 11:488–495
2. Crossley AW (1992) 6 months of shivering in a district general hospital. Anaesthesia 47:845–848
3. Horn EP et al (1997) Late intraoperative clonidine administration prevents postanesthetic shivering after total intravenous or volatile anesthesia. Anesth Analg 84:613–617
4. Witte JD, Sessler DI (2002) Periop Shiv Anesthesiol 96:467–484
5. Sessler DI (2008) Temperature monitoring and perioperative thermoregulation. Anesthesiology 109:318–338

6. Nedergaard J, Cannon B (1992) The uncoupling protein thermogenin and mitochondrial thermogenesis. New Comp Biochem 23:385–420

7. Rowell LB (1981) Active neurogenic vasodilatation in man. In: Vanhoutte P, Leusen I (eds) Vasodilatation. Raven, NY, pp 1–17

8. Gruppo di studio SIAARTI per la Sicurezza in Anestesia e Terapia Intensiva (2010) Raccomandazioni per l'area di recupero e l'assistenza post-anestesiologica. SIAARTI guidelines/recommendations

9. Sessler DI (2001) Complications and treatment of mild hypothermia. Anesthesiology 95:531

10. Reynolds L et al (2008) Perioperative complications of hypothermia. Best Pract Res Clin Anesth 22:645–657

11. Frank SM et al (1997) Perioperative maintenance of normothermia reduces the incidence of morbid cardiac events: a randomized clinical trial. JAMA 277:1127

12. Lienhart A et al (1992) Frisson postoperatoire: analyse des principaux facteurs associes. Ann Fr Anesth Reanim 11:488–495

13. Sessler DI (1993) Perianesthetic thermoregulation and heat balance in humans. FASEB J 7:638–644

14. Romanovsky AA et al (1996) First and second phases of biphasic fever: two sequential stages of the sickness syndrome? Am J Physiol 271:244–253

15. Horn EP et al (1998) Non-thermoregulatory shivering in patients recovering from isoflurane or desflurane anesthesia. Anesthesiology 89:878–886

16. Nikki P, Rosenberg P (1969) Halothane shivering in mice after injection of cathecolamines and 5HT into the cerebral ventricles. Ann Med Exp Biol Fenn 47:197–202

17. Horn EP (1999) Postoperative shivering: aetiology and treatment. Curr opin Abesthesiol 12:449–453

18. Ozaki M et al (1994) Thermoregulatory thresholds during epidural and spinal anesthesia. Anesthesiology 81:282–288

19. Horn EP et al (1999) Postop Pain Facilit Nonthermoregul Tremor. Anesthesiol 91:979–984

20. Sessler DI, Schroeder M (1993) Heat loss in humans covered with cotton hospital blankets. Anesth Analg 77:73–77

21. Bräuer A et al (2007) Efficacy of forced-air warming systems with full body blankets. Can J Anesth 54(1):34–41

22. Bennett J et al (1994) Prevention of hypothermia during hip surgery: effect of passive compared with active skin surface warming. Br J Anaesth 73:180–183

23. Negishi C et al (2003) Resistive-heating and forced-air warming are comparably effective. Anesth Analg 96:1693–1697

24. Kranke P et al (2004) Single-dose parenteral pharmacological interventions for the prevention of post-operative shivering. A quantitative systematic review of randomized controlled trials. Anesth Analg 99:718–727

25. Riudeubas MJ et al (1996) Comparing pethidine to metamizol for treatment of post-anesthetic shivering. Br J Clin Pharmacol 42:307–311

26. Terasako K, Yamamoto M (2000) Comparison between pentazocine, pethidine and placebo in the treatment of post-anesthetic shivering. Acta Anesthesiol Scand 44:311–312

27. Yang CH et al (1993) Effect of intravenous clonidine on prevention of postepidural shivering. Ma Zui Xue Za Zhi 31:121–126

28. Sia S (1998) Intravenous clonidine prevents post-extradural shivering. Br J Anesth 81:145–146

29. Alfonsi P et al (2004) Nefopam, a non-sedative benzoxazocine analgesic. Selectively reduces the shivering threshold. Anesthesiology 100(1):37–43

30. Bilotta F et al (2002) Nefopam and tramadol for the prevention of shivering During neuraxial anesthesia. Reg Anesth Pain Med 27:380–384

31. Komatsu R et al (2007) Remifentanil for general anaesthesia: a systematic review. Anaesthesia 62:1266–1280

32. Podranski T et al (2012) Compartimental pharmacokinetics of nefopam during mild hypothermia. Br J Anesth 108(5):784–791
33. Bilotta F et al (2005) Nefopam or clonidine in the pharmacologic prevention of shivering in patients undergoing conscious sedation for interventional neuroradiology. Anaesthesia 60(2):124–128
34. Kurz A (2008) Thermal care in the perioperative period. Best Pract Res Clin Anaesth 22:39–62
35. Alfonsi P (2003) Postanaesthetic shivering, epidemiology, pathophysiology and approaches to prevention and management. Minerva Anest 69(5):438–442
36. Alfonsi P et al (2009) Nefopam and alfentanil additively reduce the shivering threshold in humans whereas nefopam and clonidine do not. Anesthesiology 111:102–109
37. Mohta M et al (2009) Tramadol for prevention of postanesthetic shivering: a randomized double-blind comparison with pethidine. Anesthesia 64(2):141–146
38. Elvan EG et al (2008) Dexmedetomidine and postoperative shivering in patients undergoing elective abdominal hysterectomy. Eur J Anaesthesiol 25(5):357–364
39. Bicer C et al (2006) Dexmedetomidine and meperidine prevent postanaesthetic shivering. Eur J Anaesthesiol 23(2):149–153
40. Usta B et al (2011) Dexmedetomidine for the prevention of shivering during spinal anesthesia. Clinics (Sao Paulo) 66(7):1187–1191
41. Bajwa SJ et al (2012) Reductione in the incidence of shivering with perioperative dexmedetomidine: a randomized prospective study. J Anaesthesiol Clin Pharmacol 28(1):86–91
42. Nakasuji M et al (2011) An intraoperative small dose of ketamine prevents remifentanil-induced postanesthetic shivering. Anesth Analg 113(3):484–487
43. Shakya S et al (2010) Prophylactic low dose ketamine and ondansetron for prevention of shivering during spinal anesthesia. J Anaesthesiol Clin Pharmacol 26(4):465–469
44. Norouzi M et al (2011) Optimum dose of ketamine for prevention of postanesthetic shivering: a randomized double-blind placebo-controlled clinical. Acta Anaesthesiol Belg 62(1):33–36
45. Sajid MS et al (2009) The role of perioperative warming in surgery: a systematic review. Sao Paulo Med J 127(4):231–237
46. Paris A et al (2005) The effect of meperidine on thermoregulation in mice: involvement of α_2-adrenoceptors. Anesth Analg 100:102–106
47. Kurz A et al (1997) Meperidine decreases the shivering threshold twice as much as the vasoconstriction threshold. Anesthesiology 86:1046–1054
48. Takada K et al (2002) Meperidine exerts agonist activity at the α_{2B} adrenoceptor subtype. Anesthesiology 96:1420–1426
49. Pawar MS, Suri N (2011) Hydrocortisone reduces postoperative shivering following day care knee arthroscopy. Can J Anesth/J Can Anesth 58:924–928
50. Gozdemir M et al (2010) Magnesium sulfate infusion prevents shivering during transurethral prostatectomy with spinal anesthesia: a randomized, double-blinded, controlled study. Journ of Clin Anesth 22:184–189
51. Kizilirmak S et al (1997) Magnesium sulfate stops postanesthetic shivering. Ann NY Acad Sci 813:799–806
52. Hwang J-Y et al (2010) I.V. infusion of magnesium sulphate during spinal anesthesia improves postoperative analgesia. Br J of Anaesthesia 104(1):89–93
53. Ryu J-H et al (2008) Effects of magnesium sulphate on intraoperative anesthetic requirements and postoperative analgesia in gynaecology patients receiving total intravenous anaesthesia. Br J of Anesth 100(3):397–403
54. Powell RM, Buggy DJ (2000) Ondansetron given before induction of anesthesia reduces shivering after general anesthesia. Anesth Analg 90:1423–1427
55. Kelsaka E et al (2006) Comparison of ondansetron and meperidine for prevention of shivering in patients undergoing spinal anesthesia. Reg Anesth Pain Med 31:40–45

56. Dal D et al (2005) Efficacy of prophylactic ketamine in preventing postoperative shivering. Br J Anaesth 95:189–192
57. Sagir O et al (2007) Control of shivering during regional anaesthesia: prophylactic ketamine and granisetron. Acta Anaesthesiol Scand 51:44–49
58. Kose EA et al (2008) The efficacy of ketamine for the treatment of postoperative shivering. Anesth Analg 106:120–122
59. Torossian A (2008) Thermal management during anesthesia and thermoregulation standards for the prevention of inadvertent perioperative hypothermia. Best Pract Res Clin Anaesth 22:659–6

Epidemiology, Etiopathogenesis, Diagnosis, and Treatment of Postoperative Paralytic Ileus in Intensive Care

11

Marco Dei Poli

A recent paper has proposed a score for the assessment of the inadequacy of the digestive tract [1]. It might be, at first sight, the umpteenth rating scale to be inserted in the staging of how critical is a patient in Intensive Care: actually, for the first time, this yardstick puts the digestive tract and its function among the elements that affect the outcome of the hospital stay.

We now know how much the SOFA score (Simplified Organ Failure Assessment) underscores the hepatic, renal, circulatory, respiratory, as well as the neurological, and hemostatic failures: it is since 10 years that an expert Consensus [2] stated that the intestinal function is a primary determinant in the outcome of critically ill patients, and is therefore necessary to pay great attention to the dysfunctions of this apparatus.

The parameters that enter in the evaluation of the Gastrointestinal Failure(GIF) () score are: the truly administered percentage of the prescribed enteral nutrition, the duration of fasting, and the ileum or the diarrhea (as intolerance to nutrition), the abdominal hypertension, and the abdominal compartment syndrome.

It is well known how intolerance to nutrition is expressed as high gastric stagnation, vomiting, bowel distension, and altered transit time. The GIF score measured in the first 3 days after admission to intensive care shows a strong prognostic value.

The aim of the critical care nutrition is to minimize the malnutrition associated with the acute illness: it considers the influence of the current illness, the therapeutic interventions, the organ dysfunctions with the nutritional care, and measures risks and benefits of the nutritional care itself.

M. Dei Poli (✉)
Intensive Care Unit, IRCCS Policlinico San Donato, Piazza Malan 1, 20097,
San Donato Milanese, Italy
e-mail: deipolimd@gmail.com

B. Allaria (ed.), *Practical Issues in Anesthesia and Intensive Care 2013*,
DOI: 10.1007/978-88-470-5529-2_11, © Springer-Verlag Italia 2014

In a recent report on "nutritional risk in critical area" [3] the weight loss related to hospitalization reaches prevalence between 35 and 41 % [4]. The loss of lean body mass is related to the functional state prior to the acute episode, to the severity of the injury/illness, to the intensity of the inflammatory response, to the restoration of physiologic enteral nutrition, and the balance between loss and protein synthesis.

Any patient who remains in Intensive Area for more than 2 days in the absence of a close to normal oral intake can be considered at risk of malnutrition.

The motility disorders of the digestive tract play a central role in reducing or delaying the "normal" nutrient intake.

The postoperative ileus (POI or PI is, unfortunately, very common after major abdominal surgery (but even in other or minor surgical procedures).

An acceptable definition may be "transient cessation of coordinated motility of the digestive tract, following an abdominal surgical procedure, which effectively prevents the transit of intraluminal content and tolerance to food intake."

There are clear implications of an abnormal postoperative ileus on the poor quality of hospital stay for the patient, the increase in costs and occupation of beds in acute care areas due to increase of length of stay(LOS). In a recent review of patients undergoing colectomy, a postoperative ileus lengthened hospital stay of 8 days on average, with an additional cost of approximately $15,000 per patient [5].

The set of symptoms is variable: some patients remain largely asymptomatic, while others complain of cramps, nausea, vomiting and pain from distension. Occasionally, gaseous distension and biliary vomiting occur.

Anorexia is evident, the flatus almost always absent.

At the physical exam abdominal distention and tympanism are typically found: the tenderness is not specific and is more often correlated to wound or underlying disease.

The absence of bowel sounds typically defines paralytic ileus, which is specific and necessary to define the syndrome: on the contrary the recovery of a normal GI motility is heralded by bowel sounds reappearance.

A modern clinical approach cannot find a close link between gastrointestinal function and audible noise: the clinical decisions cannot be entrusted based on this finding.

Not even the imaging helps to establish with certainty the diagnosis of postoperative ileus: an anteroposterior or tangential X ray of the abdomen, an abdominal ultrasound or CT scan only help to deepen a causal diagnosis when the ileum does not resolve after five or 6 days (search for abdominal abscesses or anastomotic dehiscence, evidence of adhesions, volvulus, and other).

Moreover, using the resumption of bowel sounds or passage of air as the criterion to define the functional recovery of the gastrointestinal tract (GI) is irrespective of the GI physiology.

Experimental measurements of the motility of the GI show that the activity in the small intestine is reestablished in 12–24 h, after 24–48 h in the stomach and after 3–5 days in the colon.

Waiting for proofs of colon motility (flatus and noise) to restart feeding means underestimate the ability of the stomach to tolerate feeding and of the small intestine to perform the functions of digestion and absorption.

Another questionable indicator of the end of ileum is the amount of gastric residual volume, based on the assumption that a normal function of GI allows the distal transit of a higher amount of secretions. Clinical evidences show the unreliability of this parameter: more usefully, the shift of color of nasogastric secretion from green to almost colorless can be employed. It is good to remember that the nasogastric drainage should be removed as soon as possible to make room for an early feeding.

The best proof for the end of ileus is the patient's ability to tolerate oral feeding without pain, gaseous distention, bloating, or vomiting, with appropriate caution, small meal testing should be performed as soon as possible, that must be promptly increased as soon as the tolerance of the patient is demonstrated.

In the discussion that follows, the specific motility disorders of the postsurgical phase (postoperative ileus per se) will often intersect with chronic disorders of transit. Similarly, considerations of gastroparesis (limitation of the proximal portions of the GI disorders), and disorders of the ileal and colonic transit will overlie.

The discussion of remedies has been intentionally kept in its totality, leaving to the reader the placement of the various concepts in a sectorial scheme.

11.1   Anatomy and Physiology of the Digestive Tract Motility

To fulfill its task of digesting food and to promote the absorption of nutritive substance in blood, the gastrointestinal (GI) tract performs three distinct activities:
- motility;
- secretion;
- digestion and absorption.

For the purposes of our discussion, we will examine as first item the anatomical structure of the gastrointestinal tract, and then the physiology of motility.

Despite the peculiar structural changes in the different sections of the GI tract, there are common characteristics in all segments (stomach, small intestine, colon).

From the lumen to the outside we always find the mucosa, consisting of:
- the epithelium, single layer of specialized cells, characteristic of the GI tract in question;
- the lamina propria, layer of loose connective tissue containing capillaries, lymphatic cells, and glands;
- the muscularis mucosae, where the innermost layer of the smooth muscle of the GI tract is structured in two thin muscular foils, the circular one innermost and the longitudinal one outermost;
- the submucosa layer of connective, crossed by nervous trunks and blood vessels of greater dimensions;

- the muscularis externa, muscular layer consisting of smooth muscle, with internal circular fibers and external longitudinal ones. These muscle fibers are responsible for the actions of mixing and propulsion of the contents of the GI tract;
- the serosa (adventitia), a connective tissue one.

The rich innervation of the wall of the GI tract, very interconnected, is called the enteric nervous system: within its scope two plexiform structures are particularly relevant:

- the submucosal plexus of Meissner;
- the myenteric plexus of Auerbach, localized in the muscularis externa, between the two circular and longitudinal layers.

The importance of the enteric nervous system (ENS), which together with the sympathetic and parasympathetic innervation constitutes the autonomic nervous system (ANS), is proven by the large number of neurons that are involved, about 100 million, same as all the remaining ANS or the entire spinal cord.

The peculiarity of the ENS is to be able to operate entirely within the GI tract, without the involvement of the spinal cord or central nervous system (CNS). This function is strongly independent and led the English to create the term "GI minibrain", assuming that the ENS possesses a set of preprogrammed responses to afferent stimuli which can lead to similar efferent answers. For example, the mechanical distension during fasting and the presence in the same site of bacterial enterotoxin elicit both the stimulation of a profuse secretion of fluids and electrolytes, along with coordinate, propulsive, and propagating muscle contraction.

Across the whole GI tract the action of parasympathetic NS is activatory and excitatory, while the one of the sympathetic NS is inhibitory. Moreover, it is intuitive that in all stages of stress activity sympathicotonic digestive processes are downregulated and, at the same time, are dysfunctional: furthermore, isn't it common to say, "I have everything left on the stomach…" when you are subjected to stress or tension?

In effect, despite the ability of the GI tract to work with "local" reflections, which take place entirely in the ENS, nervous control of the digestive system is also a function of extrinsic nerves, parasympathetic extrinsic pathways, and to a lesser extent, sympathetic, under the control of brainstem and autonomic centers.

Acetylcholine (ACh) is the main neurotransmitter that regulates the secretory and contractile activity of smooth muscle in the GI tract while the vasoactive intestinal peptide (VIP), has an important muscular and prosecretive inhibitory role. The field of neurotransmitters of the ENS is under heavy development: in addition to enkephalin, somatostatin, substance P, serotonin, and nitric oxide (NO), the list of agonists is growing, along with new developments in the understanding of their functions.

In addition to local control and the activity carried out by the sympathetic NS and parasympathetic NS, the upper control is present, localized in the central brain structures (for example, the response of "flight or fight" which drastically reduces the blood flow to the GI tract, or the response "sight and smell" for food, which increases the gastric secretion).

This communication is bidirectional, so even local secretions send signals to the center: it's the case of cholecystokinin (CCK) that, in part, mediates the feeling of satiety.

Thus, a real "cerebro-neuro-intestinal" axis is created, that acts as a bidirectional system of functional control through the autonomic nervous system, hormones, gastrointestinal peptides, and the immune system.

The latter is, in fact, an essential component of "neuro-digestive" communication, in particular thanks to the neuroimmune regulatory action of the mast cells of the intestinal lamina propria: sensitive to neurotransmitters, they process the information from the CNS to the ENS and respond to interneurons of ENS itself; they send sensory input from the intestinal lumen when in contact with antigens, and regulate the activity of smooth muscle by their chemical mediators.

The motor activity of the GI tract, which is regulated by the ENS and the activity of smooth muscle, complies with three main functions:

- segmental contractions associated with non-propulsive movements of the intraluminal content: their effect is the mixing and blending of content and secretion, to promote digestion and absorption of nutrients;
- contractions generating propulsion: the movements that with their propagation transport the food and the products of digestion in the caudal direction, toward the disposal sites;
- in some hollow organs (stomach and intestines in particular) an activity of "reservoir" is present, to contain and hold a temporary luminal contents: this function is achieved through the coordination of motor function of other structures—the sphincters—that separate the different structures of the GI tract [6].

In all these activities we recognize a central role to the coordinated GI smooth muscle activities.

The meccano electric properties of intestinal smooth muscle necessary for this purpose are of two types:

(1) tonic contractions (sustained);
(2) rhythmic contractions (alternance of contraction and relaxation).

The smooth muscle cells of the gastrointestinal tract are long (about 500 μm) and narrow (5–20 μm), organized in bundles, separated, and defined by connective tissue.

The intrinsic rhythmic contractility is a function of membrane voltage (V_m) of the single myocell.

V_m can swing in two ways:

- in a low frequency range below the threshold, many times in a minute, known as slow-wave activity (slow-wave activity, or Basic electric rhythm);
- reaching the threshold of generation of a real action potential.

The integrated effect of slow waves and action potentials determines the muscular activity of the GI tract.

On the contrary to what happens in most excitable tissues, the membrane potential at rest of the smooth muscle cell of the GI tract varies significantly over time, giving rise to slow waves, in measure of 3 (stomach) to 12 (duodenum) per minute.

These waves, thanks to the "gap junctions" between adjacent muscle cells, propagate rapidly along entire sections of the intestine.

The width and frequency of slow waves can be modulated by neuronal intrinsic and extrinsic activity (e.g., sympathetic activity decreases in the amplitude or abolishes the waves) or by hormones.

At the exceeding of the threshold of the cell excitability, slow wave generate one or more action potentials (1–10/s).

While the slow waves in the absence of action potentials lead to weak contractions of the gastrointestinal tract, bursts of action potentials, grouped at the peak of slow waves, produce vigorous contractions: the higher the frequency of action potentials, the greater is the force of the smooth muscle cell contraction, with the individual contractions of each potential that add up to produce global and progressive tension increase.

During the interval between discharges, the voltage level never drops to zero even in case of considerable reduction: this tension is the basal tone, modulated by drugs, hormones, and neuroeffectors.

For the understanding of the subject we are dealing with, it is necessary to deepen the physiology of the motility in stomach and intestines, leaving at separate in-depth analysis the esophageal motility, the swallowing, vomiting, and defecation, as well as the important activities reflected between distant segments of tract digestion (e.g., the gastrocolic reflex).

11.2 The Stomach

The basic functions of gastric motility are:
- to allow the function of container for even large amounts of food that can be ingested in a meal;
- to fragment the food and mix the particles obtained with gastric secretions;
- to empty the stomach contents into the duodenum.

It all starts when, as a result of esophageal peristaltic wave, the lower esophageal sphincter is released, which corresponds to the relaxation—so-called receptive—of the fundus and body of the stomach. The latter allows increases in volume of more than 1.5 l without inducing significant increases of intragastric pressure (reservoir function): very weak contractions occur, which induce a negligible mixing of the food in this location.

The antrum instead, produces vigorous contractions that effectively mix chyme and gastric juice, as well as divide the antral content in smaller particles. These "jet" contractions push the gastric contents into the duodenum, with a speed finely regulated by multiple mechanisms that should prevent the chyme to be sent to the duodenum in an amount greater than its boarding capacity.

Because of the scarcity of strength of the contractions of the bottom of the gastric body, the content of the stomach tends to be arranged in layers of different density, and this arrangement does not undergo stratiform remixing for periods of 1 h.

The oily layer of food fats goes on the surface, and is transferred to the duodenum at last; liquids flowing around the solid mass are rapidly emptied into the duodenum. Particles of large volume or not digestible remain in the stomach for longer time.

The stomach contracts at a rate of about 3/min: the contractions start in the middle of the body and, heading toward the pylorus, progressively increase of strength and speed: therefore in the antrum there is the highest intensity of fragmentation and remixing.

Obviously, this description is valid for the phase during which the stomach takes food from swallowing and esophageal peristalsis: different story for fasting stomach motility (consistent with such an attitude of the intestine).

In a subject having a fasting, the antrum is dormant for a period of 75–90 min, which is followed by a phase of intense electrical and motor activity lasting about 10 min, in which the antrum contracts vigorously, and pylorus releases: in this way the stomach expels caudal parts of food or other material left over from the previous meal, followed by a new period of quiescence of 75–90 min.

This cyclic alternation of contractions and quiescence is part of a more complex transverse mechanism, called migrating myoelectric complex (MMC).

Antrum and duodenum are well coordinated with each other, so when the antrum shrinks the duodenal bulb is released. The gastroduodenal junction, in whom the pylorus functions as a true sphincter, must:

- enable the tightly regulated emptying of gastric contents, with a speed that commensurate with the ability of the duodenum to digest the chyme;
- prevent the reflux of duodenal contents into the stomach.

The stomach has a rich innervation (parasympathetic from vagus nerve and sympathetic from the celiac plexus) which presides over the activation or inhibition of motility and secretion (shared with hormones and neuropeptides) in the same way the pylorus receives stimulus to contract from sympathetic fibers and by hormones such as gastrin, CCK, secretin, and gastroinhibitory peptide (but also by vagal fibers employing ACh), while induction of relaxation is given by the parasympathetic that uses the VIP as a neurotransmitter.

11.2.1 The Small Intestine

The mucosa of the duodenum and jejunum is equipped with receptors and sensors for osmolarity, pH, some lipids, amino acids, and peptides.

Taking advantage of a complex physical and neurohormonal signaling:

- the fats do not empty into the duodenum at a speed higher than that of emulsion of bile acids and lecithin;

- the hydrochloric acid (HCl) passes into the duodenum at a speed lower than that necessary to pancreatic and duodenal secretions for buffering it;
- the speed with which the other components of the chyme are transferred from the stomach into the duodenum never exceeds the capacity of the latter to digest them;

(...in summary... the presence of fats, acidic pH and hypertonicity/hyperosmolarity in the duodenum, all slow the gastric emptying, through a decrease in the contractile force of the antrum and an increase in the contractile power of the smooth duodenal muscle).

Almost 5 m of small intestine are traversed by the chyme in a time ranging from 2 to 4 h.

It is in the 25 cm of the duodenum and in about the 2 m of the jejunum—the two proximal portions—that most of the digestion and absorption of nutrients occurs, and it is here, therefore, that the motility assumes preponderant significance, to enhance the functions of mixing chyme and secretions, contact with the microvillus and propulsion toward the colon.

The most represented movement is the segmentation, close contractions of contiguous segments of the circular muscle layer of the small intestine: the alternating contractions and relaxations of the circular wall optimizes mixing and contact with the mucosa.

Short peristaltic waves, and long ones to a lesser extent, promote the contraction of successive segments of the intestine with peristaltic progression toward aboral direction (or orocaudal).

As in most proximal segments of the stomach and duodenum, also in the small intestine there are slow waves with a progressively smaller frequency, from 11–13 of the duodenum to 8–9 in the distal ileum. The release of action potentials that are inscribed on the tonic phenomena activate contractions of the circular muscle, limited to short bowel tracts, so performing an highly localized activity.

As elsewhere, the basic electrical rhythm originates in the intrinsic innervation (ENS), while frequency and intensity of bursts of action potentials are influenced by ANS and neurohormones.

Anyway, the motion of a bolus of chyme within the intestine, result of an upstream contraction and a downstream relaxation, follows the "law of the intestine", that fix the movement direction in the aboral sense.

Compared to what happens after the ingestion of food and the production of a bolus of chyme, intestinal motility of a fasting individual is completely different, characterized by discharges of intense electrical and contractile activity, separated by long periods of quiescence: in analogy as what described for the stomach, this activity is called migrating myoelectric complex (MMC).

The MMC has the periodicity of about 75–90 min, and only when a complex reaches the terminal portion of the ileum the next complex is generated in the stomach, with contractions of greater intensity than those recorded in an intestine containing chyme: it is an activity of cleaning and emptying toward the distal portions (colic).

Another type of intestinal motility is that of the muscularis mucosae, which contract irregularly, about three times per minute: the profile of ridges and folds of the mucous membrane is modified to increase contact of the continuously stirred nutrients with secretions and their absorption. Similarly, the villous contract probably optimizing the lymphatic flow.

11.2.2 The Colon

The role of the colon is to transform 500–1,500 ml of chyme into feces containing the equivalent of only 50–100 ml of water: this action of reabsorption takes place thanks to a mixing movement, slowly progressing (5–10 cm/h), of the chyme that gradually becomes more and more solid. In fact caecum and colon work primarily as mixing machines, with little segmental propulsive movements, in reverse peristalsis, all aimed at promoting the reabsorption of water and salts. It is only with a frequency of one/three times per day that in the colon a peristaltic wave of contraction is produced, in which the segments involved remain contracted a long time: it is the peristaltic wave of mass, which has the function of advancing the semi-solid mass in a long section of the colon, in the direction of the evacuation tract. Because of the greater consistency of the luminal contents, the need for a greater contractile developed force is guaranteed by teniae coli (specialized external muscle layer), and by greater vigor contractile layers concentrated in the rectum and in the anal canal. The complex system of neural and hormonal control of gastrointestinal motility operates in the state of fasting and food intake by managing physical and secretive activities.

Talking about the "perioperative motility disorders" of the gastrointestinal tract, we talk about a system (digestive) artificially inactivated: the digestive tract is in fact structured to deal with boluses of ingested nutrients, and during fasting only plays auto cleansing activity. You must therefore remind the concept of the migrating motor complex(MMC).

During fasting, MMC characterizes the contractile pattern of the GI tract, in its entirety [7]. In men the contraction frequency is every 1/2 h, and this "house-cleaning" is developed in four phases.

The first (lasting about 60 min) is characterized by oscillatory potentials of the membrane of the smooth muscle without development of contractions, which instead appear in the transition to phase II.

In stage III there is an increase of frequency of contractions up to the maximum allowed by the slow underlying wave (3/min in the stomach and 11/min in the duodenum). In this stage the contraction migrates from the stomach to the ileo-caecal (thanks to "gap junctions" between myocytes), moving distally the entire luminal residual.

Phase IV sees the cessation of contractions, with the return to the quiescent phase of the GI tract.

Typically, the introduction of food (fed state) interrupts the MMC, and gives rise to the characteristic phasic pattern.

11.3   The Reasons of Postoperative Ileus

The pathogenesis of any transit disorder is multifactorial, with direct, indirect, local, and systemic factors, and its arbitrary establish a priority order among these mechanisms [8]. The description of the different contributions, proven or hypothetical, studied in humans and in animals, will be useful in understanding how to approach the postoperative ileus and other motility disorders.

11.3.1 Surgical Manipulation

The surgical manipulation of the abdominal organs makes the dysmotility of the digestive tract inevitable, with a relative contribution of local inflammatory reaction, loss of mucosal integrity and translocation of luminal contents, and alteration of the neural and neurohumoral signaling [9].

11.3.2 Intestinal Injury

The intestinal mucosa is particularly susceptible to any proinflammatory stimulus, of traumatic, postischemic reperfusive type, or infectious, and each of these can produce organic damage and dysmotility. The transition outward the lumen of the intestinal contents inevitably activates all paths of systemic inflammation. The direct surgical trauma is directly involved in this process.

11.3.3 Inflammation

The intestine is a really peculiar site for the immune response: it is a powerful interface with the external world, which interacts with food, toxins, living ecosystems. The villi are extremely sensible to exogenous stimuli, the muscularis externa is covered by leukocytes and in particular macrophages: any proinflammatory stimulus combines these defensive positions to release interleukins, prostaglandins, nitric oxide, and reactive oxygen species. Sepsis and surgery trauma on the digestive tract are described in the literature as typical inducers of gastrointestinal dysmotility [10, 11].

11.3.4 Hypoperfusive Damage

The gastrointestinal tract is particularly susceptible to decrease of cardiac output: while the macrohemodynamics (systemic arterial pressure and heart rate) does not change for bleeding up to 30 % of the blood volume, the gastrointestinal splanchnic is already suffering at 10–15 % [12].

The hypoperfusive damage is easily revealed by the organ dysfunction that ensues, mostly the gastroparesis and the increase of intra-abdominal pressure. The hypoperfusive damage is easily revealed by the organ dysfunction that ensues, mostly the gastroparesis and the increase of intra-abdominal pressure.

11.3.5 Systemic Hypoxia and Hypercapnia

Hypoxia—in animal models—induces mucosal acidosis in the intestine, even with maintained perfusion [13]. Respiratory acidosis alters, in an inhibitory mode, the gastropyloric motility.

11.3.6 Neurogenic Inferences

Surgical manipulation of the intestine can alter the neuronal and neurohormonal balance in different ways, all explored only in form of hypotheses. One of these involves the release of hypothalamic corticotropin releasing factor(CRF) useful to activate inhibitory adrenergic efferent pathways destined to intestinal smooth muscle [14]. Another hypothesis invokes a local release, following hypoxia and hypoperfusion, of 5-hydroxytryptamine three with a close link between induction of vomiting and disturbance of motility.

Other inhibitory neurotransmitters locally released include nitric oxide (NO), VIP, substance P, and prostaglandins.

11.3.7 Metabolic Disorders

The altered motility of the GI may be motivated by any disorder of acid-base balance, blood glucose, and electrolyte homeostasis, particularly by hypokalemia, by hypomagnesemia and hyponatremia.

Hyperglycemia and metabolic acidosis both slow emptying of the stomach [15].

11.3.8 Fluid Balance

We will discuss when treating the postoperative ileus the importance of intraoperative fluid restriction. Like any parenchyma or tissue, even the intestinal wall may experience edema, as stressed in a fundamental work on Lobo about salt and water balance during the intraoperative period of colonic surgery [16].

11.3.9 Hypothermia

Hyperthermia and hypothermia are both associated with dysfunction of GI motility. It is not clear whether the redistribution of blood flow, especially in the context of hypothermia, plays a primary role, nor if the delays in recovery of motility of cardiac surgery patients can only be attributed to the role of induced hypothermia.

11.4 Anesthetic Drugs and Ileum

Virtually any anesthetic drug has an effect on motility of the GI tract.

The action of anesthetic drugs is exercised mainly on the intestinal tracts which is directly regulated by neuronal integration. In particular the colon, where the tight junctions between myocells (gap junctions) are under-represented, is particularly sensitive to the inhibitory action of anesthetic drugs.

The effects of gastroparesis are dangerous in the context of anesthesia since they may lead to regurgitation and subsequent inhalation, and are also critical in the induction of PONV (post operative nausea and vomiting) and interference with the absorption of per os drugs.

11.4.1 Propofol

Numerous reports are available in literature on the effects of propofol on gastrointestinal motility. At intravenous subhypnotic doses (0.5 mcg/ml) and hypnotic (sleepy but arousable on command) propofol slows mildly orocecal transit [17].

At high doses, even the fat emulsion of the drug (Intralipid) may adversely affect gastric emptying.

The mechanisms of the inhibitory effect of propofol (and midazolam) on the alterations of motility are not yet clarified. It is possible (but not proven) an activation of GABAa receptors, widely present in the CNS, and therefore also in the dorsal vagal nuclei, which send cholinergic fibers in the GI tract [18].

At ENS level the answer is bivalent, activating and inhibiting motility, and it is supposed that the one induced by propofol (and midazolam) is inhibitory.

11.4.2 Nitrous Oxide

Despite being an anesthetic gas in disuse, like enflurane and halothane, the characteristic of nitrous oxide to be delivered electively in the structures containing gas (such as the gastrointestinal tract) remains well known, with the result of an expansion of these spaces many times the initial volume. This has led to contraindicate the use of nitrous in all situations of intestinal surgery in which a volvulus or occlusion with gaseous distension are proven.

Nitrous oxide, however, does not disturb by "itself" the gastrointestinal motility, with negligible effects compared to other inducers of postoperative ileus.

11.4.3 Inhalation Anesthetics

The effects on colonic motility of inhaled anesthetics are well highlighted in work on the animal: the administration of enflurane and halothane was known to cause the cessation of the contractile activity in the right and left colon, and the suppression of motor activity lasted for the whole period of administration of the gas, normally recovering at the complete elimination of the same in the expired gas. The recovery of peristaltic activity was earlier in the right colon than the left [19].

11.4.4 Morphine and Opiates

Opioids play a primary role in the genesis of postoperative ileus, because of their depressant effects on motility in the digestive tract.

The pharmacological action involves receptors, locally in the digestive tract, with a minimal contribution of spinal and brain receptors.

Among the classes of receptors for opiates (κ, δ and μ), the one implicated in the effects on the gastrointestinal system is the μ: μ receptor action on the CNS is kind of analgesic.

The action of morphine and derivatives on intestinal motility is ubiquitous, and include inhibition of gastric motility, antrum, and first portion of the duodenum hypertonia. The action of opiates is biphasic, initially causing a contractile stimulus for the ileal activation of MMC, which is subsequently inhibited, with induction of atony and slow transit. At colonic level, morphine reduces the propulsive waves, and increases the tone and amplitude of non-propulsive contractions.

Alongside the action and the effects of opioids administered for therapeutic purposes, in the context of surgical trauma there is an increase in endogenous opiates (endorphins), with obvious relapse and amplification of the effects on transit [20].

The relationship between the analgesic effect and the constipating one is about 4:1, that means that it takes doses ×4 to obtain analgesia compared to the alteration of motility.

Moreover, while it easy to induce tolerance to the analgesic effect for repeated doses of morphine, it is impossible to induce tolerance to the constipating effects.

The antagonism of the effect of μ receptor by administration of naloxone has limited effectiveness, and in any case, it induces partial or complete loss of analgesia [21]. We will discuss later the use of the most modern and selective μ receptor antagonists in the treatment of postoperative ileus.

It is stimulating to reconsider the whole context of the motility disorders of the GI tract as the consequence of a hypersympathetic tone, due to surgical stress and pain, a condition known to induce inhibition of contractile activity.

Experiments on animal models have demonstrated an increase in serum levels of catecholamines after laparotomy and manipulation of the intestinal loops and, in mice, the depletion of the intestinal deposits of norepinephrine after laparotomy [22].

The blockade of sympathetic reflexes by resection of the splanchnic innervation or by chemical sympathectomy reduces postoperative ileus significantly [23]. The change of priorities in the homeostatic control systems regarding the digestive apparatus is well demonstrated by changes in perfusion and redistribution of cardiac output in the states of stress and hyperdynamics: it is not surprising that the loss of parasympathetic dominance modulating digestion and absorption amplifies the motility disturbances seen at the bedside.

11.5 The Therapeutic Approach

The strategies for the prevention and treatment of gastrointestinal dysmotility include the use of prokinetic molecules stimulating motility.

Among these there are the central and peripheral antagonist's dopamine-2 receptors, the motilin agonists and the agonists of serotonin-4 and -3 receptors.

It is clear that improvements in understanding the mechanisms of neurohumoral control of gastrointestinal motility will enable the development of new molecules, and their application in critical and non-critical patients.

As already mentioned in the section devoted to the physiology of gastrointestinal motility, there is a complex receptor activity spread throughout the ENS in and out of the myenteric plexus and intestinal smooth muscle: the beginning and propagation of the contractile activity of GI are mostly based on this activity [24].

The main excitatory neurotransmitters are acetylcholine and tachykinins released by motor neurons in the myenteric plexus, active on M2 and M3 muscarinic receptors for tachykinins of the smooth muscle.

Dopamine inhibits the release of acetylcholine from these neurons by binding to D2 receptors, with a reductive effect on gastric emptying and intestinal peristalsis.

The motilin, a peptide secreted by enteroendocrine cells of the GI tract, amplifies and induces phase III of the MMC.

The serotonin (5-hydroxytryptamine or 5-HT) is located all along the GI tract, regulating motility, secretion of the electrolytes, and the visceral perception of intestinal distension and pain. Of particular interest is the pharmacological modulation of 5HT3 receptors (contraction and relaxation of smooth muscle) and 5HT4 (chloride secretion and increase of ileal and colonic transit).

The cholecystokinin (CCK) is secreted from the duodenal mucosa in response to the presence of free fatty acids in its lumen: the effect is a slowing of gastric emptying and colonic transit mediated by CCK-1 receptors distributed throughout the GI tract.

We mentioned above the control of motility mediated by opiates receptors, and we will see the therapeutic implications in the next section.

11.5.1 Targeted Drug Therapy

The depressant effect of the hypersympathetic tone on the GI motility has justified the use of antagonists or blockers of the sympathetic activity to reduce the duration of postoperative ileus.

The results of the administration of **propranolol** (4 or 10 mg twice per day) showed significant effects only in some studies [25] but not in others [26].

The role of the **postoperative epidural analgesia** finds an excellent explanation in the decrease of hypersympathetic tone associated to pain.

The many benefits of postoperative epidural analgesia are:
- greater pain control and more space for mobilization;
- dose reduction of opioid analgesia, with secondary reduction of side effects;
- blockade of nociceptive afferents from the wound with reduction of the effects induced by surgical stress.

The shortening of ileus duration after thoracic epidural analgesia, compared to intravenous treatment with opiates, is well documented and proven [27].

Epidural analgesia with local anesthetics and of opiates may modestly lengthen postoperative recovery of motility.

The reason for the shortening of ileus must be found in the block of sympathetic inhibitory reflexes, originating from the viscera and surgical wound: this explains why a thoracic but not a lumbar block leads to the favorable effects in colon surgery.

The role of pain itself in the genesis of postoperative ileus has not been fully clarified, and the pain level of Visual Analogic Score (VAS) is not directly related to the intensity of ileus when studied in multimodal programs of postoperative intervention [28].

The same results are seen during balanced anesthesia in protocols of opioids restriction, in which paracetamol and NSAIDs were included (in some studies paracetamol and NSAID seem to reduce per se the time of ileus through effects on inhibitory prostaglandin synthesis) [29].

In an extensive meta-analysis of 2008 [30], the effect of continuous intravenous infusion of **lidocaine** significantly correlated with the shortening of postoperative ileus.

Since the first report in the literature in 1954 [31], lidocaine was used as intraoperative analgesia to cover the first postoperative phase. Almost the total absence of PONV did suggest a positive action on the GI transit, which later addressed some targeted research protocols.

In these studies (8 RCT, randomized controlled studies) a bolus of lidocaine (1.5–2 mg/kg) was administered before surgical incision, followed by continuous infusion (in one study the infusion was started without bolus). In the eight studies the infusion lasted for the entire surgery and up to 24 h postoperatively.

The meta-analysis showed Forrest plots in favor of lidocaine versus placebo for reduction of postoperative ileus duration, pain, nausea, and vomiting after surgery, as well as for hospital LOS.

Evidence supports that lidocaine suppresses some neural inhibitory activity of ENS.

Known the simplicity and the low cost of the technique, this results support a wider diffusion of lidocaine.

Neostigmine is an acetylcholinesterase inhibitor: its administration causes an increase in cholinergic activity (for reduced esterification of ACh) in the wall of the intestine, with a resulting increase in motility.

Despite proofs of a significant increase in activity of the colon in the early postoperative ileus (colorectal surgery) [32], the clinical utility of neostigmine in the postoperative phase may be limited by frequent side effects such as cramping, salivation, vomiting, and bradycardia. Particularly feared by the surgeon is the possibility of stress exerted on the anastomosis by a perking up of contractile activity.

Among the most studied and diffuse prokinetics, **metoclopramide** acts as a cholinergic agonist and dopaminergic antagonist (central and peripheral D2 receptor). It starts the phase III of the MMC antagonizing the action of endogenous dopamine.

This drug has been the subject of numerous prospective randomized and placebo-controlled studies. Although some of these have demonstrated an earlier tolerance to solid foods, in general they did not show advantages compared to placebo regarding the transit of gas or of bowel movements.

Although with different end points, at least six controlled clinical trials of abdominal surgery have not been able to demonstrate the advantages of metoclopramide in the treatment of postoperative ileus [33].

Like **domperidone** (a peripheral dopamine D2 receptor antagonist) metoclopramide is associated with adverse arrhythmic effects (torsades de pointe, ventricular arrhythmias and cardiac arrest) correlated with prolongation of QTc (corrected QT): moreover metoclopramide inhibits dopaminergic transmission in the basal ganglia and causes significant extrapyramidal disorders, including dystonic reactions and tardive dyskinesia [34]. The short-term administration of metoclopramide (10 mg 4 times daily) is certainly more effective than the placebo in promoting the transit [35], but the desired prokinetic effects decrease rapidly after 3 days, opposite to the risk of irreversible tardive dyskinesias, which are related to the duration and the amount of the drug administered, and the presence or absence of previous extrapyramidal disorders .

Erythromycin exerts its prokinetic effect through a motilin agonist action: the stimulation occurs only at ileal level, where the action of motilin itself is maximum. The lack of influence of the drug on the duration of the ileus (highlighted in the majority of studies) can be explained by the paucity of effects on colonic tract, whose inertia is more relevant to the duration of the postoperative ileus [36].

Azithromycin stimulates the activity of the gastric antrum in a way similar to erythromycin, and presents a more lasting effect (104 vs. 136 min) [37].

In addition, unlike erythromycin, interactions with other drugs are fewer and less significant

Cisapride has played an important role among the prokinetics until it has been withdrawn from the commerce because of the severity of cardiac side effects.

It is a serotonin 5-HT4 receptor agonist.

The **N-methylnaltrexone** is a quaternary derivative of the opioid antagonist naltrexone.

Similar to its precursor, peripherally blocks the effect of morphine and similar compounds, but being unable to cross the blood–brain barrier, does not affect the central analgesic effect of it.

It is mainly used in oncology and algology to combat constipation from opiates: numerous studies demonstrate its usefulness in the treatment of postoperative ileus.

The **almivopan** is a powerful μ receptor antagonist, acting purely at the periphery. Intended for oral administration, it is available for the treatment of morphine-induced bowel dysfunction (oncology!) and postoperative ileus.

Its exclusive peripheral action, absolutely localized in the intestine, is due to almost zero penetration through the brain–blood barrier [38]. The duration of its action is greater than that of already available μ antagonists (naloxone, n-methylnaltrexone), thanks to the kinetics of receptor binding of the drug (high affinity but slow dissociation).

The drug has an overall positive effect in restoring motility in the context of postoperative ileus, meanwhile leaving some doubt because of an increased need of opiates to maintain the analgesic effect.

Tegaserod is a 5-HT4 partial receptor agonist, acting peripherally, and at the same time a strong 5-HT2B receptor antagonist.

Many clinical studies have demonstrated the effect of tegaserod on GI motility: the series were of 24 cases of irritable bowel syndrome [39], 12 [40], and 40 [41] healthy subjects.

The effects on gastric emptying and ileal and colonic transit were significant and mainly localized in the upper GI tract.

Diarrhea and headache are not rare side effects with the use of this medication, and 1 of 250 patients has severe forms of hypotension, hypovolemia, and syncope, with recourse to hospitalization and infusion therapy [42].

Especially when used in critically ill patients, tegaserod exposes to the potential risk of ischemic colitis, particularly if there is a preexisting defect of mesenteric flow.

Loxiglumide and **dexloxiglumide** are two isomeric molecules with a strong, effective and specific antagonism of receptors for cholecystokinin 1.

They are drugs studied for irritable bowel syndrome, non-ulcer dyspepsia, disorders of delayed gastric emptying.

In human studies [43], infusion of loxiglumide increased gastric motility by shortening the time of stomach emptying in comparison to placebo.

The accelerated emptying was associated with increased amplitude and frequency of contractions, toward the distal stomach (antrum).

Nowadays, no studies on critically ill patients are available.

Among other drugs that have been proposed or experimentally used in treating motility disorders of the GI tract—and in particular the postoperative ileus—we must also mention:

- **dihydroergotamine**
- **vasopressin**
- **prucalopride** (5-HT4 receptor agonist]
- **bisacodyl** (magnesium salt)
- **prostaglandins**
- **edrophonium** (inhibition of adrenergic and cholinergic activation)
- **bethanechol** (inhibition of adrenergic and cholinergic activation)
- **NSAIDs**
- **ceruletide** (antagonist cholecystokinin)
- **Octreotide** (somatostatin analogue)
- **atilmotina** (analogue of motilin)
- **lubiprostone** (bicyclic fat acid, the active secretion of intestinal water).

To shed light on such a vast number of proposals and studies, was published in 2009 a number of the Cochrane Library entitled "Systemic prokinetic pharmacologic treatment for postoperative adynamic ileus following abdominal surgery in adults" (Review).

The authors' conclusions are the following:

Drugs are commonly used to reduce the impact of postoperative ileus. The evidence for the majority of these drugs is based on small trials of limited methodological quality, which jeopardizes the interpretation of the provided data.

..... are necessary greater statistical power trials and greater methodological quality...

Limited evidences from a few small trials of medium-low quality indicate that the use of intravenous lidocaine and neostigmine can provide favorable effects on postoperative ileum recovery time....

For drugs acting like cholecystokinin, for cisapride, for dopamine antagonists, for pantothenic acid, for vasopressin and for propranolol the evidences are insufficient to recommend their use in the postoperative ileus. For all these agents, the effects are inconsistent when addressed to different outcomes, the sample size is insufficient for final assessments, or the methodological quality of eligible trials to test is poor.

Cisapride has been withdrawn from commerce; erythromycin has no effect on post-operative recovery of intestinal motility.

It is possible that the almivopan could reduce the recovery time of motor function of the GI tract after major abdominal surgery: the current evidence is based on six trials of reasonable size, but whose lack of adherence to reporting standards prevents to exclude potential biases...

11.5.2 Non-Pharmacological Measures

11.5.2.1 Chewing Gum

It is a simple, economic and potentially effective approach, based on the concept of "sham feeding". The sham feeding is a procedure for the study of the psychic phase of gastric secretion: in experimental animals, ingested food is brought out by a cervical esophageal fistula: the effect on gastric secretion given by chewing and swallowing is studied. The cephalic-vagal stimulation, exerted by only chew, gives rise to hormonal and propulsive activity similar to that produced by the normal power supply.

A recent meta-analysis [44] on the use of chewing gum in the postoperative abdominal shows significant results in terms of first passage of flatus, the appearance of appreciable auscultatory bowel movement, and the LOS of these surgical patients.

The use in the early postoperative phase of chewing gum (in the various studies administered in a variable manner: from 5 to 30 min 3 or 4 times a day) has the advantage of availability, absence of costs, and tolerability.

11.5.2.2 Laxatives

The use of laxatives in the treatment of constipation is widespread and supported by evidence. Broadly speaking, they are divided into osmotic (lactulose, sorbitol, polyethylene glycol) and non-osmotic (salt: magnesium salts; bulking: methylcellulose, psyllium, agar agar, etc.; irritants: senna, sodium pyrosulfate, bisacodyl). They all may be usefully and successfully employed even in critically ill patients, where the transit of fecal material and bowel cleansing are often crucial.

Numerous protocols in the field of intensive care provide at the entrance, or at the most within 72 h, defecation, in particular with laxative action to increase the intestinal water content and soften the stool consistency.

It is clear that these principles do not apply in the narrow context of postoperative ileus.

11.5.2.3 Acupuncture

There are numerous studies that approach the effects of Chinese acupuncture on the gastrointestinal tract.

The stimulation of the Neiguan point (volar forearm) significantly inhibits the frequency of the rhythmic relaxation of the lower esophageal sphincter, frequent cause of delay in the beginning of enteral nutrition in critically ill patients and/or discontinuation of mechanical ventilation [45]. Even in neurosurgery patients the Neiguan point shows a prokinetic gastric effect superior to pharmacological treatment [46].

11.5.2.4 Minimally Invasive Surgery

Laparoscopic surgery and minimally invasive surgery have been proposed to reduce local inflammation at the site of surgical trauma, which finally leads to postoperative ileus.

There is a body of literature supporting this approach, in at least four randomized clinical trials: the lack of perioperative protocols exposes these studies to the risk of bias in the evaluation of the most favorable outcomes.

11.5.3 The Multimodal Approach

A systematic view of the causes and remedies of the postoperative ileus inevitably leads to confusion and uncertainty.

Which is the best of all available treatments?

Nowadays the best treatment is a multimodal regimen.

It has been evaluated [47] a multimodal rehabilitation regimen for postoperative ileus built up with continuous epidural analgesia, early enteral nutrition and mobilization, (cisapride) and laxative treatment with magnesium salts. The authors observed a shorter transit recovery (48 h), compared with the control group.

Another protocol—enrolling patients undergoing segmental colectomy—included thoracic epidural analgesia for 48 postoperative hours, early removal of nasogastric tube or other drains, 1 l of fluids orally on the surgery day, mobilization within 8 h of surgery, the modification of the incision line from longitudinal to transverse (to reduce pain and respiratory dysfunction) and the use of magnesium laxatives [48]. 95 of 100 patients resumed intestinal activities in 48–72 h of postoperative time.

Preliminary results about the multimodal approaches suggests that programs that incorporate continuous epidural analgesia with local anesthetics, early enteral nutrition and early mobilization may reduce the postoperative ileus duration to 24–48 h in the context of colorectal surgery.

Probably these encouraging results should be limited to situations in which there is a limited inflammatory component [49].

All the contribution of the early 2000 about multimodal postoperative rehabilitation programs were reviewed in recent years by the so-called ERAS (Enhanced Recovery After Surgery) protocol.

It consists of 20 elements that strongly influence the duration of treatment and hospital stay, and incidence of complications. It is easy to see how many of the topics covered in this session are reflected in several steps of ERAS in the postoperative ileum.

11.6 Conclusions

The postoperative ileus is still a tangible problem in surgical patients and in particular in the critically ill.

The etiology is certainly multifactorial, with different mechanisms working together or at different times: sympathetic inhibitory input, secretion of hormones and neurotransmitters, inflammatory reaction, effects of opiates, or other drugs. Many different approaches have been used to reduce the impact of postoperative ileus and clinical problems arising therefrom, with variable outcomes.

So far, the best suggestion is to minimize the impact of the factors underlying the phenomenon.

Among these, the reduction of opioids and the use of alternative NSAIDs, acetaminophen, and local anesthetics in epidural analgesia.

The selective use of nasogastric decompression, the correction of electrolyte imbalance, and a cautious policy of restriction of perioperative fluids all play an important role in multimodal management of the ileum.

The promises of the future will be found in laparoscopic and minimally traumatic surgery, in superselective opiate antagonists and in pharmacological manipulation of local factors, neurotransmitters and stress hormones.

References

1. Reintam A et al (2009) Gastrointestinal failure score in critically ill patients: a prospective observational study. Crit Care 12(4):R90 (online edition)
2. Ronbeau JL (1997) Summary of round table conference: gut dysfunction in critical illness. Intensive Care Med 23:476–479
3. Hiesmayr M (2012) Nutrition risk assessment in ICU. Curr Opin Clin Nutr 15:174–180
4. Fruhwald S et al (2010) Effect of ICU interventions on gastrointestinal motility. Curr Opin Crit Care 16:159–164
5. Salvador C et al (2005) Clinical and economic outcomes of prolonged postoperative ileus in patients undergoing hysterectomy and hemicolectomy. Pharm Ther 30:590–595
6. Berne R, Levy MN (2006) Principi di fisiologia: la motilita' del tratto gastrointestinale. Casa Editrice Ambrosiana, Chapter 12, Milano
7. Szurszewski JH (1969) A migrating electric complex of the canine small intestine. Am J Physiol 217:1757–1763
8. Mythen MG (2005) Postoperative gastrointestinal tract dysfunction. Anesth Analg 100:196–204
9. Kalff JC et al (1998) Surgical manipulation of the gut elicits an intestinal muscularis inflammatory response resulting in postsurgical ileus. Ann Surg 228:652–663
10. Hassoun HT et al (2001) Postinjury multiple organ failure: the role of the gut. Shock 15:1–10
11. Mythen MG et al (1993) The role of endotoxin immunity, neutrophil degranulation and contact activation in the pathogenesis of postoperative organ disfunction. Blood Coagul Fibrin 4:999–1005
12. Hamilton Davies C et al (1997) Comparison of commonly used clinical indicators of hypovolemia with gastrointestinal tonometry. Intensive Care Med 23:276–281
13. Moretti EW et al (2003) Intraoperative colloid administration reduces postoperative nausea and vomiting and improves postoperative outcomes compared with crystalloid administration. Anasth Analg 96:611–617
14. Tache Y et al (1993) Role of CRF in stress related alteration in gastric and colonic motor function. Annals NY Acad Sci 697:233–243
15. Tournadre JP et al (2003) Metabolic acidosis and respiratory acidosis impair gastropyloric motility in anesthetized pigs. Anesth Analg 96:74–79
16. Lobo DN et al (2002) Effect of salt and water balance on recovery of gastrointestinal function after elective colonic resection: a randomised controlled trial. Lancet 359:1812–1818
17. Takefumi I (2004) Propofol and midazolam inhibit gastric emptying and gastrointestinal transit in mice. Anesth Analg 99:1102–1106
18. Greenwood-Van MB et al (1998) Tonic GABA(A) receptor-mediated neurotransmission in the dorsal vagal complex regulates intestinal motility in rats. Eur J Pharmacol 346:197–202
19. Condon RE et al (1987) Effects of halothane, enflurane and nitrous oxide on colon motility. Surgery 101:81

20. Yoshida S et al (2000) Effect of surgical stress on endogenous morphine and cytokine levels in plasma after laparoscopic or open cholecystectomy. Surg Endosc 14:137–140
21. Livingstone EH et al (1990) Postoperative ileus. Dig Dis Sci 35:121–131
22. Dubois A et al (1974) Chemical and histochemical studies of postoperative sympathetic activity in the digestive tract in rats. Gastroenterology 66:403–407
23. Nilsson F et al (1973) Gastric evacuation and small bowel propulsion after laparotomy. A study with a double isotope technique in rat. Acta Chir Scand 139:724–730
24. Hansen MB (2003) Neurohumoral control of gastrointestinal motility. Phisiol Res 52:1–30
25. Hallerback B et al (1987) Beta-adrenoceptor blockade in the treatment of post operative adynamic ileus. Scand J Gastroenterol 22:149–155
26. Ferraz AA et al (2001) Effects of propranolol of human post operative ileus. Dig Surg 18:305–310
27. Jorgensen H et al (2002) Epidural local anesthetics versus opioid based analgesic regimens on postoperative gastrointestinal paralysis, PONV and pain after abdominal surgery (Cochrane review). In: Cochrane Collaboration, The Cochrane library, Issue 1. Update software, Oxford
28. Werner MU et al (2001) Does postoperative pain influence gastrointestinal recovery and hospital stay following colonic resection in an accelerated multimodal program? Anesthesiology 26:95: A 821
29. Kelley MC (1993) Ketorolac prevents postoperative small intestine ileus in rats. Am J Surg 165:107–111
30. Marret E et al (2008) Meta analysis of intravenous lidocaine and postoperative recovery after abdominal surgery. Br J Surg 95:1331–1338
31. de Clive Lowe SG et al (1954) Succinyldicholine and lignocaine by continuous intravenous drip: report of 1000 administrations. Anesthesia 9:96–194
32. Kreis ME et al (2001) Neostigmine increases postoperative colonic motility in patients undergoing colorectal surgery. Surgery 130:449–456
33. Jepsen S et al (1986) Negative effect of metoclopramide in postoperative adynamic ileus: a prospective, randomized, double blind study. Br J Surg 73:290–291
34. Pasricha PJ (2006) Treatment of disorders of bowel motility and water flux; antiemetics; agents used in biliary and pancreatic disease. In: Brunton LL, Lazo JS, Parker KL (eds) Goodman and Gilman' s the pharmacological basis of therapeutics, 11th edn. McGraw-Hill, New York, pp 983–1008
35. MacLaren R et al (2008) Erythromycin versus metoclopramide for facilitating gastric emptying and tolerance to intragastric nutrition in critically ill patients. J Parenter Enteral Nutr 32:412–419
36. Woods JH et al (1978) Postoperative ileus: a colonic problem? Surgery 84:527–533
37. Moshiree B et al (2010) Comparison of the effect of azithromycin versus erythromycin on antroduodenal pressure profiles of patients with chronic functional gastrointestinal pain and gastroparesis. Dig Dis Sci 55:675–683
38. Camilleri M (2005) Almivopan, a selective peripherally acting mu opioid antagonist. Neurogastroenterol Motil 17:157–165
39. Prather CM et al (2000) Tegaserod accelerates orocecal transit in patients with constipation-predominant irritable bowel syndrome. Gastroenterology 118:463–468
40. Degen L et al (2001) Tegaserod, a 5-HT4 receptor partial agonist, accelerates gastric emptying and gastrointestinal transit in healthy male subjects. Aliment Pharmacol Ther 15:821–822
41. Degen L et al (2005) Effect of tegaserod on gut transit in male and female subjects. Neurogastroenterol Motil 17:1745–1751
42. Wooltorton E (2004) Tegaserod (Zelnorm) for irritable bowel syndrome: reports of serious diarrhea and intestinal ischemia. CMAJ 170:1908
43. Kunz P et al (1998) Gastric emptying and motility: assessment with MR imaging—preliminary observation. Radiology 207:33–40

44. Fitzgerald JEF et al (2009) Systematic review and meta analysis of chewing gum therapy in the reduction of postoperative paralytic ileus following gastrointestinal surgery. World J Surg 33:2557–2566

45. Zou D et al (2005) Inhibition of transient lower esophageal sphincter relaxation by electrical acupoint stimulation. Am J Gastrointest Liver Physiol 289:197–201

46. Pfab F et al (2011) Acupuncture in critically ill patients improves delayed gastric emptying: a randomized controlled trial. Anesth Analg 112:150–155

47. Basse L et al (2001) Normal gastrointestinal transit after colonic resection using epidural analgesia, enforced oral nutrition and laxative. Br J Surg 88:1498–1500

48. Basse L et al (2000) A clinical pathway to accelerate recovery after colonic resection. Ann Surg 232:51–57

49. Holte K, Kehlet H (2002) Postoperative ileus. Progress toward effective management. Drugs 62:2603–2615

Which Adult Patients Undergoing Noncardiac Surgery Should be Monitored Postoperatively in ICU?

12

Franco M. Bobbio Pallavicini

"The surgical event", understood in its entirety as the joint intervention of the surgeon and of the anesthetist, inevitably inflicts the organism with aggression of variable violence, which in turn triggers a variably severe alteration in the patient's physiological functions; said alterations persist, for variable periods, in the postoperative phase. Over the last three decades, the literature has specifically and amply demonstrated the scientific validity of these observations.

Surgery-induced tissue damage, loss of blood, neuroendocrine response to stress, the generally depressing effect of anesthetic and analgesic drugs on vital functions and on the organism's capacity to react, changes in body temperature: all these events are correlated with surgery, are able to affect outcome negatively, are not completely avoidable (e.g., the effect of anesthetic-analgesic drugs and surgical tissue damage), but they are almost always recognizable and/or predictable, and thus largely preventable and/or remediable.

Numerous studies have specifically demonstrated that a high percentage of perioperative complications, which vary from 5 to 30 %, occur within the first few hours of the patient's dismissal from the operating theater [1–5]. In their analysis of almost 200,000 people submitted to anesthesia, Tiret et al. [2] found that 52 % of the observed complications manifested during surgery itself, but that 42 % occurred within the first 24 postsurgery hours, and that 75 % of these observations were recorded in the first 5 h after surgery. The same study also found that postoperative exceeded intraoperative mortality.

Other researchers [6] have claimed and produced evidence that in-depth assessment of the state of the patient's health prior to surgery, the characteristics and course of the operation itself, and postoperative assistance that is attentive,

F. M. Bobbio Pallavicini (✉)
Intensive Care Unit and the Trauma Center, San Martino University Hospital, Genoa, Italy
e-mail: fmbp43@gmail.com

B. Allaria (ed.), *Practical Issues in Anesthesia and Intensive Care 2013*,
DOI: 10.1007/978-88-470-5529-2_12, © Springer-Verlag Italia 2014

timely, and well informed of the previous phases, can reduce morbidity and mortality by as much as 50 % if circumstantial knowledge of the case in question is shared by the entire health team appointed to manage the pre-, intra-, and postoperative phases. In their examination of almost 85,000 patients who underwent general and vascular surgery in diverse hospitals, Ghasperi et al. [7] found that perioperative mortality varied substantially from hospital to hospital (3.5–6.9 %), while the percentage of complications was almost uniform. They concluded that the incongruity between variable mortality rates and uniform complication rates was associated with variability in awareness of the patient's characteristics and surgical background, in responsiveness to the appearance of complications and in the timeliness and quality of treatment.

Published in 2009, these recent studies [6, 7] clearly and incontrovertibly demonstrate at least three central postoperative ICU issues:

- Above all that, the problem exists and it is real. Even in the countries that lead technical development and invest most substantially in all research areas, and particularly in that of medicine, the incidence of perioperative complications and mortality remains a considerable problem that is far from being reduced to acceptable levels.
- Up to 50 % of instances of perioperative complications and mortality derive from "a lack of attention" toward the patient. In turn, this lack is due to superficiality, negligence, or haste and above all to a failure to ensure "explicitly coordinated team work" throughout the pre-, intra-, and postoperative phases.
- A holistic vision, whereby the health team perceives clinical events, from assessment to surgery to postsurgical/anesthesiological effects on the patient's vital functions, as an unbroken continuum will be the key to maximal reduction of perioperative morbidity and mortality, especially in the postoperative stage.

This is the argument presented by Allaria, Dei Poli et al. in their recent article "Monitoring the vital functions in postoperative non-cardiosurgical patients" [8], in which they not only describe assessment systems for the vital functions, but also emphasize the holistic vision that appraises the patient's organism in its entirety, as well as the specific features of varying types of surgery (general, vascular, pulmonary) and of the patient's clinical characteristics (cardiopathic, obese nephropathic).

This book was written for doctors directly involved in surgery, but above all for Intensive Care Anesthetists, to whom the whole world attributes the task of (and responsibility for) dispensing "clinical treatment" to the surgical patient.

Since the current text will not deal exhaustively with this issue, interested parties are encouraged to read Allaria and Dei Poli [8] for an in-depth analysis. The continuous advancement of scientific knowledge and the subsequent improvements in drug therapies and available technologies have increasingly extended the respective indications for emergency and elective surgery in patients who are increasingly compromised and hence more susceptible to operative, and especially postoperative, complications. This assertion is all the more valid if we consider the growth in human life expectancy and the exponential increase in surgery performed on aged patients, especially on very old patients who generally bear one or more chronic pathological alteration(s) and whose physiological reserves are markedly diminished.

On the basis of current evidence, I believe we can confidently assert that:

- surgery as a whole subjects the organism to a "situation of systemic fragility" that extends to the postoperative phase and facilitates complications of varying types, some of which can even lead to death;
- various types of surgery and anesthesia can induce not only systemic but also treatment-specific repercussions;
- the systemic and specific repercussions of surgery in all the given phases, particularly those that characterize the postoperative phase, are known to be predictable and detectable, and hence to be preventable/treatable preemptively, by means of competent management both of vital function monitoring and of "holistic clinical assessment" of the patient;
- said repercussions are associated with numerous variables inhering to the types of surgery and anesthesia applied to the specific operating conditions and to the clinical characteristics of the patient. Accordingly, the entity of such repercussions can vary widely;
- the level of postoperative care varies widely too, from a few hours of observation prior to discharge (Day Surgery) to return to the ward, to admission to the Intensive Care Unit on the basis of a predictably prolonged threat to vital functions;
- the doctor in charge of the patient's "clinical performance" is by common consent and by specific competence the Intensive Care Anesthetist, who by definition must possess both a deep knowledge of all the issues at play and the ability to choose the optimal postoperative procedure for each patient.

In the attempt over recent decades to avoid/minimize the specific and systemic repercussions of surgery, research has experimented on numerous fronts: new and ever less invasive and traumatizing surgical techniques; drugs and anesthesiological methods that lessen the neuroendocrinal stress induced by surgery, and whose collateral effects are nullified or increasingly reduced; and monitoring systems that assess the efficiency of vital functions with increasing immediacy and accuracy, and diminishing invasiveness.

At the same time, since the issues, equipments, and behaviors inherent to the pre- and intraoperative phase have been defined and codified into appropriate guidelines, attention has turned to the definition of:

- the minimum levels of assistance required for the postoperative phase, on the basis that said levels depend on the type and complexity of surgery and on the patient's clinical conditions;
- the infrastructure, instrumentation, and human resource investment required for the delivery of appropriate postoperative care;
- criteria for the access of patients to the various levels of postoperative assistance, with particular emphasis on the level of monitoring/treatment required in Intensive Therapy.

We have already noted that the variables which condition the postoperative phase are numerous, and that they reflect the specificities both of surgery (choice and execution of operation and anesthesia) and of the patient's clinical characteristics. Definition of the reciprocal interplay between these variables is very elusive.

It follows that the immediate outcome of surgery varies: if recovery of the patient's functional autonomy is timely and reliable, he/she will be discharged from the hospital or returned to the given ward; alternatively, circumstances may require higher level and more prolonged care, or lead to full admission to the ICU for preventive or therapeutic care.

It is thus evident that all patients discharged from the operating theater require admission to what we may term an "area of attentive observation" until the recovery of autonomy in the vital functions is complete. However, it is similarly evident that the time scales, monitoring systems, and therapeutic schemes required for the "attentive observation" phase vary considerably, and that, fortunately, the percentage of cases requiring admission to the ICU is low.

12.1   Recovery Room, Postanesthesia Care Unit, Subintensive Postanesthesia Care Unit, Intensive Care Unit

The postoperative phase is by definition critical, and as such requires infrastructure, equipment, and staffing levels that exceed those generally required by other hospital divisions. Although the origins of intensive care date back to more than two centuries ago, current funding problems, especially as regards specialized medical staff, are stimulating substantial debate on postoperative care issues.

The first Recovery Room (RR) was instituted in England in 1801; its USA analog came into being in 1873 at the Massachusetts General Hospital [9, 10]. And yet, still today (at least in Italy), confusion and disagreement persist as to the entity, characteristics and nomenclature of units entrusted with the treatment of postoperative patients.

In regulatory terms, provision in Italy is defined by the DPR (Presidential Decree) of 14/1/1997 [11], in which the definition of the minimum requisites of an accredited hospital includes a "user re-awakening zone."

The term "re-awakening" is inappropriately limiting, in that it refers exclusively to the regaining of consciousness after general anesthesia, and neglects the recovery both of vital functions and of organic defense mechanisms, the latter being prone to surgery- and anesthesia-induced alterations (whether general or locoregional).

Hence the profusion of terminology, from Recovery Room to Postoperative Subintensive Care Unit (SICU) to Post Anesthesia Care Unit (PACU) to Postoperative Intensive Care Unit.

The opinion of the Italian Society of Anesthesia, Analgesia, and Intensive Care (SIAARTI) , as specifically expressed in its Guide Lines [1], is that it is appropriate to designate a "Recovery Room" (an "Area of Postanesethesia Recovery") and a Postoperative Intensive Care Unit (PICU).

The Recovery Room can be correctly defined as "an area" to which patients from the operating theater are admitted and in which they remain until consciousness and vital (circulatory) functions are regained [12].

It must be located within the same building as that of the operating theater, or within its immediate vicinity, and it must be staffed with specialized health workers and endowed with monitoring and therapeutic equipment for patients who have undergone surgery (including that of Day Surgery) and anesthesia, in whatever form, until the stability of the vital parameters is re-established.

The RR must be able to offer temporary admission to all patients from the operating theater, with the exception of those judged not to need anesthesia; in its capacity as the area in which operated patients recover functional stability, and are subsequently discharged to a ward or to the homeplace, or are admitted to the Intensive Care Unit (ICU), this area is a cardinal area in perioperative medicine.

The Anesthesiological Societies of numerous countries have sought over the years to rationalize and to regulate the organization and management of RRs by issuing specific, dedicated Guidelines to hospital administrators and to pertinent medical staff, and in particular to Intensive Care anesthetists [9].

In Germany, the first Guidelines were issued in 1967, and have since been regularly modified. In France, the Sociètè Francaise d'Anesthesie et de Rèanimation (SFAR) published its Guidelines in 1990 and reviewed them in 1994, the year in which they became a State law; in 1994, analogous Guidelines were published in Italy in the form of "recommendations" by the SIAARTI. [9, 13, 14].

In the USA, the American Society of Anesthesiologists (ASA) devised Guidelines in 1988 and updated them in 1994, in the wake of a review of the "standards" required for postoperative care of patients:
- all patients submitted to general, locoregional, or other forms of anesthesia must undergo appropriate postoperative examination;
- patients must be accompanied to the RR by a member of the anesthesia team;
- transport must be overseen and the appropriate therapy applied;
- handover to the RR staff must be accompanied by full clinical, and especially operative, documentation;
- the patient's conditions must be constantly monitored;
- the patient's discharge from the RR must be authorized by a medical doctor.

In France, Canada, and the USA, the RR is an obligatory facility wherever surgery is performed; in Germany, Australia, and Italy, the facility is provided for but not obligatory.

The RR must be located near to the operating theaters to enable rapid transfer of patients upon completion of surgery.

With regard to the admission capacity of RRs, standards vary widely: the USA and Canada do not prescribe a minimum number of beds; in contrast, France requires at least four RR beds per hospital and Australia 1.5 beds per operating theater. In Italy and Germany, bed numbers are determined on the basis of the surgical activities performed by each single hospital.

Italian regulation does not require a specific RR medical history sheet, but it is the doctor's duty to annotate clinical data continuously on the anesthesiological or the patient record sheet.

The quality and timing of monitoring is not regulated and is left entirely to the doctor's discretion.

RR equipment is regulated in France and Australia, whereas other nations leave this issue to the discretion of hospitals, which in turn base procurement on the basis of the entity and nature of the patient population upon which they operate.

Italian Guidelines list the minimum recommended equipment levels for RRs and specify which instruments are immediately obligatory [1, 13], but without establishing a ratio to the number of beds in the given RR.

12.2 SIAARTI: Recommendations for the Recovery Area and Postanesthesiological Care

12.2.1 Equipment Recommended for Each Recovery Area Bed

- Monitoring system with ECG, heart rate, invasive and noninvasive BP, SpO2.
- O_2 therapy systems (flow meters, humidifiers, masks).
- Breathing systems.
- Manual ventilation system.
- Peripheral and central temperature measurement system.
- Stretcher/bed with rigid mattress and removable lateral protection.

12.2.2 Readily Available Equipment

- Patient heating system.
- Mechanical ventilator, preferably with NIV function.
- Defibrillator.
- Systems for CPAP and NIV.
- Bronchoscope.
- Capnometer with a connector for endotracheal tubes and with nasal pipes.
- Syringe pumps.
- Monitor neuromuscular transmission (NMT) and antagonistic drugs to reverse the effects of neuromuscular blocker drugs.
- Cardiac stimulator.
- Drugs and apparatus for emergencies and management of compromised air flow.
- Transportable ventilator.

When it is declared, the Nurse:Bed ratio is generally 1:3.

Italian Guidelines do not specify this ratio and allow health units to decide on the basis of local circumstances.

All Guidelines attribute RR management to the Intensive Care Anesthetist, whose responsibility covers clinical, organizational, and administrative functions and who as a result has to coordinate with senior hospital management in order to create a service that corresponds in all senses (location, dimension, equipment, staff, timetables) to the needs of the given hospital.

The RR is generally open for 6–12 h on the basis of the timetable of the operating theaters. The "Postoperative Intensive Therapy" unit generally (but not necessarily) functions independently of surgical activities and is open 24/24 (generally from Monday to Friday) for the admission of patients requiring prolonged intensive care on the basis of clinical severity and/or surgical invasiveness.

The unit is required to conform to the space ratios and instrumentation levels expected of Intensive Therapy units, along with a Nurse:Patient ratio of 1:4; the number of beds obviously depends on local needs.

The unit Head is generally an Intensive Care Anesthetist (in rare instances, the role can be fulfilled by a surgeon or a Postoperative Intensive Therapy neurosurgeon) who is on call 24/24 but without having to be physically present 24/24 in the unit.

Postoperative Intensive Therapy units exist in a minority of Italian hospitals.

Subintensive Care Units (SICUs) act, in terms of care intensity, as an intermediate stage between ICU and wards. They are generally assigned to the surgery areas of what the Italian health system calls "Complex Operating Units" (General Surgery, Cardiosurgery, Thoracic Surgery, Organ Transplants, etc.), and they are frequently managed by the unit surgeons themselves. Such units do not normally avail of automatic ventilators, and they generally maintain a nurse:bed ratio of 1:6. The Health Ministry Guidelines no. 1/1996 recommend the activation in each hospital of a number of SICU beds (which are generally available for all patients in need, and not exclusively for surgery patients) that is at least equal to the number of Intensive Therapy beds.

Conformity to Ministerial recommendations in Italy is still distant, and the current status is difficult to assess, but the number of SICU beds is very low, and national distribution is uneven [15].

12.3   Which Noncardiac Surgery Patients Require Postoperative Admission to ICU?

This is the *quid* of the current conversation, but unfortunately the response to the question will most certainly be meager and disappointing: it will provide neither exact quantification, nor a precise list of clinical scenarios; nor will it define the deviation from normal physiological parameters that suggest/require admission of postoperative patients to ICU.

The fundamental issues at stake are:

(1) that surgical activity, as jointly consisting in surgery and anesthesia, invariably inflicts aggression on the organism and alters/limits the organism's vital functions and its capacity for reaction, compensation, and auto-defense. In turn, these alterations can be such that, if unchecked, they will influence the outcome of surgery itself. It is true that surgical research has generated increasingly specific and efficacious, and less invasive, surgical techniques. Diversification in anesthetic drugs and in anesthesiological techniques has likewise achieved notable progress. On a cautionary note, these advances substantially reduce, but they do not eliminate, the specific and systemic negative effects of surgery and anesthesia. However, it has been possible to substantially reduce the constraints on surgery, and thus to nurture increasing operational complexity and the deployment of surgery in increasingly compromised clinical situations; in turn, these developments have brought about a considerable increase in the number of patients who require a high level of care in the postoperative phase. Awareness of said developments has long been acute, and has spurred intense research activities that have clarified numerous features of systemic neuroendocrinal reactions to surgical stress. Light has accordingly been shed: on the variable consequences of differing types of surgery, as affected by location, complexity, and duration; on the effects of General Anesthesia (GA) and Locoregional Anesthesia (LRA) in their various forms and locations of application (e.g., spinal LRA); and on the correlation between surgical outcome and previous chronic/acute pathologies;

(2) that the effect on the organism of surgery and anesthesia persists for variable (and not infrequently considerable) lengths of time in the postoperative phase, and any lack of effective care may well permit/facilitate the development of complications. Mainly respiratory and/or cardiocirculatory, these complications can arise furtively and escape superficial observation, but they are able to prolong hospitalization and/or to compromise the final outcome;

(3) that the Intensive Care Anesthetist has to fulfill two functions simultaneously: membership of a health team; and overall responsibility for the clinical evolution of surgery in all its phases (pre-, intra-, and postoperative). It is therefore his/her institutional duty to maintain an overview of the perioperative process, to effect a detailed preoperative assessment, and to choose and implement the most effective form of anesthesia for the given patient. Finally, on the basis of all the known variables, he/she must choose the postoperative program that, allowing for unforeseen complications during surgery, will optimize the clinical path. These duties therefore include that predicting what path the patient will follow in the postoperative phase: admission to the RR for care that will suffice for the patient to be discharged or return to the ward; assessment by the RR of the patient's clinical evolution prior to the patient's return to the ward or admission to the ICU; or, finally, circumvention of the RR and immediate admission to the ICU.

12.4   Brief Observations on Monitoring and the Prevention of Postoperative Complications

This is not the occasion for exhaustive treatment of the topic, so we will simply outline the main issues, specify the essential data, and indicate where to find in-depth information in the literature [8].

Postoperative complications are associated with numerous factors that inhere to the patient's clinical profile and to the characteristics not only of surgery and anesthesia, but also of monitoring and of the care established for the immediate aftermath of discharge from the operating theater.

The incidence and gravity of these characteristics is mainly correlated to the quality of preoperative assessment and to the consequent program of intra- and postoperative care: the complications must above all be seen before they appear, by means of all possible, state-of-the-art instruments and methods.

12.4.1   Respiratory Function

The residual effect of GA, or that (whether deliberate or accidental) of high spinal anesthesia, can cause an alteration in central respiratory control and hypoventilation, and hence a more or less gradual increase in $PaCO_2$ which, if not promptly recognized can develop silently to respiratory arrest (silent death).

Mechanical obstruction by a fallen tongue, hemorrhagic complications in neck surgery, glottic edema, laryngospasm (most frequent in unweaned babies and babies in general) are all able to induce dangerous postoperative respiratory insufficiencies of variable speed and observability.

Hypoxemia (of multiple etiology, such as thoracic and supra-mesocolic surgery, obesity, a chronic lung pathology, all of which facilitate the formation of pulmonary microatelectasis) is one of the most frequent adverse events, and probably constitutes the principal cause for negative outcomes in the postoperative phase [1, 16].

Accordingly, during the awakening and recovery phase, it is necessary to monitor the respiratory pattern (respiratory frequency and thoracic excursion) and the transversability of the airways (Grade A, SIAARTI Guidelines).

The same Guidelines [SIAARTI (1)] suggest the monitoring of SpO2 with a pulse oxymeter (Grade A), which enables the rapid recognition and treatment of hypoxemia. However, there is no scientific evidence that this treatment effectively improves outcomes for operated patients [17, 18].

The availability of capnographic monitoring enables prompt recognition of hypo-apnea episodes (Grade C, SIAARTI Guidelines).

The same Guidelines [SIAARTI (1)] suggest the monitoring of SpO_2 with a pulse oxymeter (Grade A), which enables the rapid recognition and treatment of hypoxemia. However, there is no scientific evidence that this treatment effectively improves outcomes for operated patients [17, 18].

The availability of capnographic monitoring enables prompt recognition of hypo-apnea episodes (Grade C, SIAARTI Guidelines).

O_2 therapy must be guaranteed for patients with a tendency toward desaturation (Grade A, SIAARTI Guidelines), although it is not scientifically proven that systemic administration of O_2 to all patients improves their postoperative outcomes, or that this measure reduces the incidence of Post Operative Nausea and Vomiting (PONV) [1, 19–22].

Continuous positive airway pressure (CPAP) improves gas exchange, reduces atelectactic phenomena, increases residual functional capacity that develops postoperative hypoxemia, and thus reduces re-intubation in patients submitted to major abdominal surgery (Grade B, SIAARTI Guidelines) [1, 23–26].

12.4.2 Cardiocirculatory Function

For various reasons, surgery can induce an increase in sympathic activity, and may thus be the basis of postoperative cardiocirculatory complications, which generally manifest in the very first hours after surgery. These complications affect a high number (c. 7 %) [1] of patients, and primarily consist in arrhythmic (tachycardia, bradycardia) and hemodynamic (hyperhypotenstion, lung edema) phenomena [1, 8, 27].

Inadequate and/or erroneous assessment of hypovolemia can constitute a very high risk factor in the postoperative phase, and its prevention/correction can require monitoring as well as intensive and qualified care [8].

The risk inherent to such complications is decidedly higher in Chronic Heart Failure (CHF) and/or coronaropathic patients; like other risk factors, this one is correlated to the characteristics and execution of surgery and anesthesia.

The literature is currently far from convincingly identifying and quantifying the impact of clinical assessment and instrumental monitoring on the prevention of postoperative cardiocirculatory complications [1, 28].

The various Guidelines agree that, at the very least, postoperative monitoring should include heart rate, PA, and ECG. The exception to this concurrence is the American Society of Anesthesiologists' Guidelines, which maintain that ECG monitoring should not be systematic but reserved for selected at-risk patients [14, 28].

The Italian Guidelines [1] recommend systematic postoperative monitoring of FC, BP, and ECG (Grade A), as well as the availability of a defibrillator and the drugs required by the Cardio-Pulmonary Rianimation (CPR), as per the dictates of Advanced Life Support [29] (Grade A).

12.4.3 Central Nervous System and Neuromuscular Function

Reawakening and the disappearance of neuromuscular block are obviously primary functional priorities in postoperative care, in that they can differ widely in time and extent, and for varying reasons (related to the patient and to anesthesiological management); the anesthesiologist must be perfectly aware of all developments in this respect.

12.4.4 Hydroelectrolytic Equilibrium

The literature amply demonstrates that impaired hydroelectrolygic equilibrium (HEE) is frequent (affecting up to 20 % of patients submitted to major surgery) [30] and that it plays in important role in postoperative morbidity and mortality [1, 8, 30–34].

The search continues for optimal postoperative hydroelectrolytic therapy protocols, as well as for electrolytic and/or colloidal solutions that correspond better to the patient's age and clinical conditions, to the features of surgery and to intraoperative losses, and to renal function [1, 8, 31–34].

The SIAARTI Guidelines recommend (Grade B) attentive postoperative monitoring of blood volume, HEE, and dieresis in patients selected on the basis of chronic pathologies associated with the features of surgery [1].

12.4.5 Core Body Temperature (T°C)

GA invariably determines an alteration in core body temperature, which in turn reduces sensitivity to the hypothalamic centers and can induce up to a tenfold increase in the "inter-threshold range." Specifically, under normal conditions, the hypothalamic control centers vary from the central physiological temperature (36.6 °C) by 0.2–0.4 °C, whereas during GA the analogous variations are in the order of 2–4 °C.

It is therefore evident that without specific intervention by the health team, slight-to-medium core hypothermia (which is deemed to commence at less than 36 °C) is inevitable, and can be aggravated by numerous other factors: age (the elderly and infants likewise being affected), physical constitution (lean patients are more susceptible to cold conditions), endocrinal pathologies, prolonged surgery, visceral exposure, thoracic surgery, and reduced operating theater (OT) temperature [35, 38, 42].

Loco-Regional Anesthesia (LRA), especially the spinal version, likewise and invariably raises the risk of light-to-moderate hypothermia by abolishing vascular centralization reflexes in the body area affected by LRA. This effect remains throughout the operation because of exposition to the reduced temperatures of the OT [35, 38, 42].

Even slight hypothermia can induce alterations in Acido-Based Equilibrium (ABE) blood, in myocardial performance and in the Central Nervous System (CNS); it also predisposes surgical sites to infection, alters the metabolism of numerous drugs and has been recognized overall as a prominent factor in postoperative morbidity and mortality (the Killer Triad of traumatized patients: Hypothermia, Metabolic Acidosis, Coagulopathy) [1, 8, 35–45]. The SIAARTI Guidelines [1] consider the monitoring and management of core temperature to be necessary in the postoperative phase (Grade A), and suggest the use of an infrared tympanic thermometer as a reliable, minimally invasive and inexpensive tool to this end [46]. Normothermia must be re-established, and maintained by means of passive, and, if necessary, active heating (Grade A).

12.4.6 Shivering

Postoperative shivering, which is often intense and/or induces shaking, is in most cases the thermoregulatory response to hypothermia [45, 47]. Other factors that can co-occur with shivering include pain, tissue damage-related pyrogenetic cytokines, respiratory alkalosis, and vasoplegia during spinal LRA [47–49]. Shivering induces numerous effects: severe unease, agitation and fear, tachypnea, increased consumption of O_2, increased production of CO_2, increased heart rate and cardiac ouput, increased energy expenditure and metabolic demand, increased endoocular and intracranial pressure, and lactic acidosis [45–50].

Numerous studies have demonstrated the efficacy of certain drugs in the treatment of postoperative shivering (Meperidina, Clonidina, Tramadolo, Nefopam, Ketamina) [1, 51]. However, the SIAARTI Guidelines [1] argue that the cornerstone of shiver management is the maintenance of normothermia during surgery itself (Grade A), and that shiver-control drugs should only be used when shivering persists despite normothermia, normovolemia, and analgesia (Grade A).

12.4.7 Pain

The importance of the clinical and psychological implications of postoperative pain is such that discussion of the topic in the current context would be redundant.

Suffice it to observe that all Guidelines for all forms of surgery prescribe appropriate protocols for the treatment of postoperative pain and appropriate instruments for the evaluation of pain intensity as the bases of effective monitoring and treatment [1, 52, 53].

12.4.8 Postoperative Nausea and Vomit

Occurring with high frequency (10–50 %) after both GA and LRA [1, 54–56], Postoperative nausea and vomit (PONV) is a greatly feared postoperative complication. Episodes of nausea and vomit substantially affect the quality of the postoperative phase; planning, assessment, and treatment need to be timely and meticulous, and treatment should avail of efficacious antiemetic drugs (Grade A of the SIAARTI Guidelines) [1, 54, 55].

12.5 Criteria for Admission to the ICU for Postoperative Treatment

As already mentioned, one of the criteria established by the 14/12/1997 Decree issued for registration as an operating division was the existence of a "re-awakening zone," otherwise (and better) known as a "Recovery Room," which would accommodate all postoperative patients, save those deemed by the anesthetist not to need observation and/or specific treatment. Admission to RR aims to guarantee the patient's complete recovery of vital functional autonomy and to ensure that the patient's health needs will be commensurate with the ward into which he/she will subsequently be admitted.

The SIAARTI Guidelines [1] list the criteria required for the transfer of an operated patient from the RR to a ward:
- Maintenance of consciousness without excessive stimulation.
- The independent ability to preserve transversability of the airways by means of protective reflexes: swallowing and coughing.
- Satisfying expiration and oxygenation.
- Stability in the cardiovascular system. Heart rate and BP near to preoperative values, appropriate peripheral perfusion (pinkish and warm skin, capillary filling time <3 s), absence of persistent bleeding.
- Pain well under control.
- Normothermia re-established.
- Motorial activity and muscular strength re-established.

Patient assessment can be performed with a point scale, such as those respectively used by Aldrete [57] and by White and Song [58]. Originally developed for day-patient surgery, but legitimately generalizable to all RR patients, these instruments enable greater objectivity in data collection. If the patient does not demonstrate the minimum requisites for return to the ward, he/she will be sent to, and treated by, the Post Operative Intensive Therapy (POIT) unit, if there is one, or the ICU.

12.6 Which Patients Must Be Transferred Immediately to the ICU?

The literature reports numerous investigations that attempt to quantify operative risk in advance on the bases of the patient's clinical profile, of the quality of surgery and anesthesia, and of the possible intraoperative complications; treating all the risk factors as operating in isolation and/or constructing multifactorial gravity scales, research has attempted to provide a "magic number" that would enable the doctor to identify the optimal, personalized clinical path and the "therapy-care level" necessary for the patient. Managed thus, the patient's persona would be fully respected, and resources would be deployed justly.

This objective has not been reached because no Gravity or Prognostic Score would by itself be able to endow "individual choices" with certainty.

However, although these ongoing research initiatives have not achieved definitive results, they have certainly served to focus attention ever more precisely on the issue of operative risk in all its aspects. They have deepened the surgery team's, and above all the anesthetist's, knowledge of the *status quo* and of the prevailing, increasingly specific and sensitive instruments with which to defeat perioperative complications.

Without prejudice to the anesthetist's specific provisions, Guidelines specifically recommend that all patients who have undergone surgery should be admitted to a recovery zone until they have overcome such complications as may avoid detection/necessary treatment in a standard ward.

To this end, hospitals essentially have two facilities:

(1) Recovery Room, which we have already and amply discussed. This area can also accommodate other units that in some hospitals are not clearly codified, but which could be said to belong to Subintensive Care Units (SICU).

(2) ICUs, by which acronym we identify the various possible IC subunits that feature idiosyncratically in various hospitals, namely:

- POIT/PACU, rarely found in Italy, these units offer a level of care that is midway between RR and IT proper;
- Polyvalent IT units, which admit all critical patients irrespective of the nature of their pathology (managed by Intensive Care and Anesthetics specialists);
- Specialized IT units, which admit patients with specific pathologies (after neurosurgery, thoracic surgery, heart surgery), are generally but not necessarily managed by Intensive Care and Anesthetics specialists. Alternatively, such units can be managed by the Complex Operating Unit surgeons who performed surgery on the given patients.

Accordingly, patients who are admitted to the ICU in the postoperative phase can derive:

(a) **from the RR:**

- patients who in their sojourn in the RR showed persistent instability in one or more vital function(s), or who show are feared to have complications of an order that requires monitoring and treatment that is intensive and prolonged, and/or that is superior in quality and duration to what RRs can offer and is entirely unavailable in wards;

(b) **directly from the OT:**

- patients for whom admission to the ICU upon completion of surgery is already planned on the basis of the patients' clinical profile and of the type and duration of surgery and anesthesia, such that intensive, prolonged, and high-level monitoring and treatment are deemed necessary;

- patients who have undergone emergency surgery without time for sufficient prior assessment of their overall clinical profile, as frequently happens, for example, in patients who have multiple hemorrhagic lesions;
- patients who showed none of the criteria for admission to the ICU but experienced intraoperative complications of sufficient gravity to warrant prolonged intensive monitoring-treament.

In other words, the reasons for admission to the ICU distinguish between implicit/automatic and elective. Certain forms of surgery are such that "current recommendations" consider the patient's postoperative transfer to the ICU to be implicit. Likewise, when the transfer of the patient from the RR to the ICU is based on the patient's nonrecovery of functional stability, the decision is nondiscretionary. In contrast, the reasons for direct transfer of the patient from the OT to the ICU will be much more nuanced because they will depend on personal interpretations of the collective weight of the risk factors identified.

The anesthetist must therefore plan the postoperative patient's needs in advance and at the same time be prepared to adjust rapidly to unforeseen adverse events. These latter, however, are to a large degree predictable and quantifiable (albeit not exactly) on the basis of data generated by precise case histories, by exhaustive preoperative clinical examination, and by a "reasoned" use of the currently available instrumental and biohumoral methods of assessment and monitoring.

The preemptive decision to transfer the patient directly from the OT to the ICU at the end of the operation is thus necessarily based on the interpretation of numerous parameters that can co-exist and be variably associated with each other:

- personal data;
- nutritional condition;
- chronic pathologies, their possible association, and their degree of development (assessment of the patient's "physiological reserves");
- current pharmacological therapies;
- characterization of surgery: place, complexity, degree of invasiveness, length;
- description of planned anesthesia (GA, peripheral or spinal LRA) and its duration;
- degree of electiveness or urgency characterizing surgery itself;
- need for specific treatment to reduce the incidence of secondary damage (e.g., sedation and/or profound analgesia for CNS lesions, for extensive burns);
- clinical contexts with medico-legal implications (attempted suicide, psychiatric pathologies, polytraumas);
- the resources available within the hospital for care in the postoperative recovery phase (surgical RR/SICU, POIT, or merely ICU).

12.6.1 Age

With life expectancy in continuous growth and the percentage of people over the age of 65 years approaching preeminence, the Intensive Care Anesthetist's knowledge base must necessarily cover the physiopathological characteristics of aged people.

The distinctive physiology of aged patients, along with their increased susceptibility to chronic systemic pathologies (which include higher than average psychic disturbances), necessitate tailoring throughout the perioperative cycle—from preoperative assessment to monitoring of vital functions, intraoperative pharmacological treatment, postoperative recovery schedules, and the degree of care needed [59, 60]. At the highest level of generalization, it can be said that aged patients have "reduced physiological reserves" that necessarily induce "greater fragility;" in turn, said fragility is accentuated by chronic pathologies (possibly and variably inter-related) in differing stages of advancement. Old age increases operative risks and accordingly requires appropriate perioperative conduct and postoperative allocation to the hospital area that is best suited to deliver the care necessary for the prevention of complications [8, 59, 61, 62]. However, age is not an independent factor that limits recourse to surgery (Grade A recommendation) and it does not make post-OT admission to the ICU mandatory.

12.6.2 Nutritional Status

Despite the documented advances in the science of nutrition, the literature on anestheiological risk still lacks systematic assessment of the importance of the presurgery patient's nutritonal status.

Said status ranges from under nourishment (malnutrition) to excess weight to obesity.

12.6.3 Malnutrition

This condition occurs frequently and particularly affects the aged. It is identified and quantified by numerous anthropometric and biohumoral parameters; current body weight, recent (i.e., within the 3–6–months prior to surgery) body weight loss, BMI (Body Mass Index), and albuminemia are prominent and easy-to-use indicators.

Malnutrition is an additional risk factor in surgery because it is related to:
- increase in postoperative complications;
- reduction/increase in drug and other therapeutic effects;
- reduction in immune response;
- increase in surgical wound infections;
- reduction in surgical wound repair;

- reduction in organ-apparatus functioning;
- reduction in body mass and muscular strength (which in prolonged malnutrition affects the heart and the diaphragm);
- increase in psychologically damaging effects (depression, refusal of food).

Malnutrition has variously been detected in 10–80 % of hospitalized patients; it affects aged patients more than it does other classes of patient, it increases operative risk and it lengthens the average 6 days hospitalization period by 10–15 % [59, 60].

Malnutrition does not contraindicate surgery but it does necessitate attentive assessment and tailoring of the perioperative care and therapy program. In extreme cases, and when possible, surgery can be preceded by a period of artificial nutrition (enteral or parenteral) which can feature in the postoperative phase too [64, 65].

Other than in extreme cases, malnutrition does not constitute an independent factor that limits surgery and/or mandates immediate admission to the ICU.

12.7 Obesity

The worldwide percentage of obese people is now approaching 30 % and is showing the highest growth rates in infants and adolescents [8, 66–69].

By "obesity" we mean an abnormal increase in fat body mass, and categorization of its entity generally refers to the Ideal Body Weight (IBW), which can be obtained from easy formulae such as Broca's: IBW = height in cm—X (X = 100 for males and 105 for females).

BMI (ratio of body weight in Kg to body surface in m^2) is an accepted system for the assessment of a patient's nutritional status. Obesity increases morbidity and mortality, and predisposes humans to metabolic illnesses and cardiovascular and/or respiratory pathologies. It also increases operative risk (including that of intubation difficulties) both in elective and in emergency surgery; it demands in-depth knowledge of the physiopathology of obesity and of the variations in response to drug therapy, and it requires attentive monitoring of the vital functions in the postoperative period [8, 66–70].

The obesity/perioperative risk ratio is well known and has generated in-depth studies, to which readers of the current are referred for further information [8, 66–70].

Table 12.1 BMI/nutritional status ratio

BMI	Nutritional status
<18.5	Underweight
18.5–24.9	Normal
25.0–29.9	Overweight
30.0–34.9	Obesity (Class I)
35.0–39.9	Obesity (Class II)
≥40	Pathological or severe obesity

Based on data from Intensive Care Med (2004) 30:437–443

Obesity is not an independent limiting factor for surgery and it does not necessarily require postoperative admission to the ICU, not even in bariatric surgery (Table 12.1).

12.7.1 Case History and Chronic Pathologies

The cornerstone for the selection of preintrapostoperative anesthesiological itinerary is an amalgam of anamnesis enquiry, the identification of chronic pathologies and their possible mutual associations, assessment of their stage of development and of what the given stage implies in terms of quali-quantitative "pharmacological load", as collectively correlated to the specific characteristics of surgery. Said itinerary must be based on the personal experience of the anesthetist, who can/must make "reasoned" use both of the vital function data supplied by the then currently available enquiry and monitoring systems, and of specific information on operating risks reported in the (international) literature.

The ASA classification is an operative risk scoring system that is universally accepted in clinical and legal medicine. It is very generic and as such should be used as the platform for appropriate predictive assessment of operative risk, which in turn, however, will require further specification as to the characteristics of surgery [8, 61–63].

The operative risk related to the patient's clinical conditions must necessarily be correlated to the characteristics of surgery, in which numerous studies have attempted to classify. This classification attempts to provide a necessarily and highly generic "surgical grading," and aims to focus practitioners' attention on the indispensable correlation between the "patient's state of health and the impact of surgery" (Tables 12.2, 12.3).

Table 12.2 American Society of Anesthesiologists (ASA) classification of anesthesiological risk

Class	Health status
I	Patient in good health
II	Systemic pathology of medium entity
III	Systemic pathology of stabilized severe entity
IV	Systemic pathology of severe entity with constant risk of life
V	Patient moribund with life expectancy <24 h independently of surgery
Ve	Emergency surgery

Based on data from ASA Physical Status Classification System

Table 12.3 Classification of the complexity of surgical procedures (NHS, National Institute for Clinical Excellence 2003)

Grade 1: Minor complexity surgery (excision of cutaneous lesions, drainage of mammary abscesses)
Grade 2: Medium complexity surgery (inguinal hernia correction, saphenectomy, arthroscopy, tonsillectomy)
Grade 3: Medium–high complexity surgery (radical hysterectomy, total thyroidectomy, TURP)
Grade 4: High–very high complexity surgery (lung,cardiovascular, intestinal surgery…)

Based on data from Preoperative Tests. The use of routine preoperative tests for elective surgery. Evidence, Methods & Guidance. National Institute for Clinical Excellence. June 2003 Developed by the National Collaborating Centre for Acute Care

12.7.2 Patients with Chronic Heart Failure

Correct perioperative treatment of CHF patients [8, 71–73] is based both on knowledge of the physiopathology of CHF, which comprehends systolic and diastolic dysfunction, and on analysis of the characteristics of current pharmacological therapy; awareness of the repercussions on the cardiocirculatory apparatus of the various phases of surgery will likewise be crucial.

The SIAARTI Guidelines [64] offer useful recommendations for the perioperative management of the CHF surgery patient by additionally indicating the level of care needed for the postoperative phase on the basis of cardiac dysfunction grade and of the characteristics of surgery.

High-grade CHF patients, who need substantial pharmacological support in the form of substances that can interfere with compensatory mechanisms (as in, for example, hypovolemia) certainly need intense postoperative care and attentive monitoring of all vital functions, which in turn can make immediate postsurgery admission to the ICU advisable in highly complex situations and in hospitals that do not avail of the RR or of analogous facilities.

CHF induces a substantial increase in operative risk, as is well documented by Hammil [71], whose study on an approximate population of c. 160,000 operated patients found a CHF incidence of 18 % and a 63 % higher probability of mortality in the bearers of the given alteration than was found in other patients.

However, CHF does not constitute an independent limiting factor for surgery and it does not make postoperative admission to the ICU mandatory.

12.7.3 Coronaropathy

This is an extremely important issue in the field of operative risk, one that has fueled considerable research, not least on account of the availability of increasingly active and specific pharmaceutical therapies for the cardiocirculatory apparatus (e.g., β-blockers and such vasodilators as nitrates, ACE-inhibitors, and sartans). Said research has provided doctors with very effective therapeutic instruments; however, if used unknowingly, these same instruments can lead to negative consequences.

The fundamental risk facing coronaropathic patients who have to undergo surgery is that of perioperative ischemia, the genesis and gravity of which can be compounded by various factors related to the characteristics of the patient and of surgery; in this scenario, the anesthetist's specific physiopathological knowledge will play a substantial part, as will his/her perspicacity in preoperative assessment and in the consequent clinical choices regarding intrapostoperative monitoring and therapy.

Numerous initiatives and hypotheses have attempted to reduce the coronaropathic patient's operative risk: more precise gravity scores have been developed to maximize risk stratification; systematic use of β-blockers is proposed to prevent tachycardia and its highly dangerous reduction in diastolic time; systematic use of Swan-Ganz in ASA III–IV coronaropathic patients with secondary CHF has been hypothesized as providing monitoring that is capable of reducing ischemic risk; analogously, more extensive use of invasive diagnostic tests such as coronarography might also reduce ischemic risk, possibly the more so if administered in association with greater use of preoperative endoluminal revascularization techniques [8, 77–79].

The Table 12.4 is an example of gravity scoring; although dated, this Index can still play a role in clinical practice.

However, none of the innumerable studies has provided instruments that enable an exact forecast stratification of the risks incurred by the coronaropathic patient during surgery. Unfortunately, this aim may well be unachievable, given the high number and the variability of the implied causal factors.

That said, the literature has shed increasing light on certain fundamental principles that must underlie the prevention both of general operative risk and of the specific risks affecting coronaropathic patients:

- deep knowledge of the physiopathology of coronary circulation;
- deep knowledge of pharmacodynamics and of the pharmacokinetics of drugs that act on the cardiocirculatory apparatus. Particular attention should be reserved for the effect of said drugs on compensation mechanisms;
- meticulous preoperative clinical instrumental and biohumoral assessment (cTn-CK-MB-BNP) of the patient on the basis of the specific operation;
- deep knowledge of the specific possible repercussions of the given operation on the patient's cardiocirculatory apparatus;

Table 12.4 Revised cardiac risk index (Lee et al. 1999, p 77)

Known ischemic heart disease
CHF
Cerebrovascular disease
High-risk surgery
Insulin-dependent diabetes
Creatinine > 2 mg/l
Based on data from [77]

- deep knowledge of the repercussions of GA and LRA (above all, of spinal anesthesia) on the cardiocirculatory apparatus (hemodynamics and BP);
- deep knowledge of the problems inherent to infusive liquid treatment;
- choice of monitoring on the basis of prevention and rapid detection of ischemic events;
- appropriate allocation of the patient in the postoperative phase and close instrumental and biohumoral monitoring that includes "at least" 12-lead ECG and daily dosage (3–4 days) of cTn (cardiac troponine) and CK-MB;
- constant postoperative analgesia to eliminate pain and emotional stimuli, both of which can induce vascoconstriction and hence rapid reduction in myocardial perfusion.

The prevention of operative risk in the coronaropathic patient is a topic of such amplitude that thorough analysis in this chapter is not possible. The reader is accordingly invited to refer to the topic-specific chapter by Allaria [74], which summarizes the essential issues and provides the most recent and significant bibliography.

Coronaropathy does not constitute an independent limiting factor for surgery and it does not necessarily or "on principle" impose postoperative admission to the ICU.

12.7.4 Arterial Hypertension

Arterial hypertension (AH) manifests, to varying degrees, in about 50 % of patients over the age of 65 years [75].

Normally, and above all when in light-moderate form, it remains occult and only emerges during anesthesiological examination.

Not infrequently, anesthesiological examination also reveals the inappropriateness of existing pharmacological therapy relative to the clinical evolution of AH [76].

The foregoing statements indicate the importance of preoperative assessment; along with a deep knowledge of the physiopathological mechanisms underlying AH (cardiac output, peripheral resistance and aortic compliance), of the pharmacodynamics and pharmacokinetics of antihypertensive drugs, said assessment enables the optimal choice of operative procedures for hypertensive patients who have to undergo surgery.

It is obviously necessary to ascertain that the BP values obtained are authentic and not the product of an emotional reaction to medical examination (i.e., to "the white tunic effect").

The literature does not provide convincing data with which to stratify the perioperative risk of the hypertensive surgery patient; said literature is generally based on numerically limited cohorts, it is out-of-date and it does not account for the impact of recent technological and pharmacological innovation. It should accordingly be considered as barely significant.

Slight-to-moderate AH (BSP < 180 mmHg e DBP < 110 mmHg) does not constitute a perioperative risk factor and does not fall within the parameters of Lee's RCRI [77].

Severe AH (BSP > 180 mmHg e DBP > 110 mmHg) probably requires pre-operative re-assessment of pharmacological therapy and, possibly, the postpone-ment of surgery by a few days, but it does not necessarily predetermine postoperative admission to the ICU, even in the case of emergency surgery.

Singular cases of secondary AH, such as pheochromocytoma, need separate consideration and should be assessed attentively so that the patient enters surgery without pharmacological imbalances (by means of α e β-blockers) and thus avoids possibly grave perioperative complications [75, 77, 78].

Surgery for pheochromocytoma-induced AH does not necessarily impose postoperative admission to the ICU.

12.7.5 Chronic-Obstructive Bronchopneumonia

Chronic-obstructive Bronchopneumonia (COPD) is one of the commonest lung pathologies in the world [80–82].

Its incidence is very high in patients who undergo major surgery [83] and it substantially raises operative risk; positive outcomes will accordingly depend considerably on the medical profession's attention to this population [80–84].

COPD essentially reduces expiratory flow and is the expression of two principal pathologies: chronic bronchitis and pulmonary emphysema. The operative itinerary imposes numerous requirements: careful preoperative assessment of COPD gravity with recourse to all available means; the exclusion of current trends toward more acute expression; attentive monitoring of the respiratory situation (dynamic infla-tion, oxyemia, ABE...); postoperative allocation to an appropriate environment for respiratory (above all during reawakening and extubation) and cardiocirculatory monitoring; efficacious pain therapy.

The anesthetist is institutionally obliged to possess comprehensive knowledge of COPD physiopathology and its repercussions on operative risk.

Despite numerous pertinent contributions, the literature's stratification of operative risk and identification of high-risk patients is unable to satisfactorily define and resolve all the aggravating factors at play and their highly variable, reciprocal correlations.

COPDD patients who undergo major surgery, above all when thoracic or upper abdomen surgery is involved, need high-level postoperative care and an appropriate environment for the safe-guarding of vital functions. BPCO is not an independent limiting factor for surgery and does not necessarily impose postoperative admission to the ICU.

12.7.6 Asthma

Asthmatic patients who undergo surgery need: careful preoperative assessment of general clinical conditions and of the specific pathology's characteristics; particular attention during the induction (the critical phase for tracheal intubation) and the conduction of anesthesia, and careful choice of both artificial ventilation (AV) method and related drugs; appropriate monitoring of vital functions and of the parameters of respiratory mechanics; exact care in the delicate moment of awakening-extubation and in the postoperative phase.

Continuous growth in the incidence of asthma over recent years obliges the anesthetist to possess a profound knowledge of this ailment's physiopathological mechanisms, of analytical and monitoring methodologies regarding respiratory function and mechanics, and of current techniques for artificial AV. Preoperative assessment, intraoperative anesthesia, and appropriate postoperative care are indispensable for the containment of immediate and late postoperative respiratory and cardiocirculatory complications [85, 86, 95, 96].

Asthma does not constitute an independent limiting factor for surgery and does not necessarily impose postoperative admission to the ICU.

12.7.7 Diabetes

Diabetes (both Type 1, which affects 0.4–1 % of the Italian population and Type 2, which affects 3–4 %) is another highly challenging pathology for the anesthetist. Diabetic patients bear increased perioperative risk for cardiovascular, renal, and septic complications, as well as for that of surgical wound infection. Furthermore, high percentages of diabetic patients present variable Grades of coronaropathy and/or vasculopathy, renal insufficiency, and even more frequently, AH; for this latter, they typically undergo ACE-inhibitor and/or sartan therapy, which in turn can inflict substantial hemodynamic repercussions, such as conspicuous losses of blood [87].

A high percentage of diabetics (according to some surveys, as much as 90 %) presents "disautonomy" as an associated pathology; normally indicated by the acronym "CAN" (Cardiovascular Autonomic Neuropathy), this pathology is characterized by heart and vesselautonomic neuro system (ANS fiber damage.

This damage causes alterations in the control of heart rate and vascular dynamics, which typically manifest in conjunction with acute hypovolemia and insufficient compensatory response; consequently, cardiac output diminishes and AH ensues, possibly followed by myocardial ischemia and/or renal damage [87–90].

The anesthetist must possess perfect knowledge of: the physiopathology of diabetes mellito; the specific characteristics of its clinical expressions (Type 1 and Type 2); the pharmacokinetics and pharmacodynamics of endovenous and oral hypoglycemic drugs, and their possible interference with those used in the perioperative phase (anesthetics, analgesics, anti-inflammatory therapy).

Throughout their perioperative itinerary, diabetic patients require attentive monitoring of vital parameters and of glycemia to avoid complications such as ketoacidosis for Type 1 or Hyperglycemic Hyperosmolar Nonketotic Syndrome (HHNS) for Type 2 [87, 91].

Diabetes is not an independent limiting factor for surgery and does not necessarily impose postoperative admission to the ICU.

12.7.8 Neurosurgery

In neurosurgery [92] it is fundamental to maintain normal values for cerebral perfusion pressure, O_2 supply, and intracranial pressure (ICP) in order to contain immediate and secondary cerebral damage.

Accordingly, and upon scrupulous preoperative assessment, it is necessary to implement appropriate monitoring and a postoperative itinerary that provides the required level of monitoring and therapy.

Frequently, and above all in traumatologic and hemorrhagic pathologies, it is necessary to keep the patient under sedation and ventilation for variable periods that often past for several days; the patient is thus protected from pain and from the onset of alterations in the cerebral cycle (vasodilatory cascade, vasospasm), the latter being capable of inducing serious secondary lesions. Other factors for the choice of postoperative allocation are the degree of consciousness displayed by the patient on reawakening, respiratory autonomy, and ability to protect the respiratory airways.

The NCH wards of many Italian hospitals are equipped with a specific, dedicated IT, and/or neurosurgical SICU unit. Managed by anesthetists, or by neurosurgeons, or jointly by both sets of specialists, such units offer superior postoperative services by planning operations on the basis of the levels of care needed (without prejudicing the availability of emergency beds).

In hospitals that lack dedicated IT-SICU units, patients are admitted to multipurpose ICUs.

Postoperative admission to the ICU for neurosurgery patients is not automatic, but it is necessary for such pathologies as major cranial trauma and hemorrhagic stroke; it can also be considered necessary for the prevention of secondary lesions and/or for inadequate control of respiratory function and of the airways.

12.7.9 Major Vascular Surgery

Patients who undergo major vascular surgery [93] are at high perioperative risk on account of (i) the high percentage of comorbidity and (ii) of vessel clamping and declamping, with possible consequent deficits in tissue and organ perfusion.

Adverse cardiovascular events are the principal cause of perioperative complications arising from major vascular surgery. Despite important innovations in surgery (e.g., mini-invasive endoprosthesis) and in anesthesiology (LRA techniques), major vascular surgery remains subject to high morbidity and mortality. It is therefore fundamental that specific monitoring provides all the data necessary to optimize patients' hemodynamic status throughout the perioperative itinerary.

Major vascular surgery does not constitute an independent limiting factor for surgery and does not necessarily impose postoperative admission to the ICU. However, even in the postoperative phase, it does require monitoring to provide continuous assessment of the hemodynamic apparatus, as managed by staff who are expert in the interpretation of pertinent data.

12.7.10 Sepsis

Patients with severe septic shock [94] who have to undergo surgery generally require it urgently and are already admitted to an intensive care area; they may even present complications arising from previous intervention and they have generally already undergone monitoring for vital functions (cardiovascular, respiratory, renal) with more or less invasive methods. Although the literature does not specify allocation for severe septic shock patients, recommendations for monitoring and therapy levels [8, 97] and the predictably prolonged admission period make the need for admission to an intensive care area (surgical IT/ICU) explicit.

12.7.11 Hemorrhagic Patients

It is above all indispensable to "quantify" the entity of the hemorrhage, and in this regard the reader is invited to consult the literature for definitions of "massive hemorrhage" and of "post-partum hemorrhage" [98–100].

In truth, the data supplied by the literature are not exhaustive in that they derive from insufficiently large cohorts and address overly specific pathologies (polytrauma, heart surgery, liver transplant). As a result, the given findings are not extendable to general surgery.

Marietta [98] convincingly suggests the need of every Operative Unit (or perhaps, better, of each hospital or Region) for its own definition of "critical hemorrhage" and operative infusional protocol. Hemorrhagic patients present an extremely high risk of immediate (cardiocirculatory) and distant (organ/tissue perfusional deficit) complications, as determined by the entity of the hemorrhage, and by duration, treatment, and comorbidity; vital function monitoring, including that of high and qualified hemocoagulation is accordingly required in the postoperative phase [98].

Massive hemorrhage does not constitute an independent limiting factor that mandates postoperative admission to the ICU, although the clinical context in which such hemorrhages occur (polytrauma, major vascular surgery) makes such admission advisable.

12.7.12 Lung Surgery

Along with the features that it holds in common with all other forms of major surgery and anesthesia, lung surgery [101, 102] adds those regarding the site and nature of intervention, namely, the thorax, which is opened, and the lungs, which undergo resection of variable extent; arrhythmogenic manipulation of the large arteries, lateral decubitus monopulmonary ventilation—all are singular events that must be well understood, given that they are to a large extent predictable and thus preventable.

Correct preoperative assessment is indispensable and optimizes choices regarding the anesthesiological program and intra- and postoperative monitoring. Notwithstanding its need for high-level and qualified care, lung surgery, including pneuomonectomy, does not constitute an independent factor for admission to the ICU in the postoperative phase.

12.7.13 Polytrauma

Given the polymorphism of polytraumatic lesion sites, of their severity and of their associations, the present article is not the place for a complete description of the operative risk that polytraumatized patients face.

Years of study have made Severity Scores increasingly sensitive and specific [103–107], sufficiently so to enable the drafting of Guidelines on health care standards, such as, for example, the Advanced Trauma Life Support Guidelines of the American College of Surgeons [29]. Research has evidenced the importance of the timeliness of intervention (golden hour—107) and of its pertinence to the given perioperative phase. Patients who undergo emergency surgery for major polytraumatization are generally, though not necessarily, proposed for admission to the ICU in the postoperative phase, for clinical and, frequently, legal medicine issues.

12.7.14 Emergency Surgery

Emergency surgery invariably and by definition heightens operative risk since it frequently precludes not only thorough preliminary assessment, but also careful preparation of the patient and due modification of possible existing pharmacological therapies (vaso-cardioactive drugs, anticoagulants...). Surgery of this nature has to be performed in the context of severe clinical situations and of alterations in vital functions, which often forces recourse to choices of priority (as, for example, in polytrauma).

The literature has given ample space to the innumerable aggravating factors induced by emergency surgery, but has thus far been unable to provide precise and definitive information.

The additional operative risk inherent to emergency surgery justifies longer-than-average postoperative sojourns in the ICU, even when clinical conditions are less severe than those required for patients who undergo elective surgery.

12.7.15 Informed Consent

In its paper form as an Appendix to medical records, informed consent is merely the documentation, as requested by the law, of something that should consist in a considerably deeper contract between the doctor and the patient.

A contract that should be based on the reciprocal exchange of all necessary information, such that: the doctor can acquire an in-depth and not merely physical knowledge of the patient; in turn, the patient has a clear and exact picture of his/her clinical situation, of the health itinerary that he/she will follow, and of what he/she can expect upon completion of treatment.

It is indispensable that the patient who is to undergo surgery receives from the doctor all the information necessary for the patient to understand and to quantify operative risk precisely, which he/she may with total freedom decide to accept or reject.

The doctor-patient dialog that leads to the drafting and joint signing of the paper document therefore has considerably more importance and higher priority than that of merely subscribing to a "written legal insurance."

Clearly, the patient also needs to be informed that: upon leaving the operating theater, he/she will have to spend a variable period in a protected environment (the RR) before being discharged (to Day Surgery) or returning to the ward; that, on the basis of risk levels, he/she may be or may have to be admitted to the ICU, and that such admission will not of itself mean that something has not gone well in the operation. To reawaken in an "alien and alienating environment" such as that of the ICU without preparation could indeed constitute an authentic emotional and physical shock, and generate useless and absolutely avoidable fears and suspicions.

Subject to the adult patient's consent, relatives too should be informed in advance of the possibility/certainty, and the meaning, of postoperative admission of the patient to the ICU, of alterations in vital functions, which often forces recourse to choices of priority (as, for example, in polytrauma).

12.7.16 Inappropriate Postoperative Admission to the ICU

The surgery patient's postoperative admission to the ICU normally occurs on the basis of the need for intensive monitoring that is not available elsewhere because the given hospital lacks an RR and/or a SICU. Alternatively, such admission may occur not only for the security of the patient but also for that of the anesthetist, be it on account of the emergence of medico-legal problems (accidents in workplaces or in penitentiary areas, TS) or of hypothetical future legal contestation.

Both the first case, i.e., when the ICU has to compensate for the lack of alternative units suited to postoperative management, and the second, i.e., when admission to the ICU assumes the meaning of "defensive medicine," would in theory amount to an "inappropriate admission" in that it leads to the occupation of an intensive care bed and thus denies the given bed to another patient who truly needs intensive therapy. This scenario clearly conflicts with the ethical principle that argues the need for an "equitable distribution of resources."

It is my personal opinion, however, that if the anesthetist decides it is opportune to admit the surgery patient to the ICU and, having produced pertinent reasons, agrees with the doctors on duty in the ICU, he/she is acting correctly, whatever the reasons that led to the given decision.

In general terms, anesthesia reduces the human organism's capacity for self-defense, adaptation and compensation, and the efficiency of its vital functions. The anesthetist is perfectly aware of, and must accept responsibility for, the "fragility" he/she induces in the patient for the time required and in the site best suited to the given needs.

If such use of the ICU implies a "theoretically inappropriate occupation," but demonstrably serves the safety of the patient and annuls the patient's operative risk, the problem exists but assumes an organizational character and hence is the responsibility not only of the anesthetist but of the entire hospital.

12.7.17 Judgement

Which adult patients should be admitted to the ICU in the noncardiosurgical postoperative phase?

The question is important because of the substantial clinical implications it invokes and because of the frequency with which it is addressed to the anesthetist.

Recognition of the question's importance has long stimulated international researchers and has produced a quantitatively and qualitatively sizeable literature that attempts to identify and quantify generic and specific operative risk, and thus to provide doctors with objective data upon which to base their operative decisions.

In so doing, research has analyzed both the systemic impact of surgery and anesthesia on the organism and the more specifically induced impact on patients with chronic pathologies in varying evolutionary phases (CHF, coronaropthy, COPD, polytrauma); it has analyzed the problem of operative risk in the various types of surgery (general abdominal, thoracic, vascular, NCH) and sought to interpret the pertinent physiopathological mechanisms; and it has investigated and produced technologies and drugs of increasing specificity and diminishing invasiveness.

Single independent risk factors have been identified and proposed, but above all, multifactorial risk gravity scales have been devised and validated with the intention of enabling the anesthetist to base operative decisions on objective data, including that of admitting the patient to the ICU upon completion of surgery.

Unfortunately, we still lack a system that allows the doctor to take individual decisions on the exclusive basis of said gravity scales. That said, it should be added that, taken as a whole, the research in question has been of profound importance in casting more and brighter light on the issues inhering to operative risk and on the correlation between the patient's state of health and the characteristics of surgery/anesthesia.

On the basis of data already published in the literature, we can confidently advance the following brief observations:

- surgery and anesthesia, where the latter consists in both GA and LRA, above all as regards spinal anesthesia, invariably impacts on the organism by causing alterations to one or more vital functions, alterations which can occur more or less in isolation or analogously in association;
- these alterations derive from the drugs employed, from the characteristics of the operation (e.g., prolonged lateral decubitus in thoracic surgery), from the patient's clinical characteristics and from the possible presence and evolutionary stage of comorbidity;
- the influences of all these factors can be reduced but not entirely avoided, despite the continuous improvement in surgical techniques (e.g., videolaparoscopic surgery for mini-abscesses), the availability of increasingly specific anesthesiological techniques and anesthetic and analgesic drugs, and the improvement in instruments for the assessment and monitoring of vital functions;
- emergency surgery increases operative risk because it limits preoperative assessment of the patient and of his/her state of readiness for surgery;
- the Anesthetist must ineluctably possess in-depth knowledge both of the generic physiopathological implications of anesthesia, in all its forms, in patients unencumbered by comorbidity, and of the specific implications determined by chronic pathologies that may be reciprocally associated and in variable stages of evolution.
- it is futile to insist that the Anesthetist must: be omniscient, the master of all anesthesiological techniques and assessment systems for the vital functions; possess a perfect knowledge of clinically applied pharmacokinetics and pharmacodynamics, as regards not only the anesthetic and analgesic drugs that are in his/her specific domain, but all drugs that may play a role in ongoing therapy and that can interfere with surgery. ALL of the foregoing is his/her institutional duty, and goes without saying;
- operative risk is inescapable, but it is to a great extent predictable and hence may be attenuated by means of a holistic vision of surgery as uniting 3 reciprocally influential phases (pre-intra-postoperative) into a single, collective continuum;
- operative risk is quantifiable, with reasonable accuracy, by association of data gathered at preoperative consultancy with those respectively supplied by pertinent instrumental and biohumoral surveys and by those reported in the relevant literature. This process includes the systematic use of generic and/or specific gravity scales for pathologies/clinical situations (ASA, Cardiac Risk Index, ISS);
- the postoperative phase is invariably a critical period that requires qualified, intensive monitoring and/or care, which in turn must be calibrated to the single patient, in that this is the phase of stabilization/recovery of vital function autonomy. The phase is of variable duration and highly susceptible to

complications; these latter are normally cardiocirculatory and/or respiratory, and although their arrival can be stealthy and barely apparent to superficial observation, they can be very severe;

- the postoperative phase must comply to the regulations governing OT accreditation and take place in designated intensive care areas (RRs), but in the absence of RRs and/or in specific clinical conditions recourse may be taken to POIT (if it exists) or to multi-purpose ICU;
- to date, no single independent factor has been identified, nor any gravity scale, that can of itself allow postoperative admission to the ICU on the basis of individual discretion, but current research on independent factors and gravity has provided the Anesthetist with objective data that in turn have been of considerable help in assessment of operative risk.

12.8   Reasons for Postoperative Admission to the ICU

12.8.1 Elective Surgery

- Preoperative clinical conditions of sufficient gravity that, correlated to the characteristics of the required surgery, predict with reasonable certainty the need for a prolonged postoperative phase with complex monitoring and the enactment of artificial support for vital functions (e.g., AV, substantial hemodynamic support, exact monitoring of liquid flows).

Assessment must obviously be shared by the surgeons and the entire health team, as well as being coordinated with the ICU team. Postoperative admission to the ICU in this case is necessary and appropriate since the case requires not only monitoring but also prolonged intensive therapy. Admission must be proposed in advance to, and agreed with, the patient, who is free to accept or refuse the proposal. If the patient consents, the information must also be made known to the patient's relatives.

- Surgery that leads in the postoperative phase to prolonged use of sedation/ analgesia and AV (a typical regime applied to certain NCH operations) for the prevention of secondary damage.

In this case, admission to the ICU (when neurosurgical IT is not available) is planned and agreed with surgeons, intensive care colleagues, the patient, and relatives. Said admission is dutiful and appropriate.

- Even when not forecast, adverse intraoperative events related to surgery and/or to anesthesia can create sufficient conditions of risk for the health team to request the patient's postoperative admission to the ICU for monitoring and intensive therapy.

This decision must be shared by the surgeons and their ICU colleagues, and timely notice must be given to relatives. Postoperative admission to the ICU is in this case necessary and appropriate.

- A few hours after admission to the RR, and as the closure of the unit approaches, the patient presents vital function instability that is easily discernible and that place him/her in immediate danger of complications and thus requires monitoring and intensive therapy.

Admission to the ICU for the continuation of the postoperative phase is in this case necessary and appropriate and must be agreed with surgeons and their intensive care colleagues. Explanation must be given to the patient, if his/her cognitive condition so admits and, with his consent, pertinent information must be given to relatives.

- The hospital does not have an RR or other intermediate IT areas suitable for postoperative patients who require intensive monitoring for a few hours. Accordingly, the patients are admitted to the ICU.

In absolute terms, this is an "inappropriate" admission, but one that becomes appropriate in relative terms, and is thus fully justified by the fact that the patient must be guaranteed all necessary intensive care to regain independence in his/her vital functions. This problem must be dealt with at an institutional, not an individual, level.

12.8.2 Emergency Surgery

- Emergency surgery aggravates operative risk in that it generally disallows both in-depth preoperative assessment and preparation of the patient for surgery. Additionally, such surgery often takes place in a complex and grave clinical context which includes numerous lesions (e.g., polytrauma).

The relevant literature has highlighted this additional risk, for which postoperative recourse to the ICU is justified even in the case of patients for whom it would not have been requested had surgery been elective. Accordingly, this too is a case in which postoperative admission to the ICU is appropriate.

12.8.3 Judgement

We can conclude that postoperative admission to the ICU is an important arm with which to combat operative risk in patients of high fragility or whose situations are highly complex. However, recourse to the ICU should not be indiscriminate and should follow well-defined indications in order not to contravene the ethical principle of an "equal distribution of resources" and of respect for the ill. To act correctly, the Anesthetist, who is responsible for the perioperative clinical itinerary, must avail of solid bases in applied and pharmacological physiopathology; he/she must likewise be thoroughly familiar with the pertinent literature and, obviously, must be a master of the techniques of anesthesiology and intensive therapy. However, the foregoing only describes the indispensable foundation for appropriate decisions, which will be mediated by personal clinical experience and by collective assessment of the perioperative itinerary of each single patient.

Abbreviations used in the text	
GA General anesthesia	NIV Noninvasive ventilation
LRA Loco-regional anesthesia	PACU Postanesthesia care unit
ASA American society of anesthesiologists	ICP Intracranial pressure
BMI Body mass index	PONV Postoperative nausea and vomiting
CAN Cardiac autonomic neuropathy	RR Recovery room
CHF Chronic heart failure	SIAIARTI Società Italiana di Anestesia Analgesia Rianimazione e Terapia Intensiva
HEE Hydro-electrolytic equilibrium	ANS Autonomous nervous system
HHNS Hyperglycemic hyperosmolara nonketotic syndrome	OT Operating theater
AH Arterial hypertension	ICU Intensive care unit
IBW Ideal body weight	T°c Core body temperature
ICU Intensive care unit	SPACU Subintensive postanesthesia care unit
GL Guidelines	TNM Neuromuscular transmission monitor
NS Neurosurgery	AV Artificial ventilation

References

1. Calderini E (2010) Gruppo di lavoro SIAARTI per l'assistenza post-anestiologica: Raccomandazioni per l'area di recupero e l'assistenza post- anstesiologica. WWW.SIAARTI. IT. Linee Guida/Raccomandazioni. 1–25
2. Tiret L, Desmots JM, Hatton F et al (1986) Complications associated with anesthesia: a prospective survey in France. Can Anaesth Soc J 33:336–344
3. Cotè CJ, Goldstein EA, Cotè MA et al (1988) A single-blind study of pulse oximetry in children. Anesthesiology 68:184–188
4. Zelcer J, Wells DG (1987) Anaesthetic related recovery room complications. Anaesth Intensive Care 15:168–174
5. Hines R, Barrasch PG, Watrous G et al (1992) Complications occurring in the postanesthesia care unit: a survey. Anesth Analg 74:503–509
6. Hynes BA, Weiser TG, Berry VR et al (2009) A surgery safety checklist to reduce morbidity and mortality in global population. New Engl J Med 360:491–499
7. Ghasperi AA, Birkmeyer JD, Dimik B (2009) Variation in hospital mortality associated with inpatient surgery. New Engl J Med 361:1368–1375
8. Allaria B, Dei Poli M (2011) Il monitoraggio delle funzioni vitali nel perioperatorio non cardiochirurgico. Springer, Italia, pp 1–358

9. Leykin Y, Costa N, Gullo A (2001) Analysis and comparison of the guidelines regarding recovery room management. Minerva Anestesiol 67:563–571
10. Zuck D (1995) Anaesthetic and postoperative recovery rooms. Anaesthesia 50:435–438
11. Decreto del Presidente della Repubblica 14 gennaio (1997) G.U. 20 febbraio 1997, vol 42, supplemento ordinario
12. Eltringham R, Casey W, Durkin M (1998) Postoperative recovery and pain relief. Springer, London
13. SIAARTI (1994) Raccomandazioni per la sorveglianza postanestesiologica. Minerva Anestesiol
14. ASA (1990) Standards for postanesthesia care (approved by House of Delegates on October 12, 1988 and last amended on October 23, 1990)
15. Rapporto Osservasalute (2011) Emergenza: Osservatorio Nazionale sulla Salute nelle Regioni Italiane. V&P Università, pp 245–258
16. Moller JT, Wittrup M, Johansen SH (1990) Hypoxaemia in the post-anaesthesia care unit: an observer study. 73:890–895
17. Pedersen T (2005) Does perioperative pulse oximetry improve outcome? Seeking the best available evidence to answer the clinical question. Best Pract Res Clin Anaesthesiol 19(1):111–123
18. Pedersen T, Moller AM, Hovhannisyan K (2009) Pulse oximetry for perioperative monitoring. Cochrane Database Syst Rev 7(4):CD002013
19. Scuderi PE, Mims GR III, Weeks DB et al (1996) Oxygen administration during transport and recovery after outpatient surgery does not prevent episodic arterial desaturation. J Clin Anesthesia 8:294–300
20. Morioka J, Yamamori S, Ozaki M (2006) Evaluation of a compact device for capnometry of mainsteam type compared with one of side-stream type in a postoperative care unit. Masui 55:1496–1501
21. Ramaswamy KK, Frerk C (2007) Monitoring end-tidal carbon dioxide in the recovery room. Anaesthesia 62:97
22. Orhan-Sungur M, Kranke P, Sessler D et al (2008) Does supplemental oxygen reduce postoperative nausea and vomiting ? A meta-analysis of randomized controlled trials. Anesth Analg 106(6):1733–1738
23. Societè Francaise d'Anesthesie et de Rèanimation (1996) Reccomandations concernant la surveillance et les soins postanesthesiques, 2nd edition. www.sfar.org/recompostop.html
24. Rusca M, Proietti S, Schnider P et al (2003) Prevention of atelectasis formation during induction of general anesthesia. Anesth Analg 97:1835–1839
25. Hopf HW (2008) Hyperoxia and infection. Best Pract Res Clin Anaesthesiol 22(3):553–559
26. Squadrone V, Coha M, Cerutti E et al (2005) Continuous positive airway pressure for treatment of postoperative hypoxemia: a randomized controlled trial. JAMA 293(5):589–595
27. Rose D, Keith RD, Marsha M (1996) Cardiovascular events in the postanesthesia care unit: contribution of risk factors. Anesthesiology 84(4):772–781
28. American Society of Anesthesiologists (2002) Practice guidelines for postanesthetic care. Anesthesiology 96:742–752
29. European Resuscitation Council (2005) Guidelines for resuscitation 2005. Resuscitation 67(S1):S1–S189
30. Callum KG, Gray AJG, Hoile RW et al (1999) The 1999 report of the national confidential enquiry into perioperative deaths. National Confidential Enquiry into Perioperative Deaths, London
31. Zacharias M, Conlon NP, Herbison GP et al (2008) Interventions for protecting renal function in the perioperative period. Cochrane Database Syst Rev 8(4):CD003590
32. Beers MH (2005) The Merck Manual of Geriatrics: postoperative care, Sect. 3, Chap. 26. New York 2005
33. SIGN (2004) Postoperative management in adults: a practical guide to postoperative care for clinical staff, vol 77. Scottish Intercollegiate Guidelines Network (SIGN), Edinburgh, p 5

34. Kellum IA, Decker JM (2001) The use of dopamine in acute renal failure: a meta-analysis. Crit Care Med 29:1526–1531
35. Sessler DL (2000) Perioperative heat balance. Anesthesiology 92:578–579
36. W agner VD (2006) Unp la nned p erio pera tive hypothermia. AORN J 83(2):470–476
37. Vaughamn MS, Vaughan RW, Cork RC (1981) Postoperative hypothermia in adults: relationship of age anesthesia and shivering to rewarming. Anesth Analg 60:746–751
38. Winkler M, Akca O, Birkenberg B, Sessler BI et al (2000) Aggressive warming reduces blood loss during hip arthroplasty. Anesth Analg 91:978–984
39. Melling AC, Ali B, Scott EM et al (2001) Effects of preoperative warming on the incidence of wound infections after clean surgery: a randomized controlled trial. Lancet 358:876–880
40. Insler SR, O'Connor MS, Leventhal MJ et al (2000) Association between postoperative hypothermia and adverse outcome after coronary bypass surgery. Ann Thorax Surg 70:175–181
41. Lenhard R (2003) Monitoring and thermal management. Best Pract Res Clin Anaesthesiol 17(4):569–581
42. Sessler DI, Schoeder M (1993) Heat loss in humans covered with cotton hospital blankets. Anesth Analg 77:73–77
43. Frank SM, Shir Y, Raja S et al (1994) Core Hypothermia and skin surface temperature gradients. Anesthesiology 80:502–508
44. Brauer A, Michael GM, English MJM et al (2007) Efficacy of forced-air warming systems with full body blankets. Can J Anesth 54(1):34–41
45. Sessler DI (1993) Perianesthetic thermoregulation and heat balance in humans. FASEB J 7:638–644
46. Sessler DI (1994) Temperature monitoring. In: Miller RD (ed) Anesthesia. Churchill Livingstone, New York, pp 1363–1382
47. Horn EP (1999) Postoperative shivering: aetiology and treatment. Curr Opin Anaesthesiol 12:449–453
48. Horn EP, Schroeder F, Wilhelm S, Sessler DI et al (1999) Postoperative pain facilitates normothermoregulatory tremor. Anesthesiology 91:979–984
49. Horn EP, Sessler DI, Standl T et al (1998) Non-thermoregulatory shivering in patients recovering from isoflurane or desflurane anesthesia. Anesthesiology 89:878–886
50. Ralley FE, Wynands JE, Ramsay JG et al (1988) The effects of shivering on oxygen consumption and carbon dioxide production in patients rewarming from hypothermic cardiopulmunary bypass. Can Anaesth 35(332):37
51. Kranke P, Eberhart LH, Roewer N et al (2004) Single-dose parenteral pharmacological interventions for the prevention of postoperative shivering: a quantitative systematic review of randomized controlled trials. Anesth Analg 99:718–727
52. America Pain Society Quality of Care Committee (1995) Quality improvement GL for the treatment of acute pain and cancer pain. J Am Med Ass 23:1874–1880
53. Savoia G, Ambrosio F, Paoletti F et al (2002) SIAARTI study group for acute/chronic pain: SIAARTI recommendations for the treatment of postoperative pain. Minerva Anestesiol 68:735–750
54. Macario A, Weinger M, Carney S et al (1999) Which clinical anesthesia outcomes are important to avoid ? The perspective of patients. Anesth Analg 89:652–658
55. Tramer MR (2001) A rational approach to the control of postoperative nausea and vomiting: evidence from systematic review, part II: recommendations for prevention and treatment, and research agenda. Acta Anaesthesiol Scand 45:14–19
56. Apfel CC, Laara E, Koivuranta M et al (1999) A simplified risk score for predicting postoperative nausea and vomiting: conclusions from cross-validations between two centers. Anesthesiology 91:693–700
57. Aldrete JA, Kroulik DA (1970) A postanesthetic recovery score. Anesth Analg 49:924–934
58. White PF, Song D (1999) New criteria for fast-tracking after outpatient anesthesia: a comparison with the modified Aldretès scoring system. Anesth Analg 88:1069–1072

59. ASSR (Agenzia dei Servizi Sanitari Regionali: Sistema Nazionale delle Linee Guida) 2004
60. Ministero della Salute (2007) Linee di indirizzo per la ristorazione ospedaliera ed assistenziale
61. Linee Guida SIAARTI, Biagioli B, Catena G, Clementi G et al (2000) Raccomandazioni per la gestione perioperatoria del cardiopatico da sottoporre a chirurgia non cardiochirurgica. Minerva Anestesiol 66:85–102
62. Gruppo di Lavoro dell'ASSR per le Linee Guida, Ministero della Salute (2006) Linee guida sulla nutrizione artificiale domiciliare, vol 20S5, p S11–S171
63. Agenzia Sanitaria Regionale dell'Emilia e Romagna (1999) Linee Guida per un uso appropriato degli esami preoperatori
64. British Columbia Medical Association (2000) Preoperative testing
65. Eagle KA, Bergers PB, Chatman BR et al (2002) Guideline update for perioperative cardiovascular evaluation for non-cardiac surgery: executive summary–a report of the American College of Cardiology/American Heart Association task force on practice GL. Anesth Analg 94:1052–1064
66. Dei Poli M, Alberghetti A, Caporarello S (2011) Il Paziente obeso. In: Il monitoraggio delle funzioni vitali nel perioperatorio non cardiochirurgico. Springer, Bologna, pp 73–89
67. Ahmad S, Nagle A, McCarthy MJ et al (2008) Postoperative hypoxemia in morbidly obese patients with and without obstructive sleep apnea undergoing laparascopic surgery. Anesth Analg 107:138–143
68. Chung F, Yeneshvaran B, Errera F et al (2008) Patients with difficult intubation may need referral to sleep clinics Anesth Analg 107:915–920
69. Guobaux B, Bruder N, Racaules-Aime M (2004) Prise en charge preoperatoire du patient obese. In: Encyclopedie medico-chirurgicale, anesthesie- reanimation. Elsevier, Masson, 36-650-C-10
70. Ogunnaike BO, Whitten CW (2009) Anesthesia and Obesity. In: Barash PD et al (eds) Clinical Anesthesia, 6th edn. Lippincott Williams & Wilkins, Philadelphia, pp 1230–1246
71. Hammil BG, Curtis LH, Bennet-Guerrero E et al (2008) Impact of heart failure in patients undergoing major noncardiac surgery. Anesthesiology 108:559–567
72. Allaria B (2011) La gestione perioperatoria del paziente con insufficienza cardiaca cronica. In: Il monitoraggio delle funzioni vitali nel perioperatorio non cardiochirurgico. Springer, Bologna, pp 3–19
73. Rivera R, Antognini JF (2009) Perioperative drug therapy in elderly patients. 110:1176–1181
74. Allaria B (2011) Il monitoraggio delle funzioni vitali nel perioperatorio del coronaropatico. In: Il monitoraggio delle funzioni vitali nel postoperatorio non cardiochirurgico, vol 2. Springer, Bologna, pp 21–39
75. Allaria B (2011) La gestione perioperatoria del paziente iperteso. In: Il monitoraggio delle funzioni vitali nel perioperatorio non cardiochirurgico, vol 3. Springer, Bologna, pp 41–55
76. Fleisher LA (2002) Preoperative evaluation of the patient with hypertension. JAMA 287:2043–2046
77. Lee TH, Marcantonio ER, Mangione CM et al (1999) Derivation and prospective validation of a simple index for prediction of cardiac risk of major non cardiac surgery. Circulation 100:1043–1049
78. Fleisher LA, Beckman JA, Brown Ka et al (2007) ACC/AHA guidelines on perioperative cardiovascular evaluation and care for non cardiac surgery. J Am Coll Cardiol 50:c159
79. Tricoci P, Allen JM, Kramer JM et al (2009) Scientific evidence underlying the ACC/AHA clinical practice guidelines. JAMA 301:831–841
80. Caironi P (2011) Il paziente affetto da BPCO. In: Il monitoraggio delle funzioni vitali nel postoperatorio non cardiochirurgico, vol 6. Springer, Bologna, pp 91–110
81. Rabe KF, Hurd S, Anzueto A et al (2007) Global strategy for the diagnosis, management, and prevention of chronic obstructive pulmonary disease: GOLD executive summary. Am J Respir Crit Care Med 176:532–555

82. Buist AS, McBurnie MA, Vollmer WM et al (2007) International variation in the prevalence of COPD (the BOLD study): a population-based prevalence study. Lancet 170:741–750
83. Menezes AM, Perz-Padilla R, Jardim Jr et al (2005) Chronic obstructive pulmonary disease in five Latin American cities (the PLATINO study): a prevalence study. Lancet 366:1875–1881
84. Lickner M, Swaiser A, Ellemberger C et al (2007) Perioperative medical management of patients with COPD. Int J Chron Obstruct Pulmon Dis 2:493–515
85. Chiumello D, Coppola S (2011) Il paziente asmatico. In: Il monitoraggio delle funzioni vitali nel postoperatorio non cardiochirurgico, vol 7. Springer, Bologna, pp 111–126
86. Woods BD, Sladen NR (2009) Perioperative considerations for the patient with asthma and bronchospasm. Br J Anaesth 103(suppl I):57–65
87. Allaria B (2011) La gestione perioperatoria del paziente diabetico. In: Il monitoraggio delle funzioni vitali nel postoperatorio non cardiochirurgico, vol 4. Springer, Bologna, pp 57–71
88. Alberti KG (1991) Diabetes and surgery. Anesthesiology 74:209–214
89. American Diabetes Association (2005) Standard of medical care in diabetes. Diabetes Care 28(suppl 5–4):5–36
90. Marks J (2003) Perioperative management of diabetes. Am Family Physician 69:93–100
91. Venkatraman R, Singhi SC (2006) Hyperglycemic hyperosmolar nonketotic syndrome. Indian J pediatrics 73:55
92. Fumagalli P (2011) Il paziente neurochirurgico. In: Il monitoraggio delle funzioni vitali nel posoperatorio non cardiochirurgico, vol 13. Springer, Bologna, pp 217–231
93. Dei Poli M, Luci R, Colombo C (2011) Il paziente sottoposto a chirurgia vascolare maggiore. In: Il monitoraggio delle funzioni vitali nel postoperatorio non cardiochirurgico, vol 14. Springer, Bologna, pp 233–256
94. Giraldis M, Biagioni E (2011) Il monitoraggio perioperatorio del paziente settico. In: Il monitoraggio delle funzioni vitali nel posoperatorio non-cardiochirurgico, vol 8. Springer, Bologna, pp 127–144
95. Fanta CH (2009) Asthma. N Engl J Med 360:417–420
96. Quiroz-Martinez H, Ferguson ND et al (2009) Life Threatening asthma: focus on lung protection. In:Yearbook of intensive care and emergency medicine. Springer, Berlin, pp 372–382
97. Rivers E, Nguyen B, Habstad S et al (2001) Early goal-directed therapy in the treatment of severe sepsis and septic shock. N Engl J Med 8:1368–1377
98. Marietta M (2011) Il paziente emorragico. In: Il monitoraggio delle funzioni vitali nel postoperatorio non cardiochirurgico, vol 10. Springer, Bologna, pp 163–179
99. Sihler K, Napolitano MN (2009) Massive transfusion. Chest 136:1654–1667
100. World Health Organization (1990) The prevention and management of postpartum hemorrhage. WHO technical working group report, RepCH/90.7, Geneva
101. Haeusler EA (2011) Il Paziente sottoposto a chirurgia polmonare. In: Il monitoraggio delle funzioni vitali nel postoperatorio non cardiochirurgico, vol 15. Springer, Bologna, pp 257–271
102. Canet J, Mazo V (2010) Postoperative pulmonary complications. Minerva Anestesiol 76:138–143
103. Rambaldi M, Busani S, Baranzoni MT et al (2011) Il paziente politraumatizzato. In: Il monitoraggio delle funzioni vitali nel postoperatorio non cardiochirurgico, vol 12. Springer, Bologna, pp 195–216
104. Baker SP, O'Neill E, Haddon JR et al (1984) The ISS: a method for describing patients with multiple injuries and valuating emergency care. J Trauma 14(3):187–196
105. Champion HR, Sacco WJ, Copes WS et al (1989) A revision of trauma score. J Trauma 29(5):623–629
106. American College of Surgeon (1980) Advanced trauma life support (ATLS) guidelines
107. Gomez G, Fecher A, Joy T et al (2010) Optimizing outcomes in emergency room thoracotomy: a 20 year experience in an urban level I trauma center. Am Surg 76:406–410

Invasive Candidiasis in the Intensive Care Setting

13

Andrea De Gasperi, Paola Cozzi and Stefania Colombo

13.1 Introduction

Many species of *Candida*, and among them all pathogenic species, are very common in humans. *Candida albicans is* the most commonly isolated species in the average clinical setting: however, in the last few years new (and sometimes very aggressive) species of *Candida* (*C. glabrata*, *C. parapsilosis*, *C. tropicalis*, *C. krusei*, *C. guilliermondii*, *C. lusitaniae*, *C. kefyr*, *C. lipolytica*, *C. rugosa*) are on the rise. Deep-seated, invasive *Candida* infections (Invasive candidiasis, IC) which include *candidemia, disseminated candidiasis, peritonitis, endocarditis, endophthalmitis, and meningitis caused by Candida spp.*, have since long been a major concern in hospital wards, and the most recently published *secular trends* have highlighted their considerable growth [1–8] (*see also Marchetti O. et al. Epidemiology of candidemia in Swiss tertiary care hospitals: secular trends 1991–2000. Clin Infect Dis 2004; 38: 311–20*). Despite their low incidence, invasive *Candida* infections still are associated with prolongation of hospital stay, increased costs and high mortality, particularly in the absence of a timely and aggressive treatment [1–3]. While in the USA *Candida* ranks fourth overall among all pathogens isolated in blood cultures, according to the most recent studies in Europe it is usually between the 7th and 10th position [4].

A. De Gasperi (✉) · P. Cozzi · S. Colombo
2° Servizio Anestesia e Rianimazione, Ospedale Niguarda Ca' Granda,
Piazza Ospedale Maggiore 3, 20162, Milan, Italy
e-mail: andrea.degasperi@ospedaleniguarda.it

P. Cozzi
e-mail: paola.cozzi@ospedaleniguarda.it

S. Colombo
e-mail: stefania.colombo@ospedaleniguarda.it

B. Allaria (ed.), *Practical Issues in Anesthesia and Intensive Care 2013*,
DOI: 10.1007/978-88-470-5529-2_13, © Springer-Verlag Italia 2014

13.2 Invasive Candidiasis: Incidence and Definitions

Invasive *Candida* infections represent the most frequent nosocomial fungal infections in the ICU setting, much rarer being those caused by *Aspergillus spp. and* by rare fungi. Their overall incidence is between 1 and 2 %, with a range between 5 and 8 % in USA healthcare settings and between 0.5 and 3 % in Europe [5, 6]. A diagnosis of proven infection requires documentation of tissue invasion (biopsy or culture from a sterile site) and/or an appropriate blood collection method (ESCMID 2012) [9]. The evidence provided by both the EPIC studies of infections corresponding to 17 % is consequently influenced by the problems associated with the definitions: in fact, in the EPIC studies the reported incidence is of "*isolates*" and therefore not necessarily of infections (*Vincent JL, Bihari DJ, Suter PM* et al. *The prevalence of nosocomial infection in intensive care units in Europe. Results of the European Prevalence of Infection in Intensive Care (EPIC) study. JAMA 1995; 274: 639–44; Vincent JL, Rello J, Marshall J* et al. *International study of the prevalence and outcomes of infection in intensive care units. JAMA 2009; 302: 2323–9*).

According to Eggimann et al [1], in the absence of consensus definitions which may allow a clear and univocal identification of ICs in non-neutropenic patients, a large part of reliable and reproducible epidemiology is based on bloodstream infections. Their definition ("*blood culture positivity due to the presence of Candida*") offers no doubts and candidemias are always to be considered as pathological and to be treated.

Taking only candidemia into consideration, its incidence ranges from 2 to 10 cases per 1,000 ICU admissions [1–7]. In the EPIC 2 study [4], the reported figure was 6.8/1,000 admissions while in the most recent study on invasive fungal infections in Italian ICUs, incidence was of 10.08/1,000 admissions [8]. However, as the yeld of blood cultures ranges between 50 and 75 %, the real incidence of candidemia might be considered underestimated [1, 5]. Further critical aspects associated with blood culture results for *Candida* and able to affect the performance of "*early*" treatment and of "*appropriate*" therapeutical choices are (*a*) the lag between blood sampling and the available results (in many settings still reported beyond 48–72 h); (*b*) problems in identifying the *Candida* species responsible for the infection [1]. Candidemia usually (70–80 %) originates from intravascular catheters or devices, whereas chemotherapy, steroid therapy, and immunodeficiency or immunomodulation are conditions associated with the remaining 20–30 %. While the presence of candidemia is pathognomonic for infection, more complex is the problem when *Candida spp.* is found in other sites: among them, abdomen and airways (lungs or bronchial tract). For these sites, and particularly for the abdomen (Peritoneal Candidiasis) there is, so far, a lack of agreement on the definitions. The isolation of *Candida spp.* should be followed by an "interpretation" of its presence (pathogen, a co-pathogenic colonizer or an "*innocent bystander*"): case presentation and clinical setting, blood culture availability, diagnostic approach are to be considered when defining the case, with obvious, wide subjective interpretations and, consequently, possible overestimation of the phenomenon. A likely condition of "simple" colonization is not infrequently quoted as an infection, giving rise to an increased amount of "infections" and, consequently, to a likely useless overtreatment [1, 4].

Indeed, *colonization* should be defined as *the presence of Candida spp. in one or more non-sterile sites* [10]. Candiduria is the presence of Candida $\geq 10^4$ CFU/ml in the urine, whereas the presence of Candida in tracheal aspirate or BAL, very recently associated with increased morbidity in the ICU setting, should be considered a colonization of the respiratory tract and not an infection or pneumonia [10, 11].

13.3 Intra-Abdominal Infections

Before discussing the different types of *Candida peritonitis*, the definitions of *"peritonitis"* proposed by Eckmann et al. in 2011 [12] in the European comment on the most recent Intra-Abdominal Infections (IAI) IDSA guidelines (2010) [13] will be reported. In this paper the AAs identified IAIs as *complicated and uncomplicated; primary, secondary, tertiary; community-acquired, Health care-associated, nosocomial,* an often unclear and debated issue [12, 14–16].

Primary peritonitis (PP) (or spontaneous bacterial peritonitis, SBP) constitutes only about 1 % of all cases and is not associated with discontinuation/perforations of the gastroenteric tract: it includes distinct disease entities such as peritonitis in decompensated liver cirrhosis and peritonitis in nephrotic syndrome with ascites. These imply an intact gastrointestinal tract without overt barrier disruption. In adults, in the majority of cases (70 %), SBP is correlated with ascites and liver cirrhosis and in the remaining cases (30 %) with a reduced immune system. It is diagnosed when the ascitic fluid neutrophil count exceeds 250/μl. Peritonitis associated with peritoneal dialysis is also included in PPs and usually are caused by tube or catheter contamination. The most frequently involved pathogens are *coagulase-negative staphylococci* and *Staphylococcus Aureus*. Other less frequently agents are *E. Coli, Enterococci, Enterobacteriaceae, Pseudomonas aeruginosa,* anaerobes. *Candida* is not frequent at all [12, 14, 15].

Secondary peritonitis **refers to a localized or generalized peritoneal inflammation and abscess formation due to disruption of the anatomical barrier (e.g., perforated appendicitis or diverticulitis). Surgical intervention is required in large part of the cases** *Community-acquired secondary peritonitis* is always an infection of mixed etiology. It does not usually imply a risk of IC, as the most frequently involved bacteria are *Enterococci, E. Coli, Bacteroides fragilis,* and other anaerobes. The perforation site, however, affects the presence of pathogens: *Candida spp.,* together with Gram-positives microorganisms, are mainly represented in gastroduodenal perforations, while Gram-negatives and anaerobes are prevalent in case of colorectal pathology [16].

Postoperative peritonitis is a form of nosocomial secondary peritonitis and is defined as an infectious abdominal complication usually due to anastomotic leak following a surgical intervention: it requires a surgical approach. The majority of patients are usually under antibiotic therapy when diagnosed. Among the responsible pathogens are MRSA (*Methicillin Resistant Staphylococcus Aureus*), *Enterococci* (including VREF, *Vancomycin resistant Enterococcus Faecium*) and now also multi drug resistant gram-negative microorganisms. *Candida spp.*, also according to local epidemiology, may be present with variable incidence [12].

Tertiary peritonitis is referred to as a nosocomial intra-abdominal infection, not solved by a single or even sequential surgical intervention, in combination with often sequential courses of antimicrobial therapy, either with or without antifungal coverage. It is at the highest risk of *Candida* infection (40–50 %) [12, 14–16].

True peritoneal *Candida spp.* infections (*Candida peritonitis*) are the second most important clinical entities among ICs: in surgical patients *Candida* is isolated at the peritoneal level in 5–40 % of cases and is responsible for 3–12 % of community-acquired or nosocomial abdominal surgical infections. Mortality is reported between 20 and 70 % [12–18]. This entity, however, is often overreported, due to the lack of uniformity in the definition (see above) and the diagnostic approach [12, 14–17]. According to Blot et al. [14], *Candida peritonitis is definitively diagnosed* with perioperatively documented *Candida* plaques on the peritoneum, or on histology. The value of a direct examination positive for Candida in a general population with peritonitis remains uncertain, as is the value of microbiological peritoneal findings (and therefore of the interpretation of *Candida* as of an infectious or colonizing agent): however, an association between the isolation of *Candida* in a peritoneal site (in samples either collected during surgery or by direct interventional procedure and not drawned by percutaneous drainage in place for days) and a poor prognosis is frequent, even if not univocal [12–17].

For a diagnosis of *Candida* peritonitis (whose consequences are fundamental to decide whether and how to treat) it is necessary, beside the above-mentioned points, to classify IAI as

(i) *uncomplicated* (appendicitis) or *complicated* (with diffuse peritonitis);
(ii) *community-acquired or nosocomial* (in some cases, *Health care-associated infection, HCAI*, should also be taken into consideration*); if nosocomial or HCAI,* as early- or late-onset.

As specified in the IDSA 2010 guidelines for intra-abdominal infections [13], the detection of *Candida* in community-acquired acute perforations of the GE tract is close to 20 %, but treatment is unnecessary. Indeed, in community-acquired peritonitis, mortality among subjects with or without isolation of *Candida spp.* is identical [14]. In such a context, antifungal treatment is mandatory only in case of

(i) immunosuppressed or organ transplanted patients,
(ii) cancer patients,
(iii) patients with inflammatory disease,
(iv) abdominal reoperations,

(v) patients coming from chronic care settings or with an in-hospital stay >48 h, in whom MDR microorganisms may be recovered ("*Health care-associated infections*" [13] (*see below*).

In these cases, the isolation of *Candida spp.* from surgical or interventional samples freshly taken *from the* peritoneal collection is associated with a worse prognosis and an increase in mortality (20–70 %). As highlighted by Carneiro et al [17], perioperative surgical risk factors are associated with *Candida* peritonitis.

In 2003 a score was proposed by Dupont et al. based on four factors (female gender, intraoperative cardiovascular failure, upper gastrointestinal tract origin of peritonitis, antimicrobial therapy in the 48 h prior to the onset of peritonitis) associated with the presence of yeasts in the peritoneal fluid. In the presence of three or more factors, sensibility and specificity were 84 and 50 %; positive and negative predictive values were 67 and 72 %, respectively. However, these figures, while interesting, are not able to confidently support a clinical decision. Such an approach, seldom if ever used, might be considered to start an early empirical treatment in a critically ill patient [19].

A new alternative categorization, not yet prospectively validated, has very recently been proposed by Blot et al [16]: it includes the elimination of the concept of tertiary peritonitis and the terms "*complicated and uncomplicated*" and the introduction of a new grid of classification based on severity of sepsis, presence of perforation and diffusion or not of peritonitis [16]. In the figure, the "grid" [16], proposed to ease the start of a protocolized antiinfective treatment (Table 13.1).

Indeed, if the role of *Candida* as a pathogen may be considered uncertain, the presence of *Candida* is very often associated with a complicated course and an increased mortality rate, particularly in the presence of diffuse peritonitis, multisite colonization, severe sepsis/septic shock, and immunosuppression or immuno-modulation. As a consequence, despite the difficulty in classifying the role of

Table 13.1 Classification of intra-abdominal infections

	Disease expression		
	Mild (sepsis)	Moderate (severe sepsis)	Severe (septic shock)
Community-acquired or early onset healthcare-associated IAI <7 days after hospital admission)			
Without perforation	1	1	2
Localized peritonitis	1	1	2
Diffuse peritonitis	1	2	2
Late-onset healthcare-associated IAI (≥7 days after hospital admission) and or recent antimicrobial exposure			
Without perforation	2	2	2
Localized peritonitis	2	2	3
Diffuse peritonitis	2	3	3
IAI = intra-abdominal infection			

Reproduced from Blot S. Drugs 2012; 72: e17–32 with permission

Candida, the current widely accepted position [12–17] is to consider the detection of *Candida* in cases of *"persistent or severe"* peritonitis [14] as significant, and to start an antifungal treatment with antifungal drugs [12–17, 19] (a decisional algorithm was proposed by Blot et al. in 2007 [14] and, very recently, was redesigned by the same group [16].

13.4   *Candida spp.* in the Respiratory Tract

As already underlined for peritonitis, an overestimation of the phenomenon of *"pulmonary Candida infection"* is evident. Differently from peritoneal Candida, the presence of *Candida* in the respiratory tract is almost always classifiable as *colonization*. Indeed, the characteristics of the bronchial epithelium and of alveoli make the adhesion of yeasts very unlike [1, 4]. Pulmonary candidiasis is therefore quite rare, usually associated to an hematogenous spread and in this case responsible for micro-abscess formations. It does not mean that the detection of *Candida* on bronchoaspirate on BAL is not to be considered [20], but it should not necessarily be assumed as an infection and in any case it should not be treated as such. On the contrary, it has to be considered, as very recently demonstrated, the association between *Candida* colonization in the respiratory tract [20] and an increase in the incidence of VAP (Ventilator-associated pneumonia) caused by MDR bacteria (mainly by *Pseudomonas Aeruginosa*) with a worse prognosis. Further studies on this specific item are awaited.

The consequences of an overestimation of the phenomenon are, as already stated, the higher than real reports of *"candida pneumonitis,"* an unjustified treatment of a simple colonization, an overuse of antifungal drugs with possible emergence of resistance due to overexposure, a significant (and unjustified) increase in costs.

13.5   Epidemiology of Invasive Candidiasis

The distribution of *Candida* infections today may roughly be considered as identical in medical and surgical wards and in the ICUs: in some settings, IC proved to be even less represented in ICUs than in medical and surgical wards. Indeed, it has to be stressed the importance of focusing not only on ICUs, but also on medical and surgical units [21], where infections from *Candida*, when properly defined and monitored, are on the rise: such settings may represent a "reservoir" of those severe infections (severe sepsis/septic shock), later cared for in the ICU setting.

The case mix of ICUs, local epidemiology, the presence of risk factors, the use of prophylactic, empirical or targeted antimicrobial treatments, the surveillance measures, but also the non-univocity of definitions, and the different diagnostic approach are in different ways, factors able to impact on the IC in each single setting [1]. Diagnostic problems, delay in IC recognition and high mortality, (30–60 % according to the *Candida* species but heavily influenced by the therapeutic delay) are among the major challenges clinicians have to face when dealing with ICs [1–3, 22].

An issue rapidly gaining relevance is the possible modification in the epidemiology (*epidemiological shift*) of *Candida spp.* infections. According to the most recent studies carried out in Italy (the "real" epidemiology Italian clinicians have to consider), prevalence of *C Albicans* is still around 60 % and for the large part still fluconazole-susceptible. *C Glabrata and C Parapsilosis* account for about 13 % [8].

There are however European (Spain) or Italian settings where an increase in IC caused by *non-albicans Candida* has been or is being observed [22, 23].

According to Tortorano et al, in comparison to studies performed in the late 90s, there has indeed been a decrease in the incidence of *C Albicans* and an increase in *C Parapsilosis and C Glabrata* % [8].

Excessive pharmacological pressure, inappropriate antifungal prophylaxis (or, if appropriate, carried out using subtherapeutic doses of drugs), selection of *Candida* species resistant to triazole agents, are among the major causes at the basis of this epidemiological shift. The knowledge of the center own epidemiology (*Candida* species and their susceptibility to antifungal agents, the so-called Candida *phenotype*) is pivotal for an appropriate management of IC in any setting. As a matter of fact, *Candida* species responsible for infections impacts on mortality: in the most recent observations, *C. tropicalis* has been associated with higher mortality (*C. tropicalis* 41 vs. other species 29 %). On the contrary, infections caused by *C. parapsilosis* showed lower mortality (*C. parapsilosis* 22.7 vs. other species 33.0 %) [24].

13.6 Invasive Candidiasis: Pathogenesis

In the critical care setting, ICs are associated with specific risk factors closely correlated with procedures and/or therapeutics: among them, central venous catheters (CVCs), total parenteral nutrition (TPN) and/or absence of enteral nutrition, prolonged and/or multiple antibiotic therapies for the presence of severe sepsis/septic shock. Alternatively, postsurgical complications are quite frequently reported as risk factors, (particularly in the case of relaparotomy for anastomotic leaks or in cases of complicated transplant surgery) in patients admitted in the ICU for severe sepsis/septic shock and multiorgan failure. Diabetes, acute or chronic renal failure, prolonged mechanical ventilation and use of steroids constitute [1–5] or become risk factors for *Candida* infections caused by particular species [18]. Multiple site colonization is frequent in this specific clinical setting.

The origin of invasive *Candida* infections is by now widely recognized as being *endogenous* and correlated to *Candida spp.* colonization after suppression of the normal intestinal flora associated to a discontinuation of physiological barriers (gastroenteric tract surgery, necrotizing pancreatitis, chemotherapy, ischemia—reperfusion injury). A bloodstream invasion thus may follow colonization [1]. This concept, well described by Eggimann et al, [1] explains the greater propensity to Candida infections of immunomodulated/immunosuppressed individuals, not necessarily neutropenic.

The source of infection, however, might not be always endogenous, but correlated to the presence of biofilms on CVCs or intravascular prostheses, able to interfere with the action of some antifungals [25].

Biofilm production is frequent with *C. tropicalis* (71.4 % of isolated strains), *C. glabrata* (23.1 %), *C. albicans* (22.6 %), *and C. parapsilosis* (21.8 %): the presence of biofilm, if not properly managed, prevents eradication and increases mortality, as recently demonstrated by Tumbarello et al. [25].

The immune response which follows the invasion by *Candida spp.* involves both the humoral and the cellular component of immunity. Of the latter, a relevant role is played by monocytes, macrophages, and dendritic cells. In particular, the role of *Toll-like receptors 2 and 4* must be stressed, both for the recognition of fungal cell wall structures (in particular mannans) and for their proinflammatory response, associated with the synthesis of cytokines and chemokines (TNF, IL1). An interferon (IFN) γ-mediated response able to evoke the synthesis of anti-Candida immunoglobulins has recently been demonstrated [1]. Interestingly enough, the synthesis of Procalcitonin (PCT) in case of fungal infections is reduced, if compared to the response documented during bacterial infections [26], and may recognize, as a mechanism, the inhibition of PCT synthesis secondary to the increase in γ INF. In most cases, a Candida infection is maintained because of a state of immunodeficiency and/or due to resistant bacteria selection following antibiotic treatments.

While principles of therapeutic approaches will be discussed later, it is pivotal to acknowledge since now that universal prevention measures, such as hand hygiene and adequate CVC management (see for example the recently published IDSA 2012 CVC management guidelines) are be considered as effective tools able to contribute, together with a rational management of the antibiotic therapy, to a decrease in nosocomial *Candida spp.* infections.

13.7 The Problem of Diagnosis

13.7.1 Conventional Diagnosis

As already underlined, the problem of a diagnosis of IC is pivotal. According to Eggimann et al. [1], from 5 to 15 % of patients admitted in the ICU are colonized by *Candida*, but only 15–30 % are later found to be affected by IC and often, as already mentioned, it is difficult to differentiate colonization from infection. Positivity of blood cultures still ranges between 50 and 75 % and mean time to positive cultures may ranges from 48 to >72 h.

The most recent EFIGS (European Fungal Infection Study Group (EFISG) of the ESCMID) guidelines (2012) [9] recommend in case of suspected IC
- Blood cultures
1. Three venous blood samples (from 2 to 4), in a single 30 min session;
2. Total blood volume, for adult patients, of 60 ml;
3. Daily frequency;
4. 5-day incubation period;
5. Species identification.
- Tissue or "significant" fluid collection using
1. Aseptic technique for sample collection from usually sterile sites
2. Imaging- guided needle aspiration (not via drainages)
3. Prompt transportation to the laboratory, rapid fixation
4. Use of selective media for cultures
5. Candida species identification
6. The presence of positivity in samples from deep-seated tissues or from collection adequately performed from a usually sterile site typically indicates a deep-seated infection (IC)
   Negative cultures do not exclude infection (see blood cultures)
   It has to be stressed that microscopic examination requires expertise for interpretation, and morphology cannot be used for definitive identification.

Positive cultures for Yeasts should be followed by identification of the species. In comparison to conventional methods, usually taking from one to three days, new technologies should be preferred today if available, such as FISH (*Fluorescent* in situ *hybridization*) or MALDITOF-MS (*Matrix assisted laser desorption ionization time of flight mass spectrometry*), which allow rapid identification of the species and therefore a prompt and targeted therapeutic approach.

13.7.2 Non-microbiological Diagnosis: Serological and Molecular Approach

Today non-culture based procedures have been added to culture based methods and are gaining relevance [1, 9, 27]. Research studies aim now at the detection of metabolites, antigens, antibodies, DNA, able to provide earlier diagnosis in the absence of culture data but in presence of biological markers. The EFIGS guidelines [9] still express caution toward these techniques, particularly for PCR techniques, even if the near future of diagnostics: in particular at the moment there is no standardization and reproducibility of these procedures. The use of one of them (*Septifast Roche*), is increasingly applied in critically ill patients: however a word of caution has to be expressed and EFIGS 2012 does not recommend its use for *Candida* [9]. Ever increasing importance and significant evidence are being achieved by blood tests able to detect circulating fungal cell wall components, in particular *mannan and β-D-glucan*, as biological markers for fungal infection. The use of Anti-Candida Albicans IgG (*C albicans germ tube antibody*, CAGTA) is reported in Spanish studies, but seldom applied elsewhere.

Mannans are components of the fungal cell wall. They are similar to glucan but show higher antigenicity. They are rapidly eliminated from the serum, thus a dosage of the antigen–antibody complex is suggested. This test has been used for about 10 years, but it has never received much attention: its use is in any case not advisable for the critically ill patient (EFIGS 2012) [9].

1-3 β-D-glucan is an element of the fungal cell wall: it is not specific for *Candida*, as it is common to many fungi (including *Aspergillus, Scedosporium, Fusarium, Pneumocystis Jirooveci*). Sensibility and specificity range between 70 and 89 %. The use of of *β-D-glucan* is today increasingly considered in critically ill patients, alone or associated with rules or scores able to predict fungal infection in at-risk subjects (*predictive rules*) [1, 9, 27–31]. Dosage of *β-D-glucan*, if available, is recommended by EFIGS GLs [9]. In EORTC 2008 guidelines for hematological patients, it represents a microbiological criterion for the diagnosis of probable IC. The most recent prospective study [28] using cutoff values >80 ng/ml (using Fungitell test, Associates of Cape Cod, Inc., East Falmouth, MA USA) reports high positive and negative predictive values (>70 % and >98 %), high sensibility and specificity (>93 %), and ability to reliably guide early antifungal treatment (positive blood cultures anticipated by 24–72 h): the association with Candida Score (*see below*) further improved the performance of this test. In the commentary of this study [30], use of *β-D-glucan* is proposed as relevant, provided results are available within 24 h,

1. If positive, as a marker to start a "preemptive" antifungal treatment.
2. If negative, to discontinue the empirical treatment in the absence of positive blood cultures.
   The need for confirmation with prospective studies is obvious.
   Major concerns or doubts on *β*-D-glucan, beside its cost, are

- Cutoff value (overlapping of positive and negative patients, with cutoff >80 ng/ml for Fungitell, which is now proposed to be set much higher)
- The assay (only one of the four available, Fungitell,, has so far been validated and considered in EFIGS guidelines) [9];
- The schedule ("stand alone"; one single weekly test; twice a week)
- Alone or better in association with a score or a predictive rule

As already mentioned, *β-D-glucan*, being a fungal cell wall component, is not specific for *Candida*: it is positive also in case of *Aspergillus infections* and *false positives* are possible in case of glucans in the diet, use of Beta-lactam antibiotics, use hemocomponents or immunoglobulins; in patients undergoing hemodialysis (presence of cellulose in the filters); in the case of use of gauzes for abdominal packing; in the case of a presence of positive blood cultures for Gram-positives (Cross reactivity) [9, 27–30].

13.7.3 Procalcitonin

A small elevation of procalcitonin (PCT) has been reported during fungal infection (especially if compared with the PCT modifications in the course of septic shock secondary to bacterial infections) [26]. The reasons are not completely clear, but the increase in γ INF observed in response to a fungal infection (and its effect on PCT synthesis) may play a role. Recently, it has been demonstrated that the increase is higher in presence of infection than of colonization [31]: however, in spite of a better positive predictive value (54 %), the NPV did not change (89 %).

13.7.4 Genomic Approach

In the extreme difficulty to reliably diagnose IC (and therefore eagerly awaiting solutions able to improve an inacceptably high mortality rate, particularly in case of delayed treatment), some positive and extremely interesting results could arise from the study of genetic determinants able to modulate (or not) the host respone to *Candida* colonization or infection [31]. In hematopoietic stem cell transplant recipients a variant of the *dectin-1 gene* was associated with an increase risk of Candida colonization and infection: the in vitro inflammatory response of cells from these subjects was reduced in presence of yeast. In this line, screening this type of polymorphism in critically ill patients might help in stratifying the risk of IC [31].

13.8   Risk Factors and Predictive Rules

In the presence of difficulties and/or diagnostic delays and being aware of the high impact fungal infections have on morbidity and mortality, particularly in the absence of a prompt and correct treatment [3], efforts have for a long time been focused on the detection of conditions or factors that expose patients to a high risk of fungal infections: in these subjects, prophylactic, "*preemptive*" or empirical treatments may play a key role in limiting morbidity and mortality [1, 18], avoiding therapeutic delays and granting timely and appropriate interventions [1–4]. In case of empirical treatment, negative cultures or negative biomarkers (as β-D-glucan) require a *de-escalation* therapy, in analogy with the treatment of bacterial infections.

The risk factors associated with IC are many in the critically ill patient [17]: unfortunately the very high number of factors represents by itself a reason to limit their easy, practical and reliable use as predictors. This is the mainstay for the constant search for surrogates or markers as reliable predictors of Candida infection, with or without the use of cultures [1, 4].

Colonization Index (*CI*)—The first attempt aimed at an identification of rules able to predict ICs was based on the observation of the development of candidemia in the presence of *Candida* colonization [7]. The colonization index (*colonization index = number of body sites colonized with the same genotype of Candida over the total number of tested sites, usually 5*) was proposed in surgical patients in 1994 by Pittet et al to predict the development of IC [32]. A value >0.5 identified all patients at risk of invasive infection and therefore requiring prophylactic or preemptive therapy: sensibility and specificity were 100 and 69 %, respectively. A *corrected colonization index* (CCI) had been proposed by the same group, based only on positive cultures and calculated on the ratio "heavy colonized cultures/ positive cultures": a value >0.4 was associated with sensibility and specificity of 100 % [1, 4]. Despite having been quoted as interesting, both CI and CCI present several problems: among them, scarse specificity, difficulty of implementation, lack of reproduction of the study on a large sample of patients, costs (costs/benefits are not clear, so far), large organizational impact [1, 31]. Such an index cannot represent by itself the only predictor for IC and single positive experiences are contradicted by not yet conclusive data [1]. In such a neither simple nor always clear setting, the very recent study by Azoulay et al. concerning the use of systemic antifungal agents administered in ICUs in the absence of documented fungal infection, but only in presence of risk factors [33] might shed further light. Mortality was found to be identical in treated and not-treated subjects: however, a trend toward a lower than expected mortality (according to APACHE II score) was observed in treated subjects. Despite it did not achieve statistical significance, a "protective" effect of the antifungal therapy was hypothesized [33]. While definitive conclusions are not possible as yet, there is place for prospective studies on the clinical impact of therapy with antifungal agents (but not with fluconazole) in critically ill septic patients, colonized and with risk factors, using a Candida score cutoff superior (but not equal) to 3 (*see below*) [33].

13.8.1 Predictive Rules

Ostrozky Zeichner [34–36]—The difficulty in the implementation of the colonization index and the prediction problems without it, led Ostrozky Zeichner et al. to study and propose a rule for the prediction of *candidemia* based on the presence of risk factors independent from the presence of *Candida* colonization: this rule is based on the contemporary presence of 1 major criterion (use of antibiotics or presence of CVC) and at least two more criteria (TPN from day 1 to 3; dialysis on day 1 to 3; any major surgery on day - 7 to zero; pancreatitis on day −7 to zero; steroids on days −7 to 3; use of other immunosuppressive agents on days −7 to zero) [34]. *Ostrozky-Zeichner rule* has a high negative predictive value (97 %), but a very low positive predictive value. The incidence of IC according to this rule, in the original study applied to 34 % of the patients of the tested cohort, was 10 %. The introduction in the rule of the "*mechanical ventilation for longer than two days*" factor determined an improvement of the tool, reducing the number of "at-risk" patients to 18 %, but still maintaining the ability to identify 10 % with IC. A recent retrospective validation of this tool in a cohort of 352 patients has highlighted an incidence of Candidemia of 2.3 %. Developing a dedicated algorithm and proposing a final score (Nebraska Medical Center, NMC rule) the high negative predictive value (99 %) has been confirmed, but also the very low positive predictive value (<5 %), thus making the rule useful to identify patients unlikely to develop IC and therefore not to be treated with antifungal therapies [37]. As already stressed, all prediction rules have very low positive predictive value.

Candida Score—Candida score by Leon et al., proposed in 2006 [37] and prospectively validated in 2009 [39], has started to be properly understood only in the past 2 years (see in particular Peman and Zaragoza) [40]. Differently from the Ostrosky-Zeichner rule, colonization index has a relevant role. Four parameters, to which after a multivariate analysis a weight then transformed into a score was attributed, represent the independent predictors of IC in postsurgical patients staying in an ICU for ≥4 days. The score [38] assigns 2 points for severe sepsis, and 1 point each for recent surgery, TPN, multifocal Candida colonization. Patients with a relatively high risk of IC (7.5-fold in comparison to not at-risk patients) were those with a score >2.5 points in the first retrospective series [38], ≥3 in the second validation series [39]. Interestingly enough, in the latter series, the presence of a score ≤3 was associated to risk of IC ≤5 %, while the risk increased from 3.7-fold to 10.3-fold with scores higher than 3 (4 and 5, respectively) [38, 39].

It has to be stressed that [40] the major point is to consider as critical **not** a score equal to 3, but only higher than 3. Indeed, a score of 3 would lead to the treatment of a large number of patients, given the ease with which a score equal to 3 may be reached in postsurgical ICU patients, making large part of the empirical treatments very likely unnecessary [40]. This important point has recently been confirmed by Leroy et al. in a prospective study, in which the observation was extended to "medical" patients. This study clearly demonstrated that empirical treatment in patients with a Candida Score equal to 3 was useless, whereas Candida Score 3 or ≤3 clearly identified patients with very low risk of IC [41]. The Candida Score represents an approach of the uttermost interest: its predictive value might be even better with the use of Beta D-glucan, as pointed out both by Posteraro et al. and by Eggimann and Marchetti [28, 30].

In conclusion, the main critique to all the predictive rules is their low positive predictive value, their strength mainly residing in the very high negative predictive value. False positive results are then more than possible, making the risk of *overtreatment* and related problems, high [31]. An association with biological markers could represent an interesting future perspective.

13.9 Treatment

Treatment of IC and Candidemia includes 5 strategies [1, 4, 9, 31, 42]: *prophylaxis, targeted prophylaxis, preemptive treatment, empirical treatment, upfront treatment.*

13.9.1 Prophylaxis

Administration of an antifungal drug to all the subjects considered at risk of IC, not infected and in the absence of signs/symptoms of infection: in other words, the treatment is only due to the fact of being within a category considered at risk (e.g., solid-organ transplant recipients). The aim is to reduce morbidity and mortality by decreasing fungal load. The main concerns are the large number of treatments with the risk of overexposure and, according to some, the chance of inducing resistance and selecting *non-albicans Candida* species (therefore fluconazole-resistant). There is evidence of efficacy in surgical patients considered at high risk and in some subgroups of ICU patients [1, 4]: the drug of choice is in any case fluconazole. The quality of the pattern and the number of involved patients represent, however, the greatest critical aspects of these studies. Dosages of fluconazole were quite different in the various studies and therefore difficult to compare.

The IDSA 2009 guidelines [42] recommend in an ICU prophylaxis only in high-risk patients and in settings with high incidence of Candida infections and with an administration of fluconazole in doses of 400 mg daily. An incidence of Candida infections >10 % may be considered as high: in such a case, the number of patients to be treated to avoid infection is certainly fewer than 20, whereas it would be over 100 in the case of incidence corresponding to 1–2 % [1, 18]. Although solid-organ transplant recipients may be considered at increased risk, today among transplant recipients some high-risk categories have been identified, which lead to an exclusion of transplant per se as a condition of risk (see *targeted prophylaxis*). Other categories (details in IDSA 2009 and EFIGS 2012 GLs) [9, 42] are stem cell transplant recipients and subgroups of subjects who have undergone chemotherapy: also categories at risk are to be identified (see *Targeted prophylaxis*).

13.9.2 Targeted Prophylaxis

Administration of an antifungal drug to subjects considered at high risk of IC (presence of risk factors, either in a critical number or specific), not infected and in the absence of signs/symptoms of infection: treatment only in patients considered at high risk. This strategy reduces the number of treatments and probably better identifies patients who may benefit from the administration of antifungal agents. An example is represented by the current trend, for instance, for liver transplant recipients, in whom specific conditions able to identify patients at high risk (severe blood loss/number of transfused blood units, long duration of surgery, retransplantation, relaparotomy within 5 days from transplant, acute or chronic renal failure, use of CVVH, choledochojejunostomy, acute hepatic failure) [43]. The use of fluconazole is suggested. In specific cases, because of the risk of aspergillosis and not only of candidiasis, lipid-based or liposomal amphotericins or echinocandins, instead of fluconazole are now strongly suggested [43].

13.9.3 Preemptive Treatment

Administration of antifungal agents based on the presence of risk factors and/or the presence of (*bio*) *markers for infection* (the original definition was for CMV infection/disease and in this case adapted to fungal infection): here the colonization index or Beta -D-glucan are to be considered as markers. Patients are thus considered at (very) high risk and therefore requiring treatment: its aim is to reduce mortality associated with IC. It is often considered/described as empirical treatment [4].

13.9.4 Empirical Treatment

Administration of antifungal agents to patients with persistent signs/symptoms of infection despite optimal antibiotic therapy, at risk for IC, but in the absence of identification of IC or of a proven source: *these patients are treated on a clinical (empirical) basis.*

It is the most widely used treatment, but also the most debated (*see also paragraph about intra-abdominal infections*). There is considerable interest in the empirical use of antifungal agents (in particular fluconazole), opposed however by some studies [1, 4, 44] in which demonstration of benefits is absent: in such a context, the number of ICs in the healthcare setting (exposition, case mix) and the presence of risk factors play a fundamental role. Knowledge of center epidemiology and use of correct definitions allow limitation of the empirical treatment to those patients at high risk of IC and only in settings in which the risk of IC is substantial (>10 %). The clinical scenario for empirical treatment could be the presence of (i) strong clinical suspicion, despite the absence of culture data, (ii) hemodynamic instability, (iii) organ dysfunction (this profile is a temptative description of the definition of "moderately or severely critically ill patient" found in the guidelines) [45]. The empirical treatment includes, according to IDSA [42] and EFIGS [9] guidelines reccomendations, one echinocandin or, alternatively, lipid-based or liposomal formulation of amphotericin B.

The clinical setting has to be stressed again: unstable patient (severe septic/ shock and organ dysfunction) who did not respond to broad spectrum antibiotic treatment given at appropriate dosage and with correct schedule, in the absence of *Candida spp.* positive blood cultures (or of significant abdominal cultures), who has already been exposed to azoles, with presence of risk factors for IC or in the presence of multiple site colonization from *non-albicans Candida* [3, 4, 45].

In stable patients and/or non yet exposed to azoles, the use of fluconazole is instead suggested. In this setting, early and appropriate treatment is pivotal to reduce mortality. In the presence of favorable culture evidence, a *de-escalation therapy* should be taken into consideration.

The space given to echinocandins or alternatively to lipid-based formulations of Amphotericin B (Abelcet Teva; AmBisome Gilead) in the newest guidelines for critically ill patients largely depends on the increased rate of IC sustained by *non-albicans Candida* and in particular by *C Glabrata* [9, 13, 15, 42]. The problem of *Candida Parapsilosis*, on the rise in some clinical settings, and the use of echinocandins is to be considered: echinocandins might be less effective on *C Parapsilosis* than both fluconazole and amphotericin B. Then these latter drugs are to be taken into consideration in case of a therapeutic failure of previous treatment with echinocandins [45].

The use of echinocandids in subjects with tertiary peritonitis and therefore at a high risk of IC led to a significant decrease in the incidence of IC in retrospective studies [46]. This comparison is however open to criticism: prospective randomized studies are eagerly awaited to reliably answer this question.

In the presence of proven or strongly suspected CVC infection, *catheters are to be removed and replaced*: major problems may rise in oncohematologic patients, for whom such solution might be suboptimal and has to be discussed on a case-by-case basis, evaluating risks/benefits [47].

13.9.5 Targeted Treatment

Administration of antifungal agents with documented IC, giving priority to fungicidal drugs [1, 4, 45].

Susceptibility of *Candida spp.* to the different antifungal agents is reported in IDSA guidelines 2009 [42].

Therapeutic alternatives, have since the 1990s experienced an ongoing development: the therapeutic armamentarium is quite large today, (according to some, even excessive). Three main classes of drugs are available: polienes, azoles, echinocandins. Of the latter, three are nowadays available for the treatment of invasive candidiasis: *caspofungin, anidulafungin, micafungin*. Other principles are either being developed or at advanced stage of study.

13.10 Antifungal Drugs

The antifungal drugs most commonly used in the treatment of ICs will now be briefly analyzed. We suggest the paper recently published by Mazzei and Novelli [55] for the PK/PD properties of the main antifungal drugs.

In Tables 13.2 and 13.3 (Pereira et al) [48] spectrum of activity, kinetic properties and dose adjustments in case of organ dysfunction.

The choice among the various antifungal drugs is neither immediate nor obvious. Risk factors, local epidemiology, organ toxicity, pharmacokinetic and pharmacodynamic profiles, interferences with other drugs (e.g., the contemporary use of antifungal drugs and antiretroviral drugs or immunosuppressive drugs) constitute some of the several factors that should contribute to the rationale of the choice of an antifungal drug. In the case of documented equal efficacy, the pharmacoeconomic profile should deserve a weight, given the scarsity of the

Table 13.2 Antifungal spectrums of activity

Organism	Amphotericin B	Fluconazole	Voriconazole	Posaconazole	Anidulafungin	Caspofungin	Micafungin
Aspergillus species							
A. flavus	±	−	+	+	+	+	+
A. fumigatus	+	−	+	+	+	+	+
A. niger	+	−	+	+	+	+	+
A. terreus	−	−	+	+	+	+	+
Candida species							
C. albicans	+	+	+	+	+	+	+
C. glabrata	+	±	+	+	+	+	+
C. krusei	+	−	+	+	+	+	+
C. lusitaniae	−	+	+	+	+	+	+
C. parapsilosis	+	+	+	+	±	±	±
C. tropicalis	+	+	+	+	+	+	+
Cryptococcus neoformans	+	+	+	+	−	−	−
Coccidioides species	+	+	+	+	±	±	±
Blastomyces	+	+	+	+	±	±	±
Histoplasma species	+	−	+	+	±	±	±
Fusarium species	±	−	+	+	−	−	−
Scedosporium apiospermium	±	−	+	+	−	−	−
Scedosporium prolificans	−	−	±	±	−	−	−
Zygomycetes	±	−	−	+	−	−	−

+ signs indicate that he anti fungalagent has activity against the organism specified. − signs indicate that the antifungal agent does not have activity against the organism specified. ± signs indicate that the antifungal agent has variably activity against the organism specified. Amphotericin B includes lipid formulations. Reproduced from Pereira and Paiva. Annual Update in Intensive Care and Emergency medicine. Springer Berlin 2011: 516–30 with permission

Table 13.3 Doses adjustment and organ dysfunction

Organ dysfunction	AMB deo	L-AMB	ABLC	ABCD	fluconazole	Voriconazole	Posaconazole	Anidulafungin	Caspofungin	Micafungin
Moderate to severe liver dy function	No	No	No	No	No	Yes	No	No	Yes	No
Renal dysfunction	No	No	No	No	Yes	No*	No	No	No	No

*i.✓. voriconazole is contraindicated in patients with creatinine clearance <50 ml/min; AMB deo: amphotericin B deoxycholate; L-AMB: liposomal amphotericin B; ABLC: amphotericin B lipid complex; ABCD: amphotericin B colloidal dispersion. Reproduced from Pereira and Paiva. Annual Update in Intensive Care and Emergency medicine. Springer Berlin 2011: 516–30 with permission resources and the high costs of the different molecules, with the exception of fluconazole and amphotericin deoxycholate, (the latter considered by many as obsolete for its relevant side effects and seldom, if ever, used).

13.11 Polyenes [49–52]

Polyenes act by binding to sterols (ergosterol) in the fungal cell membrane, forming a transmembrane channel (hydrophilic channel) capable of determining cell death due to changes in membrane permeability and loss of potassium and cell solutes. Their mechanism of action also includes a proinflammatory stimulus that triggers innate immunity by means of *Toll-like receptors*. Their action is either fungicidal or fungistatic, depending upon the levels in body fluids and the susceptibility of the microorganism. They still represent a pivotal class for the treatment of fungal infections, although the original molecule (Amphotericin B deoxycholate, Fungizone, a polyenic macrolide produced by Streptomyces Nodosus) is by now only rarely used, at least by systemic route, due to high toxicity and the many side effects (chills, fever, myalgia, acute renal failure). They are characterized by high protein binding and long half-life. Elimination routes are still poorly understood. In the case of use in the presence of renal failure, dosage should not be modified. During continuous renal replacement therapies (CRRT, mainly CVVH, continuous venovenous hemofiltration), the dosage remains unchanged. Both lipid-based formulations have favorable profiles in terms of tolerance, biodistribution and bioavalaibility. With liposomal Amphotericin (AmBisome Gilead) blood levels are higher, whereas using Amphotericin lipid-based complexes (Abelcet,Teva), tissue (liver, spleen, lung) levels are high and blood level low [50]. The real meaning and the clinical impact of these properties are still under strong debate [51, 52].

Amphotericin B has a very large spectrum of activity, which includes both molds (including *Aspergillus, Mucor, Zygomycetes* and rare fungi) and yeasts (but *Candida lusitaniae* is intrinsically resistant, together with *C guillermondii, Aspergillis terreus, and Scedosporium*). The broad spectrum of action makes its use in empirical treatment particularly attractive: toxicity of deoxycholate formulation prevents its use, particularly in the presence of newer less toxic drugs, while lipid-based formulations have nowadays several clinical indications [50].

The new lipid-based formulations (in particular the lipid-based complex, *Abelcet Teva* and the liposomal formulation, *AmBisome Gilead*) have by now practically replaced the old deoxycholate formulation, as the side effects and the quite relevant renal toxicity, mainly at tubular level, have been considerably reduced. Liposomal formulation seems to be slightly better tolerated than the lipid-based formulation: increases in serum creatinin and BUN, or hypopotassemia and hypomagnesemia seems to be more frequent with the lipid-based formulation. Although rare, hepatic toxicity has been reported (mainly a cytolitic component). Costs (particularly for the liposomal formulation) are high.

The dosage of the liposomal formulation (AmBisome, Gilead) is 3 mg/kg/day (in case of treatment of Mucor or Zygomicetes infection dosage is up to 5 mg/kg/day and of 3–5 mg/kg/day for treatment of Visceral Leishmaniasis have been reported). The dosage in case of use of lipid-based formulation (Abelcet, Teva) is 5 mg/kg/day.

13.12 Azoles [53]

Azoles inhibit the P450-cytochrome (inhibition of C 14-alpha-demethylase) which inhibits the conversion of lanosterol to ergosterol: intracellular accumulation of methyl sterol prevents cell growth and its replication. Among Azoles, Triazoles (fluconazole, voriconazole, itraconazole, posaconazole) are those most frequently used in critical care, especially the first two.

13.12.1 Fluconazole [53]

Fluconazole is certainly the most used drug in the treatment of fungal infections. Its spectrum of action does not include *C Krusei* and, *C Glabrata.*, but covers *C Parapsilosis*. On the contrary, it includes coccidioidomycosis, cryptococcosis, blastomycosis. It shows low protein binding, optimal tissue distribution, including Cephalorachidian fluid (CFR) (levels corresponding to 70 % of the blood level). The standard intravenous dosage is 12 mg/kg loading dose, followed by 6 mg/kg/day maintenance. Elimination is renal and in the presence of glomerular filtration <60 >10 ml/min dose adjustment is needed (either the dose has to be halved or the interval of administration doubled). In the presence of CRRT the dosage should be increased, due to the substantial increased removal performed by the extracorporeal circuit (some authors suggest up to 500–600 mg every 12 h) [52]. The pharmacological interferences might include the increased blood levels of phenytoin, glipizide, glyburide, warfarin, rifabutin, ciclosporin (even if for the latter the effect is less if compared to itraconazole). Rifampicin, instead, reduces its blood levels. Low toxicity, optimal tissue penetration, formulation versatility (easy switch from intravenous to oral formulation), therapeutic drug monitoring and low cost, make this drug extremely attractive for prophylaxis in critical care. Instead, it has been replaced (as already reported) by Echinocandins and lipid (Abelcet) or liposomal(Ambisome) Amphotericin B formulations in the empirical treatment of non-neutropenic critically ill patients with severe sepsis/septic shock and/or organ dysfunction (see IDSA 2009 and EFIGS 2012 guidelines) [9, 42].

13.12.2 Voriconazole [53]

Water-soluble triazolic drug with a low molecular weight. Voriconazole has a broad spectrum of action, with specific activity for *Candida spp., Aspergillus, Fusarium, Scedosporium, and Mucor*. It is not active against Zycomycetes. Its protein binding corresponds to 50–60 %, it is well distributed at tissue level, crosses the hemato-encephalic barrier, giving CRF levels corresponding to 40–70 % of blood levels. It may be administered by intravenous route (6 mg/kg every 12 h on the first day, then 4 mg/kg every 12 h afterwards: relative contraindication in the case of renal failure, due to the presence of cyclodextrin, which accumulates at renal level). The oral route may be used for the high bioavailability at a dose of 6 mg/kg every 12 h on the first day (400 mg × 2) and of 4 mg/kg every 12 h (200 mg x 2) as maintenance. No cyclodextrin is present, consequently it has no contraindications in the case of renal failure. In the case of mild-to-moderate liver disease (CHILD Classes A–B) maintenance dosage should be halved. Voriconazole blood levels should be kept between 1 and 5 ng/ml to achieve optimal therapeutic activity: monitoring of blood levels (TDM, therapeutic drug monitoring) is critical for the broad variability of absorption among patients. Several interactions are possible: relevant are those with cyclosporine and tacrolimus. Adverse reactions have been reported as affecting visus, CNS (hallucinations), skin (cutaneous rashes) and liver (from a temporary increase in transaminases up to rare cases of liver failure). QT interval prolongation should be taken into consideration. In the case of combined administration of voriconazole and IL-2 inhibitors (cyclosporine and tacrolimus), the dosage of tacrolimus should be reduced to 1/3 of the usual dose, that of cyclosporine halved. There are significant interactions with oral anticoagulant drugs: it may in fact determine a prolongation of the prothrombin time.

It is the first choice in the treatment of cerebral and pulmonary aspergillosis. Taken from [56], the table with the most common interactions observed with azole administration.

13.12.3   Echinocandins [31, 54–56]

Used in the clinical setting since the beginning of the 2000s, the echinocandins are semisynthetic, cyclic lipopeptides: three of them are available on the market, (*caspofungin, micafungin, anidulafungin*), others are being developed [55]. They represent a new and extremely interesting class of drugs, as they target the fungal cell wall. Their activity is thus fungicidal and side effects, due to an extremely selective mechanism of action, are few. Their mechanism of action is based on the inhibition of the synthesis of 1-3 β-D glucan, an essential component of the fungal cell wall, through non-competitive inhibition of the glucan synthase: the integrity of the cell wall is modified, determining osmotic damage of the fungal cell and its death. As the target is not present in human cells, toxicity is low and tolerance is high. They are fungicidal for *Candida* (moreover showing high activity in the presence of *Candida spp.* within the biofilm) and fungistatic for *Aspergillus*. As already mentioned, they show high MICs *for C Parapsilosis and for C Guillermondii* (and therefore their use has been discouraged by many, even if favorable reports are available). Echinocandins have high protein binding and a long half-life. They are administered only by intravenous route at fixed dose

Although similar, the three echinocandins (caspofungin, micafingin, anidula-fungin) show kinetic and dynamic differences [48]. On a PK/PD base, it is possible to differentiate their use in different clinical conditions or in case of organ failure. An example is represented by *anidulafungin*, indicated for patients with altered liver function, given the absence of metabolism and the spontaneous degradation. If *caspofungin* is used in patients with moderate-severe liver dysfunction, the maintenance dose has to be halved. No modification is instead required for micafungin. An alteration in renal function and the necessity to use CRRT do not determine any modification in the dosage either for caspo-, or for mica- or for anidulafungin [52].

13.13 Conclusions

The difficulty in the treatment of IC is due, as often underlined, to diagnostic and interpretative difficulties and to the aggressiveness of infections. A wide consensus on the definitions is eagerly awaited, to reach uniformity of strategies and of clinical behaviour, particularly in those clinical presentations for which the uncertainties are greater: peritoneal Candidiasis is a significant example.

Timely, appropriate and aggressive intervention is pivotal in any form of severe fungal infection and even more in septic shock: this is why aggressive treatment becomes vital in ICUs.

Recently released guidelines might ease this problem.

References

1. Eggimann P, Barberini L, Calandra T, Marchetti O (2012) Invasive candidiasis in the ICU. Mycoses 75:65–72
2. Leroy O, Gangneux JP, Montravers P et al (2009) Epidemiology, management, and risk factors for death of invasive Candida infections in critical care: a multicenter, prospective, observational study in France (2005–2006). Crit Care Med 37:1612–1618
3. Kollef M, Micek S, Hampton N, Doherty JA, Kumar AS (2012) Septic shock attributed to Candida infection: importance of empiric therapy and source control. Clin Inf Dis 54(12):1739–1746
4. Kett DH, Azoulay E, Echeverria PM, Vincent JL (2011) Candida bloodstream infections in intensive care units: analysis of the extended prevalence of infection in intensive care unit study. Crit Care Med 39:665–670
5. Playford EG, Lipman J, Sorrell T (2010) Management of invasive candidiasis in the ICU. Drugs 70:823–839
6. Chalmer CM, Bal AM (2011) Management of fungal infections in the intensive care unit: a survey of UK practice. BJ Anesth 106:827–831
7. Echeverria PM, Kett DH, Azoulat E (2011) Candida prophylaxix and therapy in ICU. Sem Resp Crit Care Med 32:159–173
8. Tortorano AM, Dho AM, Prigitano A, Breda G, Grancini A et al (2011) Invasive fungal infections in the intensive care unit: a multicentre,prospective, observational study in Italy (2006–2008). Mycoses 55(1):73–79

9. Cornely OA, Bassetti M, Calandra T, Garbino J, Kullberg BJ, Lortholary O (2012) et ESCMID*(ESCMID Fungal Infection Study Group, EFIGS) guideline for the diagnosis and management of Candida diseases 2012: non-neutropenic adult patients. Clinical microbiology and infection: the official publication of the European Society of Clinical Microbiology and Infectious Diseases 18(Suppl 7):19–37

10. Viale PG (2009) Candida colonization and candiduria in critically ill patients in the intensive care unit. Drugs 69(Suppl. 1):51–57

11. Guzman JA, Tchokonte R, Sobel JD (2011) Septic shock due to candidemia: outcomes and predictors of shock development. J Clin Med Res 3(2):65–71

12. Eckmann C, Dryden M, Montravers P, Kozlov R, Sganga G (2011) Antimicrobial treatment of complicated intraabdominal infection and the new IDSA guidelines. a commentary and an alternative European approach according to clinical definitions. Eur J Med Res 16:115–126

13. Solomkin JS, Mazuski JE, Bradley JS, Rodvold KA, Goldstein EJC et al (2010) Diagnosis and management of complicated intra-abdominal infection in adults and children: guidelines by the Surgical Infection Society and the Infectious Diseases Society of America. Clin Inf Dis 50:133–164

14. Blot S, Vandewoude KH, De Waele JJ (2007) Candida peritonitis. Curr Opin Crit Care 13:195–199

15. Sartelli M, Viale P, Koike K, Pea F, Tumietto F, van Goor H, Guercioni et al (2011) WSES consensus conference: guidelines for first line management of intra-abdominal infections. World J Emerg Surg 6:2

16. Blot S, De Waele JJ, Vogelaers D (2012) Essentials for selecting antimicrobial therapy for intra-abdominal infections. Drugs 72(6):e17–e32

17. Carneiro HA, Mavrakis A, Mylonakis E (2011) Candida peritonitis: an update on the latest research and treatments. World J Surg 35:2650–2659

18. Mikulska M, Bassetti M, Romeo S, Viscoli C (2011) Invasive candidiasis in non-hematological patients. Mediterr J Hematol Infect Dis 3(1):e2011007. DOI 10.4084/MJHID.2011.007

19. Dupont H, Bourichon A, Paugam-Burtz C, Mantz J, Desmont JM (2003) Can yest isolation in peritoneal fluid be predictive in ICU patients with peritonitis? Crit Care Med 31:752–757

20. Hamet M, Pavon A, Dalle F, Pechinot A, Prin S et al (2012) Candida spp. airway colonization could promote antibiotic-resistant bacteria selection in patients with suspected ventilator-associated pneumonia. Intensive Care Med 38:1272–1279

21. Sobel J (2010) Changing trends in the epidemiology of Candida blood stream infections: a matter for concern ? Crit Care Med 38:990–992

22. Marriott DJE, Playford EG, Chen S, Slavin M, Nguyen Q et al (2009) Determinants of mortality in non-neutropenic ICU patients with candidaemia. Crit Care 13:R115. doi: 10.1186/cc7964

23. Bassetti M, Taramasso L, Nicco E, Molinari MP, Mussap M, Viscoli C (2011) Epidemiology, species distribution, antifungal susceptibility and outcome of nosocomial candidemia in a tertiary care hospital in Italy. PLoS ONE 6(9):e24198. doi:10.1371/journal.pone.0024198

24. Andes DR, Safdar N, Baddley JW et al (2012) Impact of treatment strategy on outcomes in patients with candidemia and other forms of invasive candidiasis: a patient-level quantitative review of randomized trials. Clin Infect Dis 54:1110–1122

25. Tumbarello M, Fiori B, Trecarichi EM, Posteraro P, Losito AR et al (2012) Risk factors and outcomes of candidemia caused by biofilm-forming isolates in Tertiary Care Hospital. PLoS ONE 7(3):e33705. doi:10.1371/journal.pone.0033705

26. Martini A, Gottin L, Menestrina N, Schweiger V, Simion D, Vincent JL (2010) Procalcitonin levels in surgical patients at risk of candidemia. J Infect 60(6):425–430

27. Eggimann P, Bille J, Marchetti O (2011) Diagnosis of invasive candidiasis in the ICU. Ann Int Care 1:37

28. Posteraro B, De Pascale G, Tumbarello M, Torelli R (2011) Mariano Alberto Pennisi MA et al. Early diagnosis of candidemia in intensive care unit patients with sepsis: a prospective

comparison of (1-3)-beta-D-glucan assay, Candida score, and colonization index. Crit Care 15:R249

29. Del Bono V, Delfino E, Furfaro E, Mikulska M, Nicco E et al (2011) Assay in early diagnosis of nosocomial clinical performance of the (1,3)-b-d-Glucan Candida bloodstream infections. Clin Vaccine Immunol 18:2113

30. Eggimann P, Marchetti O (1017) Is (1-3)-β-D-glucan the missing link from bedside assessment to pre-emptive therapy of invasive candidiasis? Crit Care 2011:15

31. Charles PE, Bruyere R, Dalle F (2012) Early recognition of invasive Candidiasis in the ICU. In: Vincent JL (ed) Annual update in intensive care and emergency medicine. Springer Berlin, pp 311–323

32. Pittet D, Monod M, Suter PM, Frenk E, Auckenthaler R (1994) Candida colonization and subsequent infections in critically ill surgical patients. Ann Surg 220:751–758

33. Azoulay E, Dupont H, Tabah A, Lortholary O, Stahl JP et al (2012) Systemic antifungal therapy in critically ill patients without invasive fungal infection. Crit Care Med 40:813–822

34. Ostrosky-Zeichner L, Pappas PG, Shoham S et al (2011) Improvement of a clinical prediction rule for clinical trials on prophylaxis for invasive candidiasis in the intensive care unit. Mycoses 54:46–51

35. Ostrosky-Zeichner L (2012) Invasive mycoses: diagnostic challenges. Am J Med 125: S14–S24

36. Ostrosky-Zeichner L, Sable C, Sobel J et al (2007) Multicenter retrospective development and validation of a clinical prediction rule for nosocomial invasive candidiasis in the intensive care setting. Eur J Clin Microbiol Infect Dis 26:271–276

37. Hermsen ED, Zapapas MK, Maiefski M, Rupp M, Freifeld AG, Kalil AC (2011) Validation and comparison of clinical prediction rules for invasive candidiasis in intensive care unit patients: a matched case-control study. Crit Care 15:R198

38. Leon C, Ruiz-Santana S, Saavedra P et al (2006) A bedside scoring system (Candida score) for early antifungal treatment in nonneutropenic critically ill patients with Candida colonization. Crit Care Med 34:730–737

39. Leon C, Ruiz-Santana S, Saavedra P et al (2009) Usefulness of the ''Candida score'' for discriminating between Candida colonization and invasive candidiasis in non-neutropenic critically ill patients: a prospective multicenter study. Crit Care Med 37:1624–1633

40. Peman J, Zaragoza R (2010) Current diagnostic approaches to invasive candidiasis in critical care settings. Mycoses 53:424–433

41. Leroy G, Lambiotte F, Thévenin D, Lemaire C, Parmentier E, Devos P, andn Leroy O (2011) Evaluation of "Candida score" in critically ill patients: a prospective, multicenter, observational, cohort study. Ann Intensive Care 1(1):50

42. Pappas PG, Kauffman CA, Andes D, Benjamin DK, Calandra TF, Edwards JE et al (2009) Clinical practice guidelines for the managementof candidiasis: 2009 update by the Infectious Diseases Society of America (IDSA). Clin Inf Dis 48:503–535

43. Grossi PA, Dalla Gasperina D, Barchiesi F, Biancofiore G, Carafiello Gp, De Gasperi A et al (2011) Italian guidelines for diagnosis, prevention, and treatment of invasive fungal infections in solid organ transplant recipients. Transpl Proc 43:2463–2471

44. Schuster MG, Edwards J, Sobel JD, Darouiche RO, Karchmer AW, Hadley S et al (2008) Empirical fluconazole versus placebo for intensive care unit patients : a randomized trial. Ann Intern Med 149:83–90

45. Garnacho Montero J, Diaz martin A, Marquez Vacaro JA (2012) Management of invasive candidiasis in the critically ill. In: Vincent JL (ed) Annual update in intensive care and emergency medicine. Springer, Berlin, pp 324–336

46. Senn L, Eggimann P, Ksontini R et al (2009) Caspofungin for prevention of intraabdominal candidiasis in high risk surgical patients. Intensive Care Med 35:903–909

47. Clancy CJ, Hong Nguyen M (2012) The end of an era in defining the optimal treatment of invasive candidiasis. Clin Inf Dis 54:1123–1125

48. Pereira JM, Paiva JA (2011) Antifungal therapy in the ICU: the bug, the drug, the mug. In: Vincent JL (ed) Annual update in intensive care and emergency medicine. Springer, Berlin, pp 516–530

49. Moen MD, Lyseng-Williamson KA, Scott LJ (2009) Liposomal amphotericin B: a review of its use as empirical therapy in febrile neutropenia and in the treatment of invasive fungal infections. Drugs 69(3):361–392

50. Chandrasekar P, Amphotericin B (2008) lipid complex: treatment of invasive fungal infections in patients refractory to or intolerant of amphotericin B deoxycholate. Ther Clin Risk Manag 4(6):1285–1294

51. Azanza Perea JR, Barberan J (2012) Anfotericina B forma liposómica: un perfil farmacocinético exclusivo. Una historia inacabada. Rev Esp Quimioter 25:17–24

52. Honore PM, Jacobs R, Spapen HD (2012) Use of antifungals during continuous hemofiltration therapies. In: Vincent JL (ed) Annual update in intensive care and emergency medicine. Springer, Berlin, pp 337–44

53. Lasse Florl C (2011) Triazole antifungal agents in invasive fungal infections. Comp Rev Drugs 71:2405–2419

54. Bal AM (2010) The echinocandins: three useful choices or three too many? Int J Antimicrobial Agents 35:13–18

55. Mazzei T (2009) Novelli apharmacological properties of antifungal drugs with a focus on anidulafungin. Drugs 69(Suppl. 1):79–90

56. Bow EJ, Evans G, Fuller J et al (2010) Canadian clinical practice guidelines for invasive candidiasis in adults. Can J Infect Dis Med Microbiol 21:e122–e150)

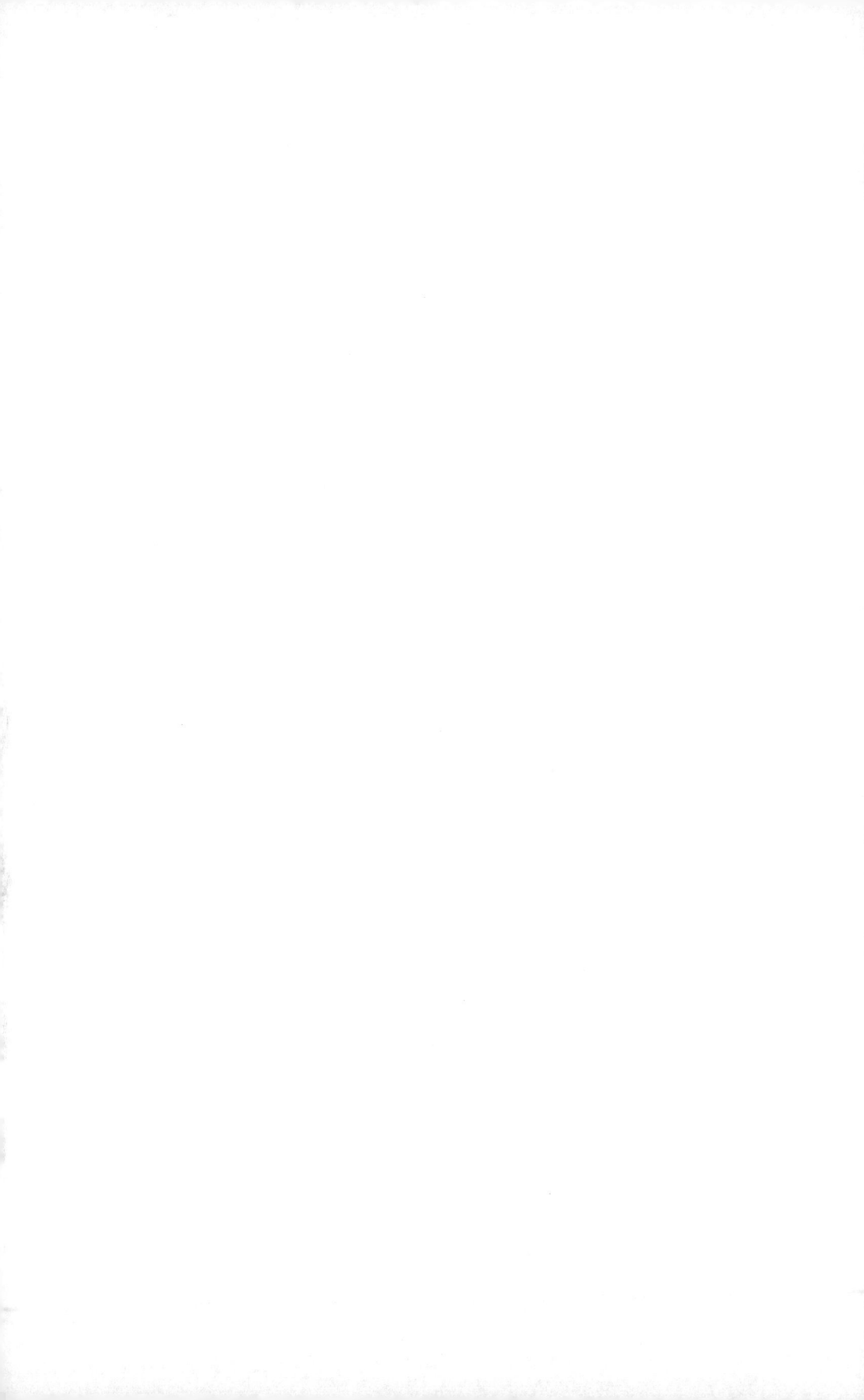

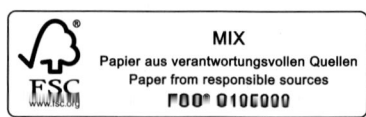

Printed by Books on Demand, Germany